PATHOLOGICAL ANXIETY

PATHOLOGICAL ANXIETY

Emotional Processing in Etiology and Treatment

Edited by
BARBARA OLASOV ROTHBAUM

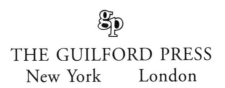

THE GUILFORD PRESS
New York   London

© 2006 The Guilford Press
A Division of Guilford Publications, Inc.
72 Spring Street, New York, NY 10012
www.guilford.com

Printed in the United States of America

This book is printed on acid-free paper.

Last digit is print number: 9 8 7 6 5 4 3 2 1

Library of Congress Cataloging-in-Publication Data

Pathological anxiety : emotional processing in etiology and treat-
  ment / edited by Barbara Olasov Rothbaum.
    p. ; cm.
  Includes bibliographical references and index.
  ISBN 1-59385-223-1 (alk. paper)
    1. Anxiety—Treatment. 2. Cognitive therapy. 3. Imagery
(Psychology)   I. Rothbaum, Barbara Olasov.
  [DNLM: 1. Anxiety Disorders—therapy. 2. Anxiety Disorders
—etiology. 3. Anxiety Disorders—physiopathology. 4. Cognitive
Therapy—methods. 5. Fear—psychology. 6. Imagery (Psycho-
therapy)—methods.   WM 172 P297 2005]
  RC531.P38 2006
  616.85'2206—dc22
                                                    2005010330

About the Editor

Barbara Olasov Rothbaum, PhD, is a tenured Professor of Psychiatry and Director of the Trauma and Anxiety Recovery Program at Emory University School of Medicine. Dr. Rothbaum specializes in research on the treatment of individuals with affective disorders, particularly anxiety and posttraumatic stress disorder (PTSD). She has won both state and national awards for her research, and is an invited international speaker within her field. She has published numerous journal articles, book chapters, and books on the treatment of PTSD, and is a Diplomate in Behavioral Psychology of the American Board of Professional Psychology. Currently, Dr. Rothbaum serves as President of the International Society for Traumatic Stress Studies (ISTSS), and is a former Associate Editor of the *Journal of Traumatic Stress*. She is a pioneer in the application of virtual reality to the treatment of psychological disorders.

Dr. Rothbaum had the pleasure of working with Dr. Edna B. Foa in Philadelphia from 1986 to 1990 and has continued to collaborate with Dr. Foa over the years.

Contributors

Laura B. Allen, MA, Center for Anxiety and Related Disorders, Boston University, Boston, Massachusetts

David H. Barlow, PhD, Center for Anxiety and Related Disorders, Boston University, Boston, Massachusetts

Evelyn Behar, MS, Department of Clinical Psychology, The Pennsylvania State University, University Park, Pennsylvania

T. D. Borkovec, PhD, Department of Psychology, The Pennsylvania State University, University Park, Pennsylvania

Shawn P. Cahill, PhD, Department of Psychiatry and Center for the Treatment and Study of Anxiety, University of Pennsylvania, Philadelphia, Pennsylvania

David M. Clark, PhD, Department of Psychology, Institute of Psychiatry, London, United Kingdom

Bruce N. Cuthbert, PhD, Department of Psychology, University of Minnesota, Minneapolis, Minnesota

Jonathan R. T. Davidson, MD, Anxiety and Traumatic Stress Program, Duke University Medical Center, Durham, North Carolina

Anke Ehlers, PhD, Department of Psychology, Institute of Psychiatry, London, United Kingdom

Norah C. Feeny, PhD, Departments of Psychiatry and Psychology, Case Western Reserve University, Cleveland, Ohio

Edna B. Foa, PhD, Department of Psychiatry and Center for the Treatment and Study of Anxiety, University of Pennsylvania, Philadelphia, Pennsylvania

Martin E. Franklin, PhD, Center for the Treatment and Study of Anxiety, University of Pennsylvania, Philadelphia, Pennsylvania

Elizabeth A. Hembree, PhD, Department of Psychiatry, University of Pennsylvania School of Medicine, Philadelphia, Pennsylvania

Jonathan D. Huppert, PhD, Department of Psychiatry and Center for the Treatment and Study of Anxiety, University of Pennsylvania, Philadelphia, Pennsylvania

Terence M. Keane, PhD, National Center for PTSD, VA Boston Healthcare System, Boston University School of Medicine, Boston, Massachusetts

Peter J. Lang, PhD, Department of Clinical and Health Psychology, University of Florida, Gainesville, Florida

Michael R. Liebowitz, MD, Anxiety Disorders Clinic, New York State Psychiatric Institute, New York, New York

John S. March, MD, MPH, Department of Child and Adolescent Psychiatry, Duke University Child and Family Study Center, Duke University Medical Center, Durham, North Carolina

Andrew Mathews, PhD, MRC Senior Scientist, MRC Cognition and Brain Sciences Unit, Cambridge, United Kingdom

Richard J. McNally, PhD, Department of Psychology, Harvard University, Cambridge, Massachusetts

Lisa M. McTeague, MS, Department of Clinical and Health Psychology, University of Florida, Gainesville, Florida

David Riggs, PhD, Department of Psychiatry and Center for the Treatment and Study of Anxiety, University of Pennsylvania, Philadelphia, Pennsylvania

Barbara Olasov Rothbaum, PhD, Department of Psychiatry and Trauma and Anxiety Recovery Program, Emory University School of Medicine, Atlanta, Georgia

Katherine Shear, MD, Bereavement and Grief Program, Western Psychiatric Institute and Clinic, Pittsburgh, Pennsylvania

Helen Blair Simpson, MD, PhD, Anxiety Disorders Clinic, New York State Psychiatric Institute, New York, New York

Preface

The understanding and treatment of anxiety disorders has advanced rapidly in the past 10 years. Particularly important advances include the comparison of psychotherapy and pharmacotherapy and, in some cases, the combination of psychotherapy and pharmacotherapy. Almost all mental health professionals come into contact with patients suffering from anxiety disorders, and this volume addresses the theoretical, assessment, and practical treatment issues likely to touch the professional lives of researchers and practitioners alike.

The considerable progress made in psychotherapy for these debilitating conditions largely hinges on Edna B. Foa's theoretical and clinical work on exposure therapy, first in obsessive–compulsive disorder (OCD), then in posttraumatic stress disorder (PTSD), and more recently in social phobia. She is a distinguished scholar, teacher, and clinical researcher in psychological science, particularly within the anxiety disorders.

This volume results in large part from a conference held in May 2004 in Philadelphia, Pennsylvania, in honor of Professor Foa. Many of the authors of chapters in this book were presenters at that meeting. However, we have included chapters by many more authors in order to round out this volume to cover all of the anxiety disorders and to present the latest in theory and treatment of pathological anxiety, especially the contribution of emotional processing theory to current thinking. The contributors collectively summarize the state of the art in the anxiety disorders field, identify gaps in our knowledge, and stimulate future steps for clinical research and the dissemination of empirically supported interventions.

Our list of authors is an international "who's who" in the field of anxiety, and we are proud to present this volume to you. As it was in large part the result of a tribute to Edna Foa's lifetime of work in the area, I begin the book with a brief history of her life.

Edna B. Foa was born in Haifa, Israel, on December 28, 1937, and received her undergraduate education in Israel, coming to the United States for her graduate education in 1966. Her entire career as an academic professional has been spent in Philadelphia, first at Temple University, then at

the Medical College of Pennsylvania, and, since 1998, at the Department of
Psychiatry at the University of Pennsylvania School of Medicine. In 1979,
she founded the Center for the Treatment and Study of Anxiety, where,
with the collaboration of many colleagues, she has been conducting her
research and clinical activities.

EARLY INFLUENCES AND EDUCATION HISTORY

Edna Foa was drawn to psychology as an adolescent, when she discovered
the writings of Sigmund Freud and became fascinated with psychoanalysis.
After graduating from high school, she went to a normal school to train to
work with delinquent children. Her teacher of psychology there was a
trained psychoanalyst who encouraged her to write her final thesis on the
Freudian explanation of childhood delinquency.

After working for 2 years in a boarding school for delinquent children,
she continued to study psychology at Bar-Ilan University, where she received her BA in 1962. At Bar-Ilan, her clinical psychology teachers all represented psychoanalytic or psychodynamic orientations; none of them
thought that psychotherapy could or should be studied empirically. However, at Bar-Ilan Foa was also exposed to research in experimental and social psychology and became extremely interested both in the science of psychology and in empirical research. This interest was fostered by her late
husband, Uriel G. Foa, who was then the chair of the university's Department of Psychology and a distinguished researcher in social psychology.

Her first contact with behavior therapy and behavior modification occurred at the University of Illinois, where she received her MA in 1970 under
the supervision of O. Hobart Mowrer. In the 1960s, the clinical program in
the Department of Psychology at Urbana was one of the strongholds of behavior therapy and modification; its faculty included Leonard Ullmann,
Leonard Krasner, and Gordon Paul, to name only a few. There, Foa first became acquainted with the work of Joseph Wolpe and with the integration of
experimental psychology concepts into psychopathology and treatment. Her
educational experience at the University of Illinois, together with Uriel Foa's
mentoring in research methodology, marked the beginning of her
professional career.

After completing her PhD in 1970 at the University of Missouri at Columbia, she was awarded a postdoctoral fellowship from the National Institute of Mental Health to work with Wolpe at Temple University, the
mecca of behavior therapy at the time. There she had the opportunity to
meet leaders in the field, many of whom influenced her conceptual and empirical work. Of particular importance for her was the influence of Peter
Lang and Stanley Rachman.

PROFESSIONAL MODELS

At the University of Illinois, Foa was introduced not only to behavior modification and behavior therapy but also to the clinician-researcher model, and it is this model that is reflected in the development of her own career. She began her research examining the efficacy of behavioral treatments for anxiety disorders and identifying the active processes involved in these treatments.

Pursuing this line, she extended her interest from the study of treatment processes to the study of what it is that treatment should correct. Hence, she has been conducting studies that aim to elucidate the mechanisms involved in pathological fear and anxiety. Her work emphasizes the relationship between three areas of research: therapy outcome, therapy processes, and psychopathology. Most recently, and continuing in the spirit of the clinician-researcher model, she has aimed to disseminate the effective treatments that she and her colleagues have developed for OCD and PTSD by means of lectures, workshops, and the systematic study of the efficacy of these treatments in the hands of clinicians in community-based clinics who are not experts in cognitive-behavioral therapy.

MAJOR CONTRIBUTIONS TO THE FIELD

Most of Edna Foa's academic activity has been concerned with research on the psychopathology and treatment of the anxiety disorders, primarily OCD, PTSD, social phobia, and, to a lesser degree, panic disorder with agoraphobia, and specific phobia. This research has been theoretically driven so that her theory has informed the direction of research, and the empirical findings have in turn led to further development of the theory.

Theoretical Work

Foa's interest in the psychopathology and treatment of anxiety has produced a number of theoretical papers that are widely cited. Perhaps the best known is "Emotional Processing of Fear: Exposure to Corrective Information" (Foa & Kozak, 1986), which develops a theory on the processes involved in pathological anxiety and its treatment. Emotional processing theory conceives of the anxiety disorders as reflecting distinct pathological fear structures that include associations among representations of the feared stimuli, the feared responses, and their meaning. Accordingly, the goal of treatment for any given anxiety disorder is to form a modified structure in which the stimuli are the same as in the original structure but in which the pathological elements have been corrected. Successful therapy achieves this goal by activating the pathological structure and at the same time introducing corrective information that can be incorporated into the modified structure. Much of this volume traces the impact of this theory on the field.

Treatment Outcome Studies

In a series of studies, Foa has been developing and systematically investigating the active ingredients of exposure and response prevention (EX/RP) for OCD. At the same time, she has been investigating the efficacy of various medications, both alone and together with cognitive-behavioral therapy, in ameliorating OCD symptoms. These studies have helped to provide the knowledge of how to conduct cognitive-behavioral therapy for OCD and how to combine such therapy with medication. The treatment program that emerged from this research has been disseminated to therapists and clients via treatment manuals (Foa & Kozak, 1997; Kozak & Foa, 1997) and even more widely disseminated via a self-help book entitled *Stop Obsessing* (Foa & Wilson, 2001). As chair of the DSM-IV Subcommittee for OCD, Foa also had the opportunity to incorporate empirical research findings into the diagnostic criteria for OCD.

Since 1983, she has been studying PTSD, pursuing both outcome studies and psychopathology research. As in her earlier work in OCD, she and her colleagues have been developing and systematically studying several different short-term cognitive-behavioral treatment programs for PTSD. This research was summarized in a book presenting the theory and practice of cognitive-behavioral therapy for PTSD titled *Treating the Trauma of Rape: Cognitive-Behavioral Therapy for PTSD* (Foa & Rothbaum, 1998). The influence of these studies on the field has been such that the treatment program she developed, known as prolonged exposure (PE), is considered by many experts to be the treatment of choice for PTSD. In 2002, this treatment was recognized by an award from the Substance Abuse and Mental Health Services Administration as a model treatment to be targeted for dissemination among clinicians.

Treatment Process Research

As a complement to her interest in developing effective treatments for pathological anxiety, Edna Foa has been systematically concerned with understanding the processes that make the treatment work. In this endeavor, she was first influenced by conditioning theory and later on by the theoretical framework of information processing. For example, in several studies she found that patients who fail to show fear activation during exposure to their feared situation or memory (with fear measured by self-report, physiological responses, and facial expressions) and who fail to habituate between sessions do not benefit from treatment as much as those who do evi-

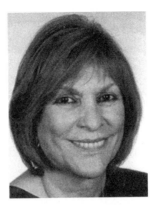

Edna B. Foa, PhD

dence this fear activation. Other process variables that she found to influence treatment outcome for PTSD include organization of the trauma narrative during repeated reliving of the trauma and changes in the schemas of "world" and "self."

Psychopathology Research

In investigating mechanisms underlying pathological anxiety, Foa has been concerned with applying methods of experimental psychology to clinical research, as well as carrying out more descriptive psychopathology studies. She has used a variety of cognitive experimental methods (e.g., dichotic listening, emotional Stroop test) in order to elucidate information-processing biases that characterize the anxiety disorders. In studying the psychopathology of these disorders, she has developed a number of measures of OCD and PTSD severity. Her self-report measure of PTSD, the Post-traumatic Diagnostic Scale (PDS), is widely used around the world.

CURRENT WORKS AND VIEWS

Edna Foa continues to conduct research on OCD, PTSD, and social phobia. In OCD, she and her colleagues are currently studying the augmentation effects of EX/RP in patients (both children and adults) who are partial responders to medication. In PTSD, she is conducting several studies that measure processes and outcome of exposure therapy. Some studies reflect her current interest in treating anxiety disorders that are comorbid with another disorder (e.g., PTSD with alcohol dependence, social phobia with depression). Other studies reflect her interest in understanding the relationship between psychological and biological factors underlying PTSD, as well as the influence of PE on each of these domains and their interrelations. Still other studies reflect her current enthusiasm for disseminating these treatments to clinicians in the community who do not have expertise in cognitive-behavioral therapy.

THIS VOLUME

The field owes a great debt of gratitude to Edna Foa and her creative research. The contributors to this volume all acknowledge the tremendous impact she has had on the field. These authors present cutting-edge conceptual and empirical knowledge regarding the psychopathology and treatment of anxiety. Chapters progress from the theoretical (Part I) to the applied (Part II) to innovations (Part III) in the study and treatment of anxiety disorders.

I want to express my deep gratitude to Elizabeth Hembree, Shawn Cahill, Marty Franklin, Norah Feeny, and David Riggs for serving on the planning committee for the May 2004 conference and for creating such a wonderful tribute to our dear friend and colleague who has had such an important impact on the field.

Submitted with respect, appreciation, and affection for Edna,

BARBARA OLASOV ROTHBAUM, PHD, ABPP

REFERENCES

Foa, E. B., & Kozak, M. J. (1986). Emotional processing of fear: Exposure to corrective information. *Psychological Bulletin, 99*, 20–35.

Foa, E. B., & Kozak, M. J. (1997). *Mastery of obsessive–compulsive disorder: Patient guide*. San Antonio, TX: Psychological Corporation.

Foa, E. B., & Rothbaum, B. O. (1998). *Treating the trauma of rape: Cognitive-behavioral therapy for PTSD*. New York: Guilford Press.

Foa, E. B., & Wilson, R. (2001). *Stop obsessing! How to overcome your obsessions and compulsions: Second edition*. New York: Bantam Doubleday Dell.

Kozak, M. J., & Foa, E. B. (1997). *Mastery of obsessive–compulsive disorder: Therapist guide*. San Antonio, TX: Psychological Corporation.

Contents

PART I

THEORETICAL CONCEPTUALIZATIONS
OF PATHOLOGICAL ANXIETY

1 Emotional Processing Theory: An Update   3
   EDNA B. FOA, JONATHAN D. HUPPERT,
   and SHAWN P. CAHILL

2 Emotional Encoding of Fear-Related Information   25
   ANDREW MATHEWS

3 Predictors of Chronic Posttraumatic Stress Disorder: 39
   Trauma Memories and Appraisals
   ANKE EHLERS and DAVID M. CLARK

4 Fearful Imagery and the Anxiety Disorder Spectrum   56
   PETER J. LANG, LISA M. MCTEAGUE,
   and BRUCE N. CUTHBERT

5 Emotional Processing Theory and the Recollection   78
   of Forgotten Trauma
   RICHARD J. MCNALLY

PART II

ASSESSMENT OF AND TREATMENTS
FOR PATHOLOGICAL ANXIETY

6 Assessment Strategies in the Anxiety Disorders   91
   DAVID RIGGS and TERENCE M. KEANE

7 Social Phobia: Then, Now, the Future   115
   JONATHAN R. T. DAVIDSON

8 Best Practice in Treating Obsessive–Compulsive Disorder: 132
   What the Evidence Says
   HELEN BLAIR SIMPSON and MICHAEL R. LIEBOWITZ

9 Cognitive-Behavioral Therapy for Pediatric   147
   Obsessive–Compulsive Disorder
   JOHN S. MARCH and MARTIN E. FRANKLIN

10 Treatment of Panic Disorder: Outcomes and Basic Processes   166
   LAURA B. ALLEN and DAVID H. BARLOW

11 The Nature and Treatment of Generalized Anxiety Disorder   181
   EVELYN BEHAR and T. D. BORKOVEC

12 Cognitive-Behavioral Perspectives on Theory and Treatment   197
   of Posttraumatic Stress Disorder
   ELIZABETH A. HEMBREE and NORAH C. FEENY

PART III
INNOVATIVE TREATMENT APPLICATIONS
AND FUTURE DIRECTIONS

13 Adapting Imaginal Exposure to the Treatment   215
   of Complicated Grief
   KATHERINE SHEAR

14 Virtual Reality Exposure Therapy   227
   BARBARA OLASOV ROTHBAUM

15 Pathological Anxiety: Where We Are and Where We Need to Go   245
   SHAWN P. CAHILL, MARTIN E. FRANKLIN,
   and NORAH C. FEENY

   Index   266

PART I

Theoretical Conceptualizations of Pathological Anxiety

1

Emotional Processing Theory

An Update

EDNA B. FOA
JONATHAN D. HUPPERT
SHAWN P. CAHILL

For nearly two decades, emotional processing theory (Foa & Kozak, 1985, 1986) has influenced the conceptualization of the nature of anxiety disorders and the psychological mechanisms of their effective treatment. This chapter discusses the basic premises of emotional processing theory as originally described by Foa and Kozak, as well as several hypotheses derived from the theory. We first describe the emotional processing conceptualization of the anxiety disorders and the mechanisms that are thought to underlie their recovery through effective treatment or natural recovery. We then discuss the current status of the theory by reviewing the relevant literature. In this review we focus on the evidence for the role of activation, within- and between-session habituation, and distraction and the relationship among these variables and cognitive, behavioral, and psychophysiological change. Next we discuss recent modifications to the theory, particularly in the areas of trauma/posttraumatic stress disorder (PTSD) and social phobia, which are based on empirical evidence, as well as learning and information processing theories. Finally, we identify a number of essential questions to guide future research in the nature and treatment of anxiety disorders.

HISTORY OF THE EMOTIONAL PROCESSING CONCEPT

The concept of emotional processing has its origin in Lang's (1977) analyses of fear-relevant imagery in the context of behavior therapy for fear reduction. In studying the procedure of systematic desensitization, Lang, Melamed, and Hart (1970) found three predictors of successful treatment: greater initial heart rate reactivity during fear-relevant imagery, greater concordance between self-reported distress and heart rate elevation during fear-relevant imagery, and a systematic decline in heart rate reactivity with repetition of the imagery. On the basis of his research, Lang (1977) suggested that "the psychophysiological structure of imagined scenes may be a key to the *emotional processing* [italics added] which the therapy is designed to accomplish" (p. 863). Although Lang did not elaborate on the term "emotional processing," subsequent papers advanced a bioinformational model of fear (e.g., Lang, 1984).

Lang's (1977, 1984) conceptual framework holds that a fear image is a cognitive structure containing stimulus, response, and meaning information that acts as a program to avoid or escape from danger. For example, the fear structure of a person with dog phobia includes representations of dogs, various physiological and behavioral fear responses (e.g., rapid heart rate, sweating, running away), and threat meanings associated with both dogs (e.g., "Dogs are dangerous") and the person's responses (e.g., "My rapid heart rate and sweating mean that I am afraid"); these representations are associated with one another. The fear structure is activated by information that matches some of the information represented in the structure and then spreads to other associated representations. Thus, in the dog-phobia example, confrontations with a dog not only activate the representation of a dog but also the danger meaning and the physiological responses of arousal and defensive behavioral responses. According to Lang (1977), "the aim of therapy could be described as the reorganization of the image unit in a way that modifies the affective character of its response elements" (p. 867). He further proposed that for image modification to occur, it is necessary for the fear structure to be activated to some extent. Accordingly, it is the necessary activation followed by image reorganization that accounts for the relationship between physiological measures (i.e., elevated heart rate reactivity followed by a decline in heart rate reactivity) and good outcome in exposure therapy for fear. However, Lang did not specify how activating the fear structure brings about changes in the response elements of the fear structure nor the nature of the changes that bring about a therapeutic outcome.

Rachman (1980) followed up on Lang's work by defining emotional processing as "a process whereby emotional disturbances are absorbed, and decline to the extent that other experiences and behaviors can proceed without disruption" (p. 51). Accordingly, successful processing would be indicated by a person's confrontation with a previously distressing stimulus or event without experiencing or exhibiting signs of distress. By contrast, clinical phenomena such as persistent fears, anxiety, or obsessions; failures to benefit from exposure therapy; and the return of fear after exposure therapy would be evidence of failed or incomplete emotional processing. Rachman's analysis provides a description of the phenomena of emotional processing but does not provide a theoretical explanation of this construct. Indeed, as noted by Foa and Kozak (1986), Rachman's definition suffers from circular reasoning: The fear reduction that is attributed to successful emotional processing is the same evidence used to infer that successful emotional processing has occurred. The task taken up by Foa and Kozak (1986) was to provide a theoretical framework to explain the phenomena of emotional processing.

FOA AND KOZAK'S EMOTIONAL PROCESSING THEORY

Fear Structures

Emotional processing theory (Foa & Kozak, 1985, 1986) builds on Lang's concept of fear structure, described previously, to explain the psychopathology and treatment of anxiety and its disorders. To this end, Foa and Kozak (1986) distinguished between normal and pathological fear structures. The former is adaptive, whereas the latter is maladaptive. In an adaptive fear structure, the associations among the representations reflect reality faithfully (e.g., a car veering toward me — danger meaning ["cars coming toward me are dangerous"] and fear [heart rate acceleration, scanning the road, veering the car off the road]). Thus, when a normal fear structure is activated by a dangerous situation (e.g., a car veering toward the person), it generates fear and leads to adaptive maneuvering by the individual (e.g., moving to safety) to avoid danger. In contrast, a pathological fear structure contains associations among the stimulus, response, and meaning representations that distort reality and includes excessive response elements (e.g., avoidance of safe situations). Foa and Kozak (1986) noted that pathological fear structures are resistant to modification but did not provide an explanation for this phenomenon. We propose that the persistence of a pathological fear structure is due to behavioral and cognitive avoidance, as well as to cognitive biases in processing information at various stages (encoding, interpretation, and retrieval). The avoidance and cognitive biases interfere with the acquisition of relevant information that is inconsistent with the existing elements of the pathological fear structure, a process that, as is discussed subsequently, constitutes the essence of recovery or emotional processing.

Foa and Kozak (1985) proposed that specific pathological fear structures underlie the different anxiety disorders and that successful psychosocial treatment modifies the pathological elements in the structures. Furthermore, each disorder contains elements common to other anxiety disorders (physiological response elements and escape or avoidance responses), as well as disorder-specific elements and associations. For example, the fear structure of patients with PTSD is characterized by a pathological association between trauma reminders, which are essentially safe situations or images, and danger or a sense of incompetence. By contrast, panic disorder is characterized by a pathological association between response elements (bodily sensations), such as shortness of breath, and threat of death or going crazy. Lang and colleagues (e.g., Lang, Davis, & Ohman, 2000; Cuthbert et al., 2003) reported differential levels of specificity and coherence of the fear structures for PTSD, panic disorder, specific phobia, and social anxiety disorder. Specifically, when imagining personally feared consequences, individuals with specific phobias had the highest magnitude of physiological reactivity, and those with panic disorder and PTSD had the lowest. Those with social phobia appeared to fall in the middle; people with generalized social phobia had somewhat less physiological reactivity, and individuals with more circumscribed fears had more physiological reactivity. These data are consistent with the contention that individuals with more discrete fears have more coherent fear structures (Foa & Kozak, 1986).

Emotional Processing: Modifying the Pathological Associations in the Fear Structures

Foa and Kozak (1985, 1986) originally defined emotional processing as the modification of the fear structure in which pathological associations among stimuli, responses, and meaning are replaced with nonpathological associations. They further suggested that this modification involves weakening erroneous associations and acquiring new associations. However, recent work on extinction and reinstatement (Bouton, 2000; Rescorla, 2001) suggests that extinction does not eliminate or replace previous associations but rather results in new learning that competes with the old information. Architecturally, it is not clear whether the new learning is best represented as the acquisition of new associations that inhibit expression of the old associations in the old structure or as the acquisition of a new fear structure that exists along with old structure (see Foa & McNally, 1996, for a discussion of the latter concept). In either case, both the old and the new information remain stored in memory. Depending on the context, either the original association/structure or the new association/structure can be activated and determine behaviors, cognitions, and emotions. Either model better accounts for spontaneous recovery in extinction paradigms and relapses after treatment than the original conceptualization by Foa and Kozak. One major therapeutic implication of this reconceptualization is that treatment should occur in multiple contexts in order to increase the likelihood that the new nonpathological fear structure or associations will be activated instead of the original pathological ones.

Foa and Kozak (1986) proposed that two conditions are necessary for emotional processing to occur: (1) activation of the fear structure and (2) incorporation of new information that is incompatible with the pathological elements of the fear structure. Activation occurs when an individual encounters stimuli or produces responses that are represented in the fear structure and that therefore are associated with danger meaning. In general, the greater the match between the fear-evoking experience and the person's pathological fear structure, the greater the activation. Although there was some suggestion of an "optimal" level of activation in the original theory, it seems that this concept requires further elaboration. Interestingly, neurobiological evidence now suggests that the amygdala needs to be activated in order to promote extinction in animals (Nader, Schafe, & LeDoux, 2000), thus indicating that some level of activation is in fact necessary. Our clinical experience suggests that an extreme level of activation (overactivation) may interfere with emotional processing, though the animal literature does not indicate such a phenomenon. It is likely that overactivation leads to a failure to incorporate new information due to inhibited attention, which diminishes encoding of the new corrective information and biases the processing of available information. Emotional processing theory posits that although activation is a necessary condition for emotional processing, it is not a sufficient condition, and that emotional processing requires the presence of information that disconfirms the erroneous elements in the structure. When such information is unavailable because the individual avoids or escapes the situation, the fear structure remains unchanged. Moreover, if the evocative situation contains information that confirms the person's feared consequences, the fear structure does not change and may even be strengthened. Even when disconfirmatory information is present during the evocative experience, emotional processing occurs only when it is encoded and incorporated into existing knowledge, that is, when new learning has occurred.

Exposure Therapy and Cognitive Modifications

Foa and Kozak (1986) suggested that certain pathological elements characterize the fear structures of individuals with anxiety disorders. The first type of pathological elements involves erroneous stimulus–stimulus associations (bald men → gun, for an individual raped by a bald man), stimulus–response associations (supermarket → heart palpitations, for an individual with panic disorder), and, most important, erroneous associations of safe stimuli with threat meanings (floors → germs → illness → death, for a person with obsessive–compulsive disorder) and responses with threat meanings (heart palpitations → heart attacks → death or danger, for a person with panic disorder). Foa and Kozak further suggested that, in addition to pathological associations, pathological elements in the fear structure involve erroneous evaluations. Three such evaluations received particular attention: exaggerated probability estimates of harm (e.g., everyone is critical), exaggerated cost associated with this anticipated harm (e.g., it is dreadful to be criticized), and the anticipation that in the absence of escape or avoidance, anxiety will remain forever and may itself cause psychological (e.g., going crazy) or physical harm (e.g., dying).

In discussing the mechanisms by which emotional processing of fear is achieved, Foa and Kozak (1985, 1986) suggested that *in vivo* exposure (real-life confrontations) to the feared stimulus (e.g., dog) in the absence of the anticipated harm corrects the exaggerated probability estimates of harm. Exaggerated cost, on the other hand, is achieved via habituation of fear during confrontation with the feared consequences, sometimes through imaginal exposure. We suggest that imaginal exposure to the feared consequences not only corrects the exaggerated cost but also strengthens the discrimination between "thoughts about harm" and "real harm," thus altering the associations between threat meaning of stimulus and/or response elements in the fear structure. A clear example is the patient with obsessive–compulsive disorder who erroneously equates thinking about harm with causing harm. Imaginal exposure to causing harm in the absence of real harm may alter the association between thinking about harm and threat. In the same vein, through repeated imaginal exposure of the traumatic memory, the patient with PTSD learns the distinction between remembering the trauma and being retraumatized, thus altering the association between the traumatic memory and threat meaning.

Exposure Therapy and Habituation

Emotional processing can occur as a result of everyday experiences (e.g., natural recovery following a trauma; see the later section on PTSD) or in the context of psychosocial treatment, such as cognitive and behavioral therapies or psychodynamic therapy. Exposure therapy involves helping people to repeatedly confront safe but feared thoughts, sensations, situations, and activities in order to promote emotional processing. Thus exposure therapy exercises are explicitly designed to activate the fear structure and at the same time provide corrective information about the nonthreat value of the stimuli, responses, and meaning elements evoked during the exercise.

Typically a decrease in fear occurs during prolonged exposure exercises (within-session habituation; e.g., Chaplin & Levine, 1981; Foa & Chambless, 1978), along with a decrease in peak intensity of fear across sessions (between-session habituation; e.g., Chaplin & Levine, 1981). Foa and Kozak (1986) identified the activation of fear followed by within- and between-session habituation as indicators of emotional processing that are related to, but conceptually distinct from, symptom reduction. In addition to being an indicator of emotional processing, habituation may be a source of disconfirming information, such as information about the *absence* of physiological responding in the presence of the targeted stimulus that is incompatible with prior response information. Habituation may also disconfirm erroneous beliefs about the consequences of intense anxiety, such as the belief that anxiety will persist unless the person escapes the fear-evoking situation.

Several studies have found a relationship of between-session habituation with symptom reduction (i.e., treatment outcome; van Minnen & Hagenaars, 2002; van Minnen & Foa, submitted; Kozak, Foa, & Steketee, 1988; Jaycox, Foa, & Morral, 1998). However, the relationship between within-session habituation and symptom reduction is more ambiguous. Within-session habituation has been positively related to longer continuous exposure (Chaplin & Levine, 1981; van Minnen & Hagenaars, 2002; van Minnen & Foa, submitted), and longer continuous exposure has been positively related to symptom reduction in some studies (Chaplin & Levine, 1981; Rabavilas, Boulougouris, & Stefanis, 1976; Stern & Marks, 1973) but not others (van Minnen & Foa, submitted). However, most studies have not found a direct relationship between within-session habituation and symptom reduction (van Minnen & Foa, submitted; Jaycox et al., 1998; Foa et al., 1983; Kozak et al., 1988; Mathews, Johnston, Shaw, & Gelder, 1974). Further evidence that within-session habituation is not a necessary condition for improvement includes the finding that people with agoraphobia who were allowed to escape from their feared situations before their anxiety decreased improved as much as those who were instructed to stay in the situations until their fear diminished (Emmelkamp, 1974; De Silva & Rachman, 1984; Rachman, Craske, Tallman, & Solyon, 1986). It is possible, then, that within-session habituation is not a reliable indicator of emotional processing. Indeed, reduction of anxiety occurring within a session may sometimes be due to factors that are hypothesized to impair emotional processing, such as distraction and cognitive avoidance. In addition, some information may take time to be processed, such that disconfirming information that had been presented during exposure is not fully incorporated until some time after the exposure exercise (i.e., between sessions) rather than within the session. In fact, this may be the case with cognitive therapy for the anxiety disorders (e.g., Clark, 2001; Rachman, 2003). That being said, it is likely that, for individuals who are fully engaged with an exposure exercise (i.e., without any avoidance) and experience within-session habituation, such habituation is still an indicator of emotional processing and may facilitate between-session habituation (Foa et al., 1983; Pitman, Orr, Altman, & Longpre, 1996). Overall, the deemphasis on the relationship between within-session habituation and outcome is not critical to emotional processing theory because the proposed mechanism underlying symptom reduction is the modification of the relevant erroneous associations through disconfirming information, not through habituation per se. In fact, Foa and Kozak (1986) proposed that within-session habituation is mainly important for patients whose core fear is the erroneous belief that anxiety "stays forever unless escape is realized." For these patients, within-session habituation provides the information that disconfirms their erroneous evaluation. In most cases, the encoding of new information that contradicts the pathological elements in the fear structure occurs both within and between sessions.

Exposure Therapy and Distraction

Foa and Kozak (1986) viewed distraction as a form of cognitive avoidance and therefore hypothesized that distraction would impair emotional processing. Theoretically, distraction could serve to limit activation of the fear structure, prevent the encoding of disconfirming information, or both. The empirical literature on the effects of distraction on fear reduction is inconsistent with regard to the relationship between distraction and habituation. A number of studies have presented data suggesting that distraction interferes with within- and between-session habituation (Grayson, Foa, & Steketee, 1986; Rodriguez & Craske, 1993; Telch et al., 2004), whereas two studies by Page and colleagues (Oliver & Page, 2003; Johnstone & Page, 2004) have suggested that distraction actually facilitates habituation in people with blood-injury and spider phobia. These inconsistencies may be due to methodological differences among studies. First, the only studies to date that have suggested that distraction may facilitate habituation and symptom reduction are for specific phobia. All studies on other anxiety-disordered populations have not found such effects, though none have attempted to replicate Page's distraction technique. Perhaps distraction facilitates partial disengagement in people with specific phobia, but it could be likely to interfere more fully in other individuals with anxiety disorders who also show less coherent fear structures (see Cuthbert et al., 2003, and previous discussion). Alternatively, it is possible that distraction and decreased attention are two different concepts. Page's method involved counting backward by various number intervals, which would still allow eye contact and some level of attentional engagement during the exposure. Many of the other studies used tasks that aimed at producing such an extensive cognitive load that virtually no attentional resources could be allocated to the threat stimuli during the exposure. If distraction is defined as complete disengagement from threat stimuli, then Page's studies do not meet such criteria. However, questions remain as to why decreased attention would be beneficial during exposure to feared stimuli, as it would presumably interfere with activation and with encoding of corrective information.

PTSD AND SOCIAL PHOBIA: THE APPLICATION OF EMOTIONAL PROCESSING THEORY TO SPECIFIC ANXIETY DISORDERS

In the original formulation of emotional processing theory (Foa & Kozak, 1986), examples from specific phobias, panic disorder with agoraphobia, and obsessive–compulsive disorder were used to explicate the model. More recently, we have focused on the psychopathology and treatment of PTSD and social anxiety disorder and have elaborated models for both disorders within the framework of emotional processing theory (Foa, Steketee, & Rothbaum, 1989; Foa & Jaycox, 1999; Foa & Cahill, 2001; Huppert & Foa, 2004). In this section we start with an application of emotional processing theory to natural recovery from trauma and treatment of chronic PTSD. Following that discussion, we describe a model of social anxiety disorder and how it may integrate well with another current conceptualization of social anxiety (Clark & Wells, 1995).

Natural Recovery from Trauma

Longitudinal studies investigating patterns of reactions following a trauma indicate that individuals differ in their abilities to successfully recover from, and therefore process, a traumatic event. Although most trauma survivors do process the trauma successfully, a substantial minority fail to do so and consequently develop chronic PTSD (e.g., Riggs, Rothbaum, & Foa, 1995; Rothbaum, Foa, Riggs, Murdock, & Walsh, 1992).

Foa (1997) identified three factors that are associated with both natural recovery from trauma and reduction of PTSD severity via exposure therapy. The first factor is emotional engagement with the trauma memory, which is equivalent to the concept of fear activation discussed earlier. In natural recovery, emotional engagement refers to fear activation that occurs when one encounters a trauma reminder in the natural environment. Given that fear activation has been found to be positively associated with treatment outcome (Foa, Riggs, Massie, & Yarczower, 1995; Pitman et al., 1996), we may hypothesize that a *lack* of emotional engagement would be associated with poor natural recovery following a traumatic event. Dissociative symptoms, such as feelings of derealization or depersonalization during or following a trauma or amnesia for information related to the trauma, have been conceptualized as strategies that reduce emotional engagement in order to avoid trauma-related emotions (Foa & Hearst-Ikeda, 1996). Consistent with the tenets of emotional processing theory, several studies have found that peritraumatic dissociation is associated with more severe PTSD (e.g., Cardena & Spiegel, 1993; Koopman, Classen, & Spiegel, 1994). Similarly, a delay in the peak reaction to a traumatic event may also be seen as initial interference in emotional engagement and thus is expected to hinder emotional processing and natural recovery. Consistent with this hypothesis, individuals whose peak symptom severity occurred within 2 weeks of the traumatic event were less symptomatic 14 weeks later than were individuals whose symptoms peaked between 2 and 6 weeks after the event (Gilboa-Schechtman & Foa, 2001).

The second factor associated with both natural recovery and treatment outcome is a change in trauma-related cognitions. Two basic meaning elements are thought to be at the core of the fear structure for PTSD: that the world is completely dangerous and that the self is totally incompetent (Foa & Rothbaum, 1998; Foa & Riggs, 1993). It follows that individuals with PTSD will exhibit more severe negative cognitions about the world and themselves than individuals who have either experienced a trauma without developing PTSD or who never experienced a trauma. This hypothesis was confirmed by Foa, Ehlers, Clark, Tolin, and Orsillo (1999). Similarly, successful emotional processing of a traumatic memory requires changes in the fear structure related to these two meaning elements such that natural recovery following trauma and recovery from chronic PTSD following treatment will both be associated with reductions in those negative cognitions. In a longitudinal study of crime victims, individuals who recovered from PTSD 3 months after their assaults exhibited fewer negative cognitions than those who continued to have PTSD (Riggs, Rauch, Moser, & Foa, 2005). Similarly, cognitions about the world and themselves decreased with treatment for PTSD, and changes in cognitions were associated with changes in PTSD severity (Foa & Rauch, 2004).

The third factor hypothesized by Foa (1997) to be associated with both natural recovery and improvement with treatment is the level of organization of the trauma narratives. This factor has also gained empirical support. Specifically, a higher degree of narrative articulation shortly after the trauma was predictive of greater recovery (lower PTSD symptom severity) 3 months later (Amir, Stafford, Freshman, & Foa, 1998). Similarly, exposure therapy for PTSD was associated with increased organization and decreased disorganization of the trauma narrative over the course of treatment, and those changes were correlated with symptom improvement (Foa, Molnar, & Cashman, 1995). The ways in which exposure therapy is thought to promote fear activation and modification of erroneous cognitions were explicated earlier. In addition, repeated recounting of the trauma memory during imaginal exposure and discussing the memory with the therapist not only alters the association between remembering the trauma and threat or danger but may also help reduce the fragmented quality of the trauma narrative. Over repetitions of the narrative, the sequence of events becomes better established, and details remembered in one recounting are incorporated into subsequent recountings, thereby helping to create a coherent narrative. It may be hypothesized that a more coherent narrative reflects a more coherent fear structure that allows more complete activation and subsequent changes in the pathological elements of the fear structure. Foa and Cahill (2001) proposed that emotional processing that leads to natural recovery occurs through repeated activation of the fear structure via the trauma memory by engaging with trauma-related thoughts and feelings, by sharing the thoughts and feelings with others, and by confronting trauma-reminder stimuli in daily life. In the absence of additional traumas, these natural exposures contain information that disconfirms the common posttrauma associations within the fear structure, such as that the world in general or specific trauma reminders are dangerous and that the person's actions during the trauma or subsequent PTSD symptoms means the person is incompetent. For example, a rape survivor may repeatedly encounter men who are physically similar to the perpetrator, thus activating the trauma memory structure. As these encounters do not lead to additional assaults, the natural initial postrape inclination to view the world (e.g., all men) as entirely dangerous is not confirmed and thus gradually subsides. In addition, repeated thinking or talking about the traumatic event promotes habituation of negative emotions and the generation of an organized trauma narrative. By contrast, individuals who avoid engaging with the traumatic memories by either suppressing related thoughts and feelings or avoiding trauma-related situations do not have the opportunity to experience the habituation of negative emotions, to disconfirm the initial posttrauma negative cognitions, or to form an organized narrative and thus develop chronic disturbances.

Consistent with the proposed conceptualization of natural recovery, Creamer, Burgess, and Pattison (1992) found, among a group of individuals who were present when a man went on a shooting spree in a crowded building, that high levels of reexperiencing shortly after the trauma were correlated with lower levels of distress 4 weeks later. Similarly, Lepore, Silver, Wortman, and Wayment (1996) found that, 18 months after the trauma of losing their babies to sudden infant death syndrome, mothers who were able to share their loss with a supportive social network had resolved their grief more than did mothers who were not able to do so. Thus avoidance of trauma memories and reminders appears to interfere with natural recovery, whereas talking about the experience with supportive others appears to facilitate natural recovery. As noted previously, a less fragmented narrative is also associated with less severe PTSD (e.g., Amir et al., 1998), but a recent study by Gray and Lombardo (2001) found that organization was no longer related to PTSD after accounting for the decreased cognitive abilities often found in patients with PTSD. To the extent that cognitive impairments seen in PTSD reflect the effects of anxiety on information processing, it is possible that increased organization is a *consequence* of emotional processing rather than a mechanism by which emotional processing occurs. More research is needed to examine the conflicting findings.

The Fear Structure of Social Anxiety Disorder

Social anxiety disorder is characterized by excessive fear of embarrassment or humiliation in interpersonal or other social situations that leads to significant distress and impairment. The core fear in social anxiety disorder is not of physical threat, but rather of criticism, isolation, ostracization, and/or rejection by others. Thus social anxiety disorder may be conceptualized as a "fear of embarrassment." Data suggest that social anxiety disorder can be clustered into specific situational fears (e.g., a fear of public speeches) or fears that vary across a number of social situations, including interpersonal and performance realms (generalized social phobia; Kessler, Stein, & Berglund, 1998). Because individuals with generalized social anxiety disorder make up the majority of the patients who seek treatment, we focus on them here. The model we present for the fear structure of generalized social anxiety disorder draws on clinical research into the psychopathology of social anxiety disorder, research in social psychology, emotion theory on embarrassment (e.g., Keltner & Buswell, 1997), and our direct clinical experience.

Stimulus Representations

By definition, the stimuli represented in the fear structure of an individual with social anxiety disorder are circumscribed to people or social situations (e.g., peers, authority figures, or individuals of the opposite sex). However, for most of these individuals, the fear structure contains a multitude of stimuli and contexts. One particular aspect of the fear structure in social anxiety disorder that has gained recent interest is images of oneself in social interactions. For example, Hackmann, Clark, and McManus (2000) found that patients with social anxiety disorder had specific recurrent images during social interactions and that these images appeared to be related to negative social interactions retrospectively reported to be related to the onset of the disorder. Furthermore, the individual views these images from the perspective of an observer (Clark & Wells, 1995; Spurr & Stopa, 2003; Wells, Clark, & Ahmad, 1998), and a consequence of these images is that they bias information processing (for a more detailed discussion of these and other findings about imagery and social anxiety, see Hirsch & Clark, 2004).

Representations of Verbal, Physiological, and Behavioral Responses

Verbal responses in the fear structure of individuals with social anxiety can have several functions: an expression of anxiety (e.g., hesitations in speech such as "ummm" or "uhhhhh"), avoidance of poor performance in a social situation (e.g., by asking questions, changing topics away from oneself, etc.), or attempts to distract others from signs of one's anxiety (e.g., saying "it's hot in here" if the person feels sweaty). Physiological responses include changes in heart rate, blushing, sweating, and trembling. Some of the physiological responses reflect anxiety (sweating, trembling or shaking), and others reflect embarrassment (blushing). Notably, anxiety is associated with increases in heart rate (Cuthbert et al., 2003), whereas embarrassment is often associated with decreased heart rate (Keltner & Buswell, 1997); and either of these experiences may occur in the individual with social anxiety disorder. Behavioral responses include various types of escape and avoidance maneuvers, which can be of a very subtle nature and may include cognitive strategies (e.g., distraction). Clark and Wells (1995) have labeled these subtle avoidance behaviors "safety behaviors" (cf. Salkovskis, 1991) and have emphasized their role in the maintenance of social anxiety disorder.

Several of the responses in social anxiety are associated with threat meaning because they are viewed as drawing criticism, thereby leading to a spiraling of anxiety in social situations. Two studies examined the hypothesis that the fear structure of social anxiety disorder contains pathological associations between response representations (e.g., heart racing, blushing, sweating) and threatening meaning (e.g., social incompetence). Roth, Antony, and Swinson (2001) found that individuals with social anxiety disorder were more likely than controls to interpret their symptoms of anxiety as pathological (i.e., intense anxiety or some psychiatric problem) and less likely to interpret them as normal. Furthermore, Wells and Papageorgiou (2001a) reported that false feedback regarding pulse rate (e.g., "your pulse has increased/decreased") influenced ratings of self-reported anxiety and the strength of beliefs about an idiosyncratic feared consequence in the expected direction in patients with social anxiety disorder. Thus perceived strength of responses influences the threat meaning of those responses.

Cognitive Biases and the Meaning Representations of Stimuli and Responses

As noted, an additional aspect of the original emotional processing theory is the central role played by two erroneous evaluations that can also be conceptualized as cognitive biases: overestimation of the probability of feared harm and exaggerated cost of the feared outcome. Both feature prominently in the pathological fear structure of social anxiety disorder (Foa & Kozak, 1985, 1986, 1993). Foa, Franklin, and Kozak (2001) elaborated on this model, proposing that the erroneous meanings associated with social stimuli and fear responses are influenced by interpretation and judgment biases. Huppert and Foa (2004) further elaborated these concepts and integrated these findings with Mathews and Mackintosh's (1998) model of information processing biases in anxiety.

Several studies provide support for the hypothesized relationship between judgment biases about social stimuli and social anxiety disorder. For example, Gilboa-Schechtmann, Franklin, and Foa (2000) found that patients with generalized social anxiety disorder had greater estimates of probability and cost for unambiguous negative events (e.g., a boss berating one in front of others), greater estimates of cost of positive events, and lower estimates of the probability of positive events than both anxious and nonanxious control participants. Similarly, Foa, Franklin, Perry, and Herbert (1996) found both cost and probability biases in patients with generalized social anxiety disorder, although changes in cost biases were more predictive of change in symptoms of social anxiety after cognitive-behavioral treatment than were changes in probability biases. Consistent with Foa et al. (1996), Uren, Szabo, and Lovibond (2004) reported that although both cost and probability bias appear to contribute to social anxiety, cost was a stronger predictor of severity, whereas probability and cost estimates equally predicted the severity of the fear of bodily sensations in panic disorder. Stopa and Clark's (2000) results further support the relationship between exaggerated cost for negative social events and generalized social anxiety disorder. The primacy of cost over probability could not be tested in their study because the latter was not examined. However, in a follow-up study, McManus, Clark, and Hackmann (2000) included both mild and severe negative social events and found that both probability and cost were related to severity of social anxiety and to treatment outcome. Voncken, Bogels, and de Vries (2003) also found that both probability and cost equally contributed to severity of social anxiety. However, Voncken et al. (2003) used only evaluation situations for the judgments, excluding physiological experiences that can be important for individuals with social anxiety.

In summary, Foa and Kozak (1985) proposed that exaggerated cost is the more prominent erroneous evaluation in social anxiety disorder, whereas overestimation of probabilities is more central to specific phobia and panic disorder. The research to date indicates that both cost and probability estimates contribute to social anxiety, but their relative contributions are not entirely clear. We suggest that for highly negative social events (e.g., being rejected by many people), probabilities are likely going to be more important, whereas for mild negative social events (which frequently occur), it is the overestimation of cost that will be more important in social anxiety. Many other anxiety disorders do not include mild negative events, thus making cost a more prominent feature in social anxiety than in other anxiety disorders. Perhaps, then, as suggested by Foa and Kozak (1985), specific fear structures underlying the anxiety disorders differ in the relative influence that probability and cost estimates have on the threat meaning associated with stimuli and responses.

THE TREATMENT OF SOCIAL ANXIETY DISORDER

In order to promote emotional processing via exposure therapy (correction of the pathological elements of the target fear structure), the situation that activates the fear structure should incorporate corrective information that is contradictory to the erroneous associations represented in the structure. Generally, the corrective information is embedded in the absence of harm during confrontation with the feared situation, object, or memory (e.g., giving a speech without the audience booing), thus leading to changes in the patient's evaluations. Indeed, Hope, Heimberg, and Bruch (1995) found that negative social cognitions decreased significantly after exposure therapy. However, for emotional processing to occur, it is essential that the person perceives that the feared consequences did not occur. In the case of a person with dog phobia interacting with a friendly dog, the absence of negative consequences is obvious. However, because of the nature of social interactions, information disconfirming the patient's belief that others are judgmental may be obscured. The ambiguity of a social situation stems from the fact that explicit negative feedback during social interactions is censored and that false praise may be offered in the name of politeness. Thus the absence of open criticism or the presence of some compliments cannot be interpreted as an indication that the individuals involved in a given social interaction unambiguously enjoyed it. Even when corrective information is available in a social interaction, a number of other factors may interfere with encoding this information: self-focus, engaging in safety behaviors, attentional bias, and overactivation. Safety behaviors (e.g., keeping hands in one's pockets to prevent people from seeing them shake; Clark & Wells, 1995; Salkovskis, 1991), also referred to as subtle avoidance behaviors (Foa & Kozak, 1986), may be performed in order to prevent the feared consequences, reinforcing the perception that criticism or rejection would have occurred had they not engaged in the safety behaviors. Attentional and interpretation biases lead to selective encoding of social situations as negative, thus further impeding opportunities for emotional processing in the natural environment of the individual with social phobia.

It follows from the preceding considerations that the goal of treatment is to set up social situations in sessions that will both activate the fear structure and provide unambiguous information that disconfirms the patient's negative perceptions and evaluations. In other words, successful treatment imposes task demands that are sufficiently strong to override the hypervigilance to negative feedback and forces the patient to incorporate evidence of his or her adequate social performance (e.g., through video feedback or feedback from others; cf. Harvey, Clarke, Ehlers, & Rapee, 2000). In this way, disconfirming evidence, either during or after the contrived social situation, is incorporated into the fear structure, thus reducing the estimated probability and cost of negative outcomes.

Accordingly, a number of techniques that have recently been introduced into cognitive-behavioral therapies for social anxiety disorder emphasize the elimination of safety behaviors, the encouragement of outward focus, and the presentation of incompatible information via video and confederate feedback (Clark, 2001). Treatments utilizing these techniques have shown a successful reduction of social anxiety (Clark et al., 2003; Wells & Papageorgiou, 2001b). To optimize emotional processing, we have combined these techniques with imaginal and *in vivo* exposure and social skills training in our individualized Comprehensive Cognitive Behavioral Therapy (CCBT; Huppert, Roth, & Foa, 2003).

After successful treatment of an individual with social anxiety disorder, there are a number of changes that indicate successful emotional processing. These include reduced (1) probability estimates, (2) cost estimates, (3) attentional biases, (4) interpretation bias, (5) beliefs that anxiety during social situations remains forever, and (6) beliefs about the consequence of social situations (e.g., being rejected). The first four indicators are changes in information processing that may mediate the changes in beliefs, as well as produce reduction in social anxiety symptoms.

DISCUSSION AND FUTURE DIRECTIONS

In this chapter we have presented an update of emotional processing theory and applied the theory to two disorders that were not discussed in great detail in Foa and Kozak's (1985, 1986) original formulation: PTSD and social anxiety disorder. Emotional processing theory appears to account quite well for natural recovery, as well as for treatment of anxiety disorders, whether by exposure therapy, cognitive therapy, or other alternatives. However, a number of questions require further examination.

1. Can emotional processing theory account for other emotions in the same way in which it accounts for fear and anxiety? Recent work by Hayes suggests that depression may be conceptualized within an emotional processing theory framework and that mechanisms similar to those underlying fear reduction operate during reduction of depression (see Hayes, Beevers, Feldman, Laurenceau, & Perlman, 2005). Data indicating that anger, guilt, and shame decrease with treatment for PTSD suggest that these emotions as well may share common mechanisms with anxiety (see Cahill, Rauch, Hembree, & Foa, 2003, Foa & Rauch, 2004; Rothbaum, Ruef, Litz, Han, & Hodges, 2003).

2. Can findings from neuroscience help clarify principles of emotional processing theory? For example, data from LeDoux's lab indicate that amygdala activation is necessary for extinction (Nader et al., 2000). This

finding is consistent with the proposition that activation of the fear structure is necessary for emotional processing to occur.

3. How can emotional processing theory be integrated with other information processing theories of anxiety (e.g., Mogg & Bradley, 1998)? How does it relate to the recent findings of training of attentional and interpretation biases (Mathews & MacLeod, 2002)?

REFERENCES

Amir, N., Stafford, J., Freshman, M. S., & Foa, E. B. (1998). Relationship between trauma narratives and trauma pathology. *Journal of Traumatic Stress, 11*(2), 385–392.

Bouton, M. E. (2000). A learning theory perspective on lapse, relapse, and the maintenance of behavior change. *Health Psychology, 19*(1, Suppl.), 57–63.

Cahill, S. P., Rauch, S. A., Hembree, E. A., & Foa, E. B. (2003). Effect of cognitive-behavioral treatments for PTSD on anger. *Journal of Cognitive Psychotherapy, 17*(2), 113–131.

Cardena, E., & Spiegel, D. (1993). Dissociative reactions to the San Francisco Bay Area earthquake of 1989. *American Journal of Psychiatry, 150*(3), 474–478.

Chaplin, E. W., & Levine, B. A. (1981). The effects of total exposure duration and interrupted versus continuous exposure in flooding therapy. *Behavior Therapy, 12*, 360–368.

Clark, D. M. (2001). A cognitive perspective on social phobia. In W. R. Crozier & L. E. Alden (Eds.), *International handbook of social anxiety: Concepts, research and interventions related to the self and shyness* (pp. 405–430). New York: Wiley.

Clark, D. M., Ehlers, A., McManus, F., Hackmann, A., Fennell, M., Campbell, H., et al. (2003). Cognitive therapy vs. fluoxetine in generalized social phobia: A randomized placebo controlled trial. *Journal of Consulting and Clinical Psychology, 71*, 1058–1067.

Clark, D. M., & Wells, A. (1995). A cognitive model of social phobia. In R.G. Heimberg, M.R. Liebowitz, D.A. Hope, & F.R. Schneier (Eds.), *Social phobia: Diagnosis, assessment, and treatment* (pp. 69–93). New York: Guilford Press.

Creamer, M., Burgess, P., & Pattison, P. (1992). Reaction to trauma: A cognitive processing model. *Journal of Abnormal Psychology, 101*, 425–459.

Cuthbert, B. N., Lang, P. J., Strauss, C., Drobes, D., Patrick, C. J., & Bradley, M. M. (2003). The psychophysiology of anxiety disorder: Fear memory imagery. *Psychophysiology, 40*, 407–422.

De Silva, P., & Rachman, S. (1984). Does escape behavior strenghten agoraphobic avoidance? A preliminary study. *Behaviour Research and Therapy, 22*, 87–91.

Emmelkamp, P. M. G. (1974). Self-observation versus flooding in the treatment of agoraphobia. *Behaviour Research and Therapy, 12*, 229–237.

Foa, E. B. (1997). Psychological processes related to recovery from a trauma and an effective treatment for PTSD. In R. Yehuda & A. McFarlane (Vol. Eds.), *Annals of the New York Academy of Sciences: Vol. 821. Psychobiology of PTSD* (pp. 410–424). New York: Academy of Sciences.

Foa, E. B., & Cahill, S. P. (2001). Emotional processing in psychological therapies. In N. J. Smelser & P. B. Bates (Eds.), *International encyclopedia of the social and behavioral sciences* (pp. 12363–12369). Oxford, UK: Elsevier.

Foa, E. B., & Chambless, D. (1978). Habituation of subjective anxiety during flooding in imagery. *Behaviour Research and Therapy, 16*, 391–399.

Foa, E. B., Ehlers, A., Clark, D. M., Tolin, D. F., & Orsillo, S. M. (1999). The Posttraumatic Cognitions Inventory (PTCI): Development and validation. *Psychological Assessment, 11*, 303–314.

Foa, E. B., Franklin, M. E., & Kozak, M. J. (2001). Social phobia: An information processing perspective. In S. Hofman & P. M. DiBartolo (Eds.), *From social anxiety to social phobia: Multiple perspectives* (pp. 268–280). Needham, MA: Allyn & Bacon.

Foa, E. B., Franklin, M. E., Perry, K. J., & Herbert, J. D. (1996). Cognitive biases in generalized social phobia. *Journal of Abnormal Psychology, 105*, 433–439.

Foa, E. B., Grayson, J. B., Steketee, G. S., Doppelt, H. G., Turner, R. M., & Latimer, P. R. (1983). Success and failure in the behavioral treatment of obsessive–compulsives. *Journal of Counseling and Clinical Psychology, 51*(2), 287–297.

Foa, E. B., & Hearst-Ikeda, D. (1996). Emotional dissociation in response to trauma: An information-processing approach. In L. K. Michelson & W. J. Ray (Eds.), *Handbook of dissociation: Theoretical, empirical, and clinical perspectives* (pp. 207–224). New York: Plenum Press.

Foa, E. B., & Jaycox, L. H. (1999). Cognitive-behavioral theory and treatment of posttraumatic stress disorder. In D. Spiegel (Ed.), *Efficacy and cost-effectiveness of psychotherapy* (pp. 23–61). Washington, DC: American Psychiatric.

Foa, E. B., & Kozak, M. J. (1985). Treatment of anxiety disorders: Implications for psychopathology. In A. H. Tuma & J. D. Maser (Eds.), *Anxiety and the anxiety disorders* (pp. 421–452). Hillsdale, NJ: Erlbaum.

Foa, E. B., & Kozak, M. J. (1986). Emotional processing of fear: Exposure to corrective information. *Psychological Bulletin, 99*, 20–35.

Foa, E. B., & Kozak, M. J. (1993). Pathological anxiety: The meaning and the structure of fear. In N. Birbaumer & A. Ohman (Eds.), *The structure of emotion* (pp. 110–121). Toronto, Ontario, Canada: Hogrefe.

Foa, E. B., & McNally, R. J. (1996). Mechanisms of change in exposure therapy. In R. M. Rapee (Ed.), *Current controversies in the anxiety disorders* (pp. 329–343). New York: Guilford Press.

Foa, E. B., Molnar, C., & Cashman, L. (1995). Change in rape narratives during exposure therapy for posttraumatic stress disorder. *Journal of Traumatic Stress, 8*(4), 675–690.

Foa, E. B., & Rauch, S. A. M. (2004). Cognitive changes during prolonged exposure versus prolonged exposure plus cognitive restructuring in female assault survivors with posttraumatic stress disorder. *Journal of Consulting and Clinical Psychology, 72*(5), 879–884.

Foa, E. B., & Riggs, D. S. (1993). Post-traumatic stress disorder in rape victims. In J. Oldham, M. B. Riba, & A. Tasman (Eds.), *American Psychiatric Press review of psychiatry* (Vol. 12, pp. 273–303). Washington, DC: American Psychiatric Press.

Foa, E. B., Riggs, D. S., Massie, E. D., & Yarczower, M. (1995). The impact of fear activation and anger on the efficacy of exposure treatment for posttraumatic stress disorder. *Behavior Therapy, 26*, 487–499.

Foa, E. B., & Rothbaum, B. O. (1998). *Treating the trauma of rape: Cognitive-behavioral therapy for PTSD*. New York: Guilford Press.

Foa, E. B., Steketee, G., & Rothbaum, B. O. (1989). Behavioral/cognitive conceptualizations of posttraumatic stress disorder. *Behavior Therapy, 20*, 155–176.

Gilboa-Schechtman, E., & Foa, E. B. (2001). Patterns of recovery from trauma: The use of intraindividual analysis. *Journal of Abnormal Psychology, 110*(3), 392–400.

Gilboa-Schechtman, E., Franklin, M. E., & Foa, E. B. (2000). Anticipated reactions to social events: Differences among individuals with generalized social phobia, obsessive–compulsive disorder, and nonanxious controls. *Cognitive Therapy and Research, 24*, 731–746.

Gray, M. J., & Lombardo, T. W. (2001). Complexity of trauma narratives as an index of fragmented memory in PTSD: A critical analysis. *Applied Cognitive Psychology, 15*(7), S171–S186.

Grayson, J. B., Foa, E. B., & Steketee, G. S. (1986). Exposure in vivo of obsessive–compulsives under distracting and attention-focusing conditions: Replication and extension. *Behaviour Research and Therapy, 24*(4), 475–479.

Hackmann, A., Clark, D. M., & McManus, F. (2000). Recurrent images and early memories in social phobia. *Behaviour Research and Therapy, 38*, 601–610.

Harvey, A. G., Clark, D. M., Ehlers, A., & Rapee, R. M. (2000). Social anxiety and self-impression: Cognitive preparation enhances the beneficial effects of video feedback following a stressful social task. *Behaviour Research and Therapy, 38*(12), 1183–1192.

Hayes, A. M., Beevers, C., Feldman, G. C., Laurenceau, J. P., & Perlman, C. A. (2005). Avoidance and processing as predictors of symptom change and positive growth in an integrative therapy for depression. *International Journal of Behavioral Medicine, 12*, 111–122.

Hirsch, C. R., & Clark, D. M. (2004). Information-processing bias in social phobia. *Clinical Psychology Review, 24*(7), 799–825.

Hope, D. A., Heimberg, R. G., & Bruch, M. A. (1995). Dismantling cognitive-behavioral group therapy for social phobia. *Behaviour Research and Therapy, 33*, 637–650.

Huppert, J. D., & Foa, E. B. (2004). Maintenance mechanisms in social anxiety: An integration of cognitive biases and emotional processing theory. In J. Yiend (Ed.), *Cognition, emotion, and psychopathology* (pp. 213–231). Cambridge, UK: Cambridge University Press.

Huppert, J. D., Roth, D. A., & Foa, E. B. (2003). Cognitive behavioral therapy for social phobia: New advances. *Current Psychiatry Reports, 5*, 289–296.

Jaycox, L. H., Foa, E. B., & Morral, A. R. (1998). Influence of emotional engagement and habituation on exposure therapy for PTSD. *Journal of Consulting and Clinical Psychology, 66*, 185–192.

Johnstone, K. A., & Page, A. C. (2004). Attention to phobic stimuli during exposure: The effect of distraction on anxiety reduction, self-efficacy and perceived control. *Behaviour Research and Therapy, 42*(3), 249–275.

Keltner, D., & Buswell, B. N. (1997). Embarrassment: Its distinct form and appeasement functions. *Psychological Bulletin, 122*, 250–270.

Kessler, R. C., Stein, M. B., & Berglund, P. (1998). Social phobia subtypes in the National Comorbidity Survey. *American Journal of Psychiatry, 155*, 613–619.

Koopman, C., Classen, C., & Spiegel, D. A. (1994). Predictors of posttraumatic stress symptoms among survivors of the Oakland/Berkeley, California, firestorm. *American Journal of Psychiatry, 151,* 888–894.

Kozak, M. J., Foa, E. B., & Steketee, G. (1988). Process and outcome of exposure treatment with obsessive–compulsives: Psychophysiological indicators of emotional processing. *Behavior Therapy, 19,* 157–169.

Lang, P. J. (1977). Imagery in therapy: An information processing analysis of fear. *Behavior Therapy, 8,* 862–886.

Lang, P. J. (1984). Cognition in emotion: Concept and action. In C. Izard, J. Kagan, & R. Zajonc (Eds.), *Emotion, cognition and behavior* (pp. 193–206). New York: Cambridge University Press.

Lang, P. J., Davis, M., & Ohman, A. (2000). Fear and anxiety: Animal models and human cognitive psychophysiology. *Journal of Affective Disorders, 61,* 137–159.

Lang, P. J., Melamed, B. G., & Hart, J. (1970). A psychophysiological analysis of fear modification using an automated desensitization procedure. *Journal of Abnormal Psychology, 76,* 220–234.

Lepore, S. J., Silver, R. C., Wortman, C. B., & Wayment, H. A. (1996). Social constraints, intrusive thoughts, and depressive symptoms among bereaved mothers. *Journal of Personality and Social Psychology, 70,* 271–282.

Mathews, A. M., Johnston, D. W., Shaw, P. M., & Gelder, M. G. (1974). Process variables and the prediction of outcome in behaviour therapy. *British Journal of Psychiatry, 125,* 256–264.

Mathews, A., & Mackintosh, B. (1998). A cognitive model of selective processing in anxiety. *Cognitive Therapy and Research, 22,* 539–560.

Mathews, A., & MacLeod, C. (2002). Induced processing biases have causal effects on anxiety. *Cognition and Emotion, 16*(3), 331–354.

McManus, F., Clark, D. M., & Hackmann, A. (2000). Specificity of cognitive biases in social phobia and their role in recovery. *Behaviour and Cognitive Psychotherapy, 28*(3), 201–209.

Mogg, K., & Bradley, B. P. (1998). A cognitive-motivational analysis of anxiety. *Behaviour Research and Therapy, 36*(9), 809–848.

Nader, K., Schafe, G. E., & LeDoux, J. E. (2000). Fear memories require protein synthesis in the amygdala for reconsolidation after retrieval. *Nature, 406*(6797), 722–726.

Oliver, N. S., & Page, A. C. (2003). Fear reduction during in vivo exposure to blood-injection stimuli: Distraction vs. attentional focus. *British Journal of Clinical Psychology, 42*(1), 13–25.

Pitman, R. K., Orr, S. P., Altman, B., & Longpre, R. E. (1996). Emotional processing and outcome of imaginal flooding therapy in Vietnam veterans with chronic posttraumatic stress disorder. *Comprehensive Psychiatry, 37*(6), 409–418.

Rabavilas, A. D., Boulougouris, J. C., & Stefanis, C. (1976). Duration of flooding sessions in the treatment of obsessive–compulsive patients. *Behaviour Research and Therapy, 14,* 349–355.

Rachman, S. (1980). Emotional processing. *Behaviour Research and Therapy, 18,* 51–60.

Rachman, S. J. (2003). Eysenck and the development of CBT. *Psychologist, 16*(11), 588–591.

Rachman, S. J., Craske, M.G., Tallman, K., & Solyom, C. (1986). Does escape behavior strengthen avoidance? A replication. *Behavior Therapy, 17*, 366–384.

Rescorla, R. A. (2001). Experimental extinction. In R. R. Mowrer & S. B. Klein (Eds.), *Handbook of contemporary learning theories* (pp. 119–154). Mahwah, NJ: Erlbaum.

Riggs, D. S., Rauch, S. A. M., Moser, J. S., & Foa, E. B. (2005). *The relationship between perceived changes in self-referential cognitions and symptoms of posttraumatic stress disorder following assault.* Unpublished manuscript.

Riggs, D. S., Rothbaum, B. O., & Foa, E. B. (1995). A prospective examination of symptoms of posttraumatic stress disorder in victims of nonsexual assault. *Journal of Interpersonal Violence, 10*(2), 201–214.

Rodriguez, B. I., & Craske, M. G. (1993). The effects of distraction during exposure to phobic stimuli. *Behaviour Research and Therapy, 31*(6), 549–558.

Roth, D., Antony, M. M., & Swinson, R. P. (2001). Attributions for anxiety symptoms in social phobia. *Behaviour Research and Therapy, 39*(2), 129–138.

Rothbaum, B. O., Foa, E. B., Riggs, D., Murdock, T., & Walsh, W. (1992). A prospective examination of post-traumatic stress disorder in rape victims. *Journal of Traumatic Stress, 5*, 455–475.

Rothbaum, B. O., Ruef, A. M., Litz, B.T., Han, H., & Hodges, L. (2003). Virtual reality exposure therapy of combat-related PTSD: A case study using psychophysiological indicators of outcome. *Journal of Cognitive Psychotherapy: An International Quarterly, 17*, 163–178.

Salkovskis, P. M. (1991). The importance of behaviour in the maintenance of anxiety and panic: A cognitive account. *Behavioural Psychotherapy, 19*, 6–19.

Spurr, J. M., & Stopa, L. (2003). The observer perspective: Effects on social anxiety and performance. *Behaviour Research and Therapy, 41*(9), 1009–1028.

Stern, R. S., & Marks, I. M. (1973). Brief and prolonged exposure: A comparison in agoraphobic patients. *Archives of General Psychiatry, 28*, 270–276.

Stopa, L., & Clark, D. M. (2000). Social phobia and interpretation of social events. *Behaviour Research and Therapy, 38*, 273–283.

Telch, M. J., Valentiner, D. P., Ilai, D., Young, P. R., Powers, M. B., & Smits, J. A. J. (2004). Fear activation and distraction during the emotional processing of claustrophobic fear. *Journal of Behavior Therapy and Experimental Psychiatry, 35*(3), 219–232.

Uren, T. H., Szabo, M., & Lovibond, P. F. (2004). Probability and cost estimates for social and physical outcomes in social phobia and panic disorder. *Journal of Anxiety Disorders, 18*(4), 481–489.

van Minnen, A., & Foa, E. B. (submitted). *The effects of long versus short imaginal exposure on treatment outcome of PTSD.* Manuscript submitted for publication.

van Minnen, A., & Hagenaars, M. (2002). Fear activation and habituation patterns as early process predictors of response to prolonged exposure treatment in PTSD. *Journal of Traumatic Stress, 15*(5), 359–367.

Voncken, M. J., Bogels, S. M., & de Vries, K. (2003). Interpretation and judgmental biases in social phobia. *Behaviour Research and Therapy, 41*(12), 1481–1488.

Wells, A., Clark, D. M., & Ahmad, S. (1998). How do I look with my mind's eye: Perspective taking in social phobic imagery. *Behaviour Research and Therapy, 36*(6), 631–634.

Wells, A., & Papageorgiou, C. (2001a). Social phobic interoception: Effects of bodily information on anxiety, beliefs and self-processing. *Behaviour Research and Therapy, 39,* 1–11.

Wells, A., & Papageorgiou, C. (2001b). Brief cognitive therapy for social phobia: A case series. *Behaviour Research and Therapy, 39,* 653–658.

2

Emotional Encoding
of Fear-Related Information

ANDREW MATHEWS

In an influential article published in 1986 titled "Emotional Processing of Fear: Exposure to Corrective Information," Edna Foa and Michael Kozak set out to challenge the (at that time) dominant view of fear and anxiety in terms of simple stimulus–response associations. Starting from Lang's (1979) conception of fear as based on a memory network of interconnected stimulus, response, and meaning propositions, Foa and Kozak (1986) proposed that increases or decreases in pathological fears depend critically on the incorporation of new information. Thus, in this view, effective behavioral treatment requires existing fear representations to be activated by a matching stimulus, followed by habituation of fear responses both within and across sessions, indicating good initial access and subsequent effective modification of the network of fear-related information in memory.

Habituation during exposure constitutes corrective information because it is incompatible with existing fear-related representations and beliefs; for example, the expectation that in a phobic situation fear will increase uncontrollably and lead to a catastrophic outcome. Attention to and encoding of new corrective information—such as that fear in fact declines over time and no catastrophic outcome occurs—was proposed to be the critical process leading to change in the fear network and reduction of anxiety.

Today, despite evolution in our conceptualization of memory networks, the core ideas about corrective information that were first developed by Foa and Kozak (1986) remain central to our understanding of processes involved in effective therapy. In the remainder of this chapter, I describe recent work that addresses closely related issues: how emotional events are encoded and how the resulting representations may play a causal role in maintaining or in recovering from emotional states.

MEMORY FOR THREATENING INFORMATION IN ANXIETY DISORDERS

The first key idea in Foa and Kozak's (1986) work is that of an interconnected network of information in memory related to feared situations that is more extensive and coherent in those with high levels of fear or anxiety. Consequently, it should be more easily accessed as a unit (a schema), and matching information should thus be more easily assimilated into the schema. Consistent with this view, high-anxious individuals are more prone to select information relevant to threat, both by perceiving the more threatening meaning of ambiguous events (Eysenck, Mogg, May, Richards, & Mathews, 1991; Foa, Franklin, Perry, & Herbert, 1996) and by attending to threatening rather than nonthreatening cues (Foa, Feske, Murdock, Kozak, & McCarthy, 1991; Mathews & MacLeod, 1994). Paradoxically, however (with the notable exception of panic disorder), demonstrating a parallel memory bias for threatening information in anxiety-prone individuals has proved much more elusive (MacLeod & Mathews, 2004).

In obsessive–compulsive disorder (OCD), for example, little evidence has been found that patients remember threatening events related to their obsessions or compulsions any better or worse than do nonobsessive controls. Tests of the hypothesis that these patients might make more source-monitoring errors—for example, by confusing whether they had actually performed an act such as turning off a light switch or merely imagined it—have been similarly inconclusive (e.g., Constans, Foa, Franklin, & Mathews, 1995). Rather, findings suggest that patients with OCD differ from controls mainly in that they lack confidence in the accuracy of their memories or that they require more evidence before they can make decisions based on the information available from memory (Foa et al., 2003).

More generally, when reviewing experimental research on memory for threatening words, pictures, or real-life events across a range of anxiety disorders, we (MacLeod & Mathews, 2004) found hardly any evidence of better memory for threatening events than in matched nonanxious controls (outside of panic disorder). If the cognitive processing underlying anxiety disorders arises from the action of a more coherent set of threatening meanings in memory, why is it so difficult to demonstrate related memory differences between anxious and control groups?

In fact, there are a number of possible reasons why such a memory bias might be difficult to demonstrate, of which I consider two in particular. First, the form in which information is encoded is critical to whether or not it can be recalled voluntarily. Highly fear-related (traumatic) information may not be encoded in verbally accessible form (cf. Brewin, 2001), so that a test involving explicit verbal memory may be insensitive to real differences in such encoded material. Öhman and Mineka (2001) have further suggested that, because the brain system specialized for processing fear-related events evolved prior to language, the fear module that has developed is largely encapsulated from and impenetrable by conscious verbally mediated processing. Again, this suggests that fear memories may not be encoded in a form that can be accessed in tests of verbal memory, whether explicit or even implicit (e.g., Foa, Amir, Gershuny, Molnar, & Kozak, 1997; Mathews, Mogg, May, & Eysenck, 1989).

Second, whether or not fear-related information can be recalled may vary greatly according to the encoding strategy adopted at the time it is encountered. For example, anxious individuals could either avoid thinking about or consciously elaborate on threatening meanings. In most of the memory experiments that we reviewed, encoding was controlled by instructions to make specific types of judgment. It is well known that semantic encoding (e.g., having participants judge the personal meaning of a word) results in better memory than does superficial encoding (e.g., counting the number of syllables), at least when explicit recall is tested. In almost all experiments that we reviewed, participants encoded both threatening and neutral words semantically, and although threat words were typically remembered better than neutral words, this finding applied equally across anxious and nonanxious groups.[1]

Interestingly, however, there were two striking exceptions—one involving generalized anxiety disorder (Friedman, Thayer, & Borkovec, 2000) and one with high- versus low-trait-anxious student groups (Russo, Fox, Bellinger, & Nguyen-Van-Tam, 2001)—in which clear group differences did emerge. Both experiments were characterized by a similar departure from the typical semantic encoding procedure. Participants were given a superficial encoding task and were also allowed much longer times to look at the words than was required to perform this simple task. They were thus free to encode the words in other ways (e.g., in terms of personal emotional meanings) if they chose, or to avoid doing so. Under these conditions, the anxious groups showed superior recall of threatening words, presumably because they had elected to encode these words in some way that assisted memory. Another study (Pury & Mineka, 2001) found that anxious individuals were faster to make emotional (negative/positive) than semantic (physical/social) judgments of words under conditions in which either judgment might be required. These data suggest that when encoding options are open, anxiety is associated with the tendency to encode words in terms of their emotional meaning rather than other, less emotional aspects of meaning.

These data converge on the conclusion that explicit memory for threatening words does not differ between groups when encoding is controlled, but it does differ when participants can choose the type of encoding they use. The most plausible conclusion is that the latter differences are due to anxiety-prone groups tending to select encoding in terms of threat value whenever more than one processing option exists. This conclusion is entirely consistent with previous findings on selective attention and interpretation, in which anxious groups have been found to select threatening meanings provided that competition exists between processing options. Thus, in real-life conditions, when encoding is unconstrained, the evidence from memory studies can readily be reconciled with the hypothesis that high levels of anxiety are associated with encoding styles that lead to more fear-related representations in memory.

NEURAL PROCESSES UNDERLYING THE COGNITIVE MODULATION OF ENCODING

So far I have argued that emotional encoding is a selective process, so that more coherent representations of fear-related information in memory may be attributable to characteristic encoding preferences in those vulnerable to anxiety. To begin investigation of this hypothesis, we (Mathews, Yiend, & Lawrence, 2004) have examined psychophysiological and neural responses to fear-related versus neutral pictures and the extent to which they can be modulated by encoding instructions. In the first study we assessed startle magnitude to a loud tone as an indirect measure of fear modulation (Lang, Bradley, & Cuthbert, 1990). In the absence of encoding instructions we expected to see greater startle magnitude while viewing a fear-related than a neutral picture (e.g., a snarling dog vs. a docile-looking dog). However, we also tested whether this difference would be increased by instructions to make an emotional judgment (i.e., "Is this picture more frightening than the previous one?"), compared with a nonemotional judgment (i.e., "Did this picture require more planning by the photographer than the previous one?").

Analysis of median startle magnitudes provided support for both suppositions. There was a main effect of picture type, with larger amplitude of startle while viewing fearful pictures, and of type of encoding, with larger amplitude associated with emotional encoding; there was also a significant interaction between the two. The form of this interaction showed that emotional encoding increased the difference due to picture type, whereas nonemotional encoding eliminated it. Because fear-related modulation of startle is controlled by the amygdala, it thus seems that encoding instructions can either increase or reduce activation of the amygdala when threatening pictures are viewed.

With the advent of brain-imaging techniques, it has become possible to investigate the nature of this modulation more directly. As before, we wanted to address the question of whether type of encoding influenced neural activation, but also to investigate whether the degree of control over encoding varied according to individual differences in fearfulness or attentional control. In a functional magnetic resonance imaging (fMRI) study, we (Mathews et al., 2004) contrasted activation to fear-related and neutral pictures, first without any encoding instructions and then while making either emotional or nonemotional judgments as before, in balanced order blocks.

Several areas thought to form part of the fear system of the brain (e.g., the amygdala and hippocampus; see Gray & McNaughton, 2000) were preferentially activated by fear-related rather than neutral pictures. This contrast was more marked in those participants having high scores on a trait measure of fearfulness, the Behavioral Inhibition Scale (BIS; Carver & White, 1994). Some differential activation across picture types persisted even when participants were making nonemotional encoding judgments. However, this difference was markedly reduced in comparison with noninstructed viewing, demonstrating the effects of encoding instructions. Most important, when the neural activation due to emotional versus nonemotional encoding was contrasted across identical sets of fear-related pictures, activation in the amygdala and hippocampus was greater during emotional than nonemotional encoding, and particularly so in high-BIS individuals. Differential activation was also observed in the anterior cingulate cortex (ACC), an area involved in the resolution of attentional and response conflict under conditions of competition. Activation in the ACC was positively correlated with scores on the Attention Control Questionnaire, but it was *negatively* correlated with BIS scores. Thus brain areas involved in attentional selection were more active in those reporting good ability to control attention but less active in those with high levels of fearfulness, as assessed by the BIS.

How are these neuroimaging data to be understood? I suggest that they are exactly in line with expectations from the model of fear and anxiety proposed by Gray and McNaughton (2000) and with the hypothesis of top-down control over encoding processes (Mathews & Mackintosh, 1998; Mackintosh & Mathews, 2003). Those reporting high fearfulness on the BIS show greater differential activation to fear-related than neutral pictures, precisely within the brain areas described by Gray and McNaughton (2000) as being responsible for variations in anxiety. In addition, these same highly fearful individuals tended to have less activation in an area involved in attentional selection (the ACC), suggesting a poorer ability to control their own encoding processes.

INSTRUCTIONAL CONTROL
OVER EMOTIONAL ENCODING

I want to turn now to the second key idea put forward by Foa and Kozak (1986): namely, that the fear-related representations in memory, once activated, can be modified by exposure to corrective information. The main source of corrective information considered in the original research was habituation of fear responses. Other research suggests that there might be various sources of corrective information, including the self-observation of different emotional consequences depending on how threat information is encoded and interpreted. However, the neuroimaging results just discussed also suggest that it may be difficult to control encoding as anxiety becomes more severe, so that control may become effectively impossible in clinical disorders.

Alternately, and as I want to argue here, it may be that at least some degree of control over emotional encoding is possible, albeit difficult, even in clinical anxiety states. At first glance, this proposal seems quite inconsistent with the observation that people with anxiety disorders believe that they cannot control how they feel. However, the perception of lack of control does not prove that such control is impossible. Indeed, the very effectiveness of cognitive-behavioral therapy shows that control can be achieved in ways that are not always anticipated by the person suffering from emotional disorders. The perception of uncontrollability may arise because the individuals concerned do not necessarily realize that the way in which they encode affective information has emotional consequences. Even if they realize that it might, they may still feel control is impossible, or they may have no knowledge about how such control can be achieved. It may be particularly difficult to learn about effective control because much of our emotional processing operates outside awareness and because achieving control over encoding requires practice before any effects can be observed.

As an example, I want to consider the case of emotional encoding in social phobia. People with social phobia often report negative self-imagery when in social situations (Hackmann, Clark, & McManus, 2000), and they seem to use such internal sources of information—rather than external cues—when judging their own performance (Clark & Wells, 1995). In addition, the positive inferences typically made about social situations by nonanxious people are conspicuously absent in social phobia (Hirsch & Mathews, 2000). We have proposed that these two findings are connected: specifically, that inappropriate attention to internal negative sources of information, such as self-imagery, effectively blocks the ability to make positive inferences based on external social cues.

To investigate this view, we (Hirsch, Clark, Mathews, & Williams, 2003) carried out an experiment in which people with social phobia were engaged in conversation with a stranger after having been instructed either to hold their usual negative self-image in mind or to replace it with a more realistic and less negative control image. Participants with phobia rated themselves as less anxious during the conversation, and their performance as being better, when they had held the less negative image of themselves in mind. Observers—who were not informed about the image content—also rated performance as better and overt anxiety as reduced when the more benign self-image was being held in mind. Thus, although the impact of differential image content was more striking in self-ratings, some beneficial effects were also apparent to an objective observer. If this simple manipulation has beneficial effects, why did the participants with social phobia not already use it spontaneously? I suggest that this is one example of how anxious individuals may be unaware that negatively biased emotional encoding may be maintaining their anxiety. Consistent with this view, some of the participants with social phobia commented that they were surprised at the contrast in their feelings between the two conditions. Under these circumstances, even a relatively simple instructional manipulation can have surprisingly powerful effects.

Further research has supported the second part of our hypothesis: that keeping a negative image in mind blocks positive inferences. Nonanxious volunteers who were required to read about and imagine themselves in ambiguous social situations were faster when identifying words that matched positive (but not negative) inferences, implying that they spontaneously infer positive outcomes. This presumably protective bias was completely absent in socially anxious individuals and patients with social phobia. Critically, when we required nonanxious volunteers to hold a negative image of themselves in mind, their normal positive inferential style was blocked also (Hirsch, Mathews, Clark, Williams, & Morrison, 2003). In a further experiment, we instructed socially anxious individuals to adopt the perspective of another, more confident person while reading about and imagining ambiguously threatening social situations. This mental set had a beneficial effect, such that they made fewer threatening inferences than they did when imagining themselves in the same situations. Finally, we have examined the effects of practice (using methods discussed in the next section) in making either negative or benign interpretations about ambiguous social situations on later self-imagery. The type of interpretations practiced influenced subsequent imagery in an emotionally congruent direction.

Thus it appears that there is a two-way interaction between interpretation bias and the content of self-image, with each influencing the other. Furthermore, quite simple experimental instructions to modify encoding style can sometimes have significant emotional consequences, even in clinical populations.

TRAINING EMOTIONAL ENCODING VIA PRACTICE

Although instructional control can sometimes have powerful effects, it almost certainly has severe inherent limitations. Because such control demands effort and draws on limited cognitive resources, when anxiety levels are high and/or cognitive resources are depleted due to other demands, it is likely to fail. Consequently, long-term control of encoding may require automating the processes involved so that minimum conscious effort is required. For example, in a series of innovative experiments, MacLeod, Rutherford, Campbell, Ebsworthy, and Holker (2002) have shown that selective attention to threat can be induced via practice in searching for a target that was always to be found in the location of the more threatening word of a displayed pair. Critically, repeated practice under the reverse condition, in which the target was always to be found in the location of the nonthreatening word of a pair, caused attention to be directed *away* from threat, even when the threatening stimuli used were new. Most important to the present discussion is the finding that, after extended practice of the latter type, anxiety under stress was reduced, even in those with initially high trait anxiety levels (for a more extensive discussion, see Mathews & MacLeod, 2002).

Analogous effects have emerged from work on the tendency to interpret ambiguous emotional events in terms of their more threatening meaning, a characteristic of encoding in anxiety-prone individuals (e.g., Eysenck et al., 1991; Richards & French, 1992). Grey and Mathews (2000) induced a similar bias by presenting volunteers with a series of threat/nonthreat homographs (e.g., BATTER, FIT, SINK), followed by a word fragment corresponding to either their threatening or nonthreatening meanings. Participants were required to complete the fragment (e.g., BATTER: ass__ult, or BATTER: panc__ke) using the preceding homograph as a clue. Thus one group was required to repeatedly generate threatening meanings, whereas the other group generated alternative nonthreatening meanings. After a large number of such trials, participants completed a test in which target fragments, or word/ nonword letter strings, followed new threat/nonthreat homograph primes. Both fragment completion times and lexical decision latencies for real words were shorter when the emotional valence of the target was the same as that practiced previously. Practice in resolving ambiguity as threatening or otherwise thus facilitates the interpretation of new ambiguous stimuli in a congruent manner. After training in this way, participants assigned to threatening interpretations resolved the meaning of ambiguous words in the same way as naturally anxious individuals (e.g., Richards & French, 1992).

However, a critical question remained unanswered in these experiments: Is an encoding bias that favors threatening meanings of ambiguous events a *cause* of anxiety? The experimental manipulation of encoding bias offers a way of directly testing this hypothesis. In a series of experiments on this issue, we (Mathews & Mackintosh, 2000) had participants read about and imagine themselves in more realistic ambiguous social situations. Groups assigned to reading descriptions that ended with negative outcomes became more pessimistic in the interpretations that they made subsequently about new ambiguous events than did those assigned to positive outcomes. Those who just passively read these descriptions did not change in anxious mood. In contrast, those who were required to actively resolve the meaning of the ambiguous passages—by completing a word fragment and answering a question that required elaborating on the assigned emotional meaning— reported mood changes congruent with training. In these experiments, therefore, active generation of emotional meaning emerged as the crucial factor in eliciting congruent changes in anxiety.

In research designed to test whether these emotional effects do indeed depend on active generation, Laura Hoppitt (2005), has contrasted training involving the active production of emotional meanings of homographs (as did Grey & Mathews, 2000) with a matched training method in which no such generation was required. In "active" training, participants saw a homograph cue and then completed word fragments as before. In the "passive" method, instead of seeing any homographs, participants saw an unambiguous synonym for the designated meaning, followed by the same fragment. Thus, although the fragment completion task remained the same, "passive" training did not require the active generation of emotional interpretations. In this case there were no effects on mood during training with homographs, even when active resolution of meaning was required, presumably because the single words used did not convey any "real" emotion. However, anxiety differences between groups did emerge later, after they had watched a mildly stressful video depicting near-fatal accidents. Participants who had received "active" training with negative interpretations reported greater increases in state anxiety in response to this video than did those who had received "passive" training. Presumably, the tendency to generate emotional meanings induced during active training influenced how the accident video was processed later, such that those in the negative group generated more threatening interpretations about the events depicted in the video.

In related research carried out by Paula Hertel (Hertel, Mathews, Peterson, & Kintner, 2003) participants were trained using a relatedness judgment task with either threat or nonthreat words, each followed by a homograph (e.g., assault: batter—related?). Then, in a purportedly unconnected experiment, new homographs were presented as cues to produce an image. After training with threatening meanings, the images produced were rated by blind judges as being more negative than after the nonthreat training, although there was no significant effect on participants' own emotional ratings.

We wondered if this apparent lack of emotional effects might reflect the fact that presenting the homograph *after* the unambiguous associate eliminated the need to actively resolve emotional ambiguity. Accordingly, in another experiment carried out by Laura Hoppitt (2005), participants were again assigned to "active" or "passive" training, either with homographs (requiring generation) or with unambiguous synonym cues (eliminating the need to generate interpretations), followed by to-be-completed word fragments. Again, there were no immediate effects on mood, but emotional effects emerged in a later test involving new ambiguous scenarios to be imagined. Following "active" negative training, state anxiety increased more during subsequent imagery than it did following "passive" negative training.

We believe that these findings converge on some important conclusions. First, exposure to emotional material, with or without active generation, induces equivalent interpretation biases when the outcome is assessed via nonemotional tasks (e.g., lexical decision or recognition memory). In contrast, when later emotional consequences are assessed, differential effects on mood emerge after training that involves the active generation of emotional meanings. This implies that an induced bias favoring valenced interpretations has an effect on mood when, and only when, that bias is actively deployed to interpret the meaning of an ambiguous emotional event.

DO THE EFFECTS OF ENCODING TRAINING PERSIST?

We are at too early a stage in this research to know how long the effects of induced processing biases will endure. Nonetheless, our original concern that they would prove extremely transitory has already been proved false. To explore durability, we began cautiously by leaving a gap of 20 minutes between the end of training and the introduction of the new ambiguous test descriptions. Somewhat to our surprise, a recognition test of how these new descriptions had been interpreted showed that effects had not dissipated at all, despite an unrelated filler task intervening between training and test items. Furthermore, effects were almost as strong when volunteers were asked to return the next day, when they read the ambiguous test descriptions for the first time (Yiend, Mackintosh, & Mathews, 2005).

Another indication of persisting effects is that, even when no emotional effects were apparent during training itself, subsequent exposure to a potentially emotional event (such as viewing an accident video) revealed an underlying vulnerability created by the prior induction. As discussed earlier, we suppose that this is due to participants' unintentionally applying the same processing style that was induced during training to potentially more emotional material such as an accident video. Unlike the persistence of interpretation bias revealed using a recognition test, later consequences for emotional vulnerability have not yet been assessed over longer periods. However, the parallel work by Colin MacLeod and colleagues on training attention bias that was described previously already suggests that emotional effects can indeed persist and accumulate over time. Students under real-life examination stress who were trained over several weeks to avoid attending to threat cues reduced their trait-anxiety scores over time more than did a matched control group (see Mathews & MacLeod, 2002). More long-term studies of this sort are a priority for future research.

CONCLUSIONS AND IMPLICATIONS

In this chapter I argued that the processing of emotional events is not a fixed and invariable process, despite often appearing that way to those prone to fear or anxiety. Anxiety-prone individuals are more likely to encode threatening aspects of ambiguous events when they are free to adopt alternative processing options, leading to better memory for threatening information. Such differences are less apparent, however, when a specific form of encoding is imposed, implying that encoding can in fact be controlled.

Similarly, neuroimaging evidence indicates that subcortical brain areas involved in fear and anxiety (such as the amygdala) are differentially activated according to the required encoding task, although such control may be less than complete, especially in highly fearful individuals. Nonetheless, even highly anxious individuals, such as those with social phobia, can sometimes exert more control over how they encode emotional events than they appear to believe, with beneficial consequences. These and other data suggest that people often fail to implement control over emotional encoding, not because it is impossible, but because they do not know how to achieve it.

To overcome the inherent limits of such effortful control methods, it is possible to modify encoding biases in both attention and interpretation by practice. Not only can such training lead to persisting alterations in encoding bias, but consequent mood changes also have provided the most convincing evidence to date that such biases play a causal role in emotional vulnerability. By bringing these emotional processes into the laboratory, we can now begin to investigate clinical hypotheses about the role of cognitive processes in therapy and the ways in which these processes can most effectively be deployed therapeutically.

I began this chapter by referring to the contribution made by Foa and Kozak (1986) in their influential research on emotional processing. I would like to finish it by citing a later article by the same authors that carried the subtitle "Cognitive behavior therapy in search of theory" (Foa & Kozak, 1997). In this article Foa and Kozak argued that progress in cognitive-behavioral therapy has been slowing, due in part to the lack of new theoretical input. In particular, although cognitive therapy has embraced some of the terminology of cognitive psychology, it has not been able to draw on experimental cognitive psychology as a basis for developing new treatment methods. I agree but hope that some of the new directions in current research, including the work on experimental modification of encoding biases, will form part of the solution to this problem.

ACKNOWLEDGMENTS

Thanks are due to David Clark, Joe Constans, Sue Grey, Colette Hirsch, Laura Hoppitt, Andrew Lawrence, Becky Lee, Bundy Mackintosh, Colin MacLeod, Jenny Yiend, and of course Edna Foa, whose work and ideas I have drawn on in writing this paper. Much of the work reported here was supported by the Medical Research Council, UK.

NOTE

1. A suggested explanation for the explicit memory bias reported in panic disorder is that some words represent threats for this group (e.g., crowds) but have a less threatening meaning for others.

REFERENCES

Brewin, C. R. (2001). A cognitive neuroscience account of postraumatic stress disorder. *Behaviour Research and Therapy, 39,* 373–393.

Carver, C. S., & White, T. L. (1994). Behavioral inhibition, behavioral activation, and affective responses to impending reward and punishment: The BIS/BAS Scales. *Journal of Personality and Social Psychology, 67,* 319–333.

Clark, D. M., & Wells, A. (1995). A cognitive model of social phobia. In R. G. Heimberg, M. Liebowitz, D. Hope, & F. Schneier (Eds.), *Social phobia: Diagnosis, assessment, and treatment* (pp. 69–93). New York: Guilford Press.

Constans, J., Foa, E. B., Franklin, M. E., & Mathews, A. (1995). Memory for actual and imagined events in OC checkers. *Behaviour Research and Therapy, 33,* 665–671.

Eysenck, M., Mogg, K., May, J., Richards, A., & Mathews, A. (1991). Bias in interpretation of ambiguous sentences related to threat in anxiety. *Journal of Abnormal Psychology, 100*, 144–150.

Foa, E. B., Amir, N., Gershuny, B., Molnar, C., & Kozak, M. J. (1997). Implicit and explicit memory in obsessive–compulsive disorder. *Journal of Anxiety Disorders, 11*, 119–129.

Foa, E. B., Feske, U., Murdock, T. B., Kozak, M. J., & McCarthy, P. R. (1991). Processing of threat-related information in rape victims. *Journal of Abnormal Psychology, 100*, 156–162.

Foa, E. B., Franklin, M. E., Perry, K. J., & Herbert, J. D. (1996). Cognitive biases in generalized social phobia. *Journal of Abnormal Psychology, 105*, 433–439.

Foa, E. B., & Kozak, M. J. (1986). Emotional processing of fear: Exposure to corrective information. *Psychological Bulletin, 99*, 20–35.

Foa, E. B., & Kozak, M. J. (1997). Beyond the efficacy ceiling: Cognitive behavior therapy in search of theory. *Behavior Therapy, 28*, 601–611.

Foa, E., Mathews, A., Abramowitz, J. S., Amir, N., Prezeworski, A., Riggs, D. S., et al. (2003). Do patients with obsessive–compulsive disorder have deficits in decision making? *Cognitive Therapy and Research, 7*, 431–445.

Friedman, B. H., Thayer, J. F., & Borkovec, T. D. (2000). Explicit memory bias for threat words in generalized anxiety disorder. *Behavior Therapy, 31*, 745–756.

Gray, J. A., & McNaughton, N. (2000). *The neuropsychology of anxiety* (2nd ed.). New York: Oxford University Press.

Grey, S., & Mathews, A. (2000). Effects of training on interpretation of emotional ambiguity. *Quarterly Journal of Experimental Psychology, 53*, 1143–1162.

Hackmann, A., Clark, D. M., & McManus, F. (2000). Recurrent images and early memories in social phobia. *Behaviour Research and Therapy, 38*, 601–610.

Hertel, P., Mathews, A., Peterson, S., & Kintner, K. (2003). Transfer of training emotionally biased interpretations. *Applied Cognitive Psychology, 17*, 775–784.

Hirsch, C., Clark, D. M., Mathews, A., & Williams, R. (2003). Self-images play a causal role in social phobia. *Behaviour Research and Therapy, 41*, 909–921.

Hirsch, C., & Mathews, A. (2000). Impaired positive inferential bias in social phobia. *Journal of Abnormal Psychology, 109*, 705–712.

Hirsch, C., Mathews, A., Clark, D. M., Williams, R., & Morrison, J. (2003). Negative self-imagery blocks inferences. *Behaviour Research and Therapy, 41*, 1383–1396.

Hoppitt, L. (2005). *Influencing vulnerability to stress through modification of emotional biases.* Unpublished doctoral thesis, University of Cambridge, Cambridge, UK.

Lang, P. J. (1979). A bio-informational theory of emotional imagery. *Psychophysiology, 16*, 495–512.

Lang, P. J., Bradley, M. M., & Cuthbert, B. N. (1990). Emotion, attention and the startle reflex. *Psychological Review, 97*, 377–398.

Mackintosh, B., & Mathews, A. (2003). Don't look now: Attentional avoidance of emotionally-valenced cues. *Cognition and Emotion, 17*, 623–646.

MacLeod, C., & Mathews, A. (2004). Selective memory effects in anxiety disorders: An overview of research findings and their implications. In D. Reisberg & P. Hertel (Eds.), *Memory and emotion* (pp. 155–165). New York: Oxford University Press.

MacLeod, C., Rutherford, E. M., Campbell, L., Ebsworthy, G., & Holker, L. (2002). Selective attention and emotional vulnerability: Assessing the causal basis of their association through the experimental manipulation of attentional bias. *Journal of Abnormal Psychology, 111,* 107–123.

Mathews, A., & Mackintosh, B. (1998). A cognitive model of selective processing in anxiety. *Cognitive Therapy and Research, 22,* 539–560.

Mathews, A., & Mackintosh, B. (2000). Induced emotional interpretation bias and anxiety. *Journal of Abnormal Psychology, 109,* 602–615.

Mathews, A., & MacLeod, C. (1994). Cognitive approaches to emotion and emotional disorders. *Annual Review of Psychology, 45,* 25–50.

Mathews, A., & MacLeod, C. (2002). Induced processing biases have causal effects on anxiety. *Cognition and Emotion, 16,* 331–354.

Mathews, A., Mogg, K., May, J., & Eysenck, M. (1989). Implicit and explicit memory bias in anxiety. *Journal of Abnormal Psychology, 98,* 236–240.

Mathews, A., Yiend, J., & Lawrence, A. D. (2004). Individual differences in the modulation of fear-related brain activation by attentional control. *Journal of Cognitive Neuroscience, 16,* 1683–1694.

Öhman, A., & Mineka, S. (2001). Fears, phobias, and preparedness: Towards an evolved module of fear and fear learning. *Psychological Review, 108,* 483–522.

Pury, C. L. S., & Mineka, S. (2001). Differential encoding of affective and non-affective content information in trait anxiety. *Cognition and Emotion, 15,* 659–693.

Richards, A., & French, C. C. (1992). An anxiety-related bias in semantic activation when processing threat/neutral homographs. *Quarterly Journal of Experimental Psychology, 45,* 503–525.

Russo, R., Fox, E., Bellinger, L., & Nguyen-Van-Tam, D. P. (2001). Mood-congruent free recall bias in anxiety. *Cognition and Emotion, 15,* 419–433.

Yiend, J., Mackintosh, B., & Mathews, A. (2005). The enduring consequences of experimentally induced biases in interpretation. *Behaviour Research and Therapy, 43,* 779–797.

3

Predictors of Chronic Posttraumatic Stress Disorder

Trauma Memories and Appraisals

ANKE EHLERS
DAVID M. CLARK

Posttraumatic stress disorder (PTSD) is a disabling condition that people may develop in response to one or more traumatic event(s), such as deliberate acts of interpersonal violence, severe accidents, disaster, or military action. The question of how we can predict who will develop PTSD after traumatic events has generated great interest among researchers and clinicians. A recent meta-analysis (Ozer, Best, Lipsey, & Weiss, 2003) established seven predictors of PTSD following trauma: (1) psychological problems prior to the trauma, (2) a history of earlier traumas, (3) psychopathology in the family of origin, (4) a high degree of peritraumatic dissociation, (5) negative emotions during the trauma, (6) high perceived life threat during the trauma, and (7) lack of social support following the event. In this chapter, we review evidence showing that the prediction of chronic PTSD can be further enhanced if characteristics of trauma memories and appraisal are taken into account.

Many of these studies arose from our inspiring collaboration with Edna Foa. It was Edna Foa's inspirational lecture on the role of uncontrollability and unpredictability in PTSD—later elaborated in her article in *Psychological Bulletin* (Foa, Zinbarg, & Rothbaum, 1992)—that kindled our interest in PTSD. We feel truly privileged that Edna Foa gave us the opportunity to join her in investigating cognitive processes that underlie the

39

symptoms of PTSD. Her work exemplifies how knowledge derived from learning theory and cognitive psychology can be integrated to formulate powerful theoretical models of anxiety disorders and how such models can then be used to develop successful treatments. The close integration of Edna Foa's theoretical and clinical work and her passion for helping patients and for developing and testing ideas are a model for anyone working in clinical psychology.

ONSET VERSUS MAINTENANCE OF PTSD SYMPTOMS

The question of who develops PTSD after trauma is not as straightforward as it sounds. Rothbaum, Foa, Riggs, Murdock, and Walsh (1992) and Riggs, Rothbaum, and Foa (1995) showed that in the immediate aftermath of traumatic events, many trauma survivors experience at least some of the symptoms of PTSD. A sizeable proportion recover in the next few weeks or months, but in a significant subgroup the symptoms persist, often for years (Kessler, Sonnega, Bromet, Hughes, & Nelson, 1995; Rothbaum et al., 1992). Factors that are responsible for the initial onset of symptoms may be different from the ones that determine whether a person with initial symptoms recovers or stays symptomatic.

Whether or not people develop intrusive memories after traumatic events depends on characteristics of their memories for the traumatic event and their appraisals at the time of the trauma. Whether the symptoms persist depends on whether or not they update the memories and their appraisals and on their interpretations and responses to the initial symptoms of PTSD and other consequences of the trauma (Ehlers & Clark, 2000; Ehlers & Steil, 1995; Foa & Riggs, 1993; Foa & Rothbaum, 1998).

CHARACTERISTICS OF TRAUMA MEMORIES: THEORETICAL BACKGROUND

"Among the anxiety syndromes, PTSD is most dramatically a disorder of memory" (McNally, 1998, p. 971). Building on Lang's (1977) network model of emotion, Foa, Steketee, and Rothbaum (1989) proposed that the trauma is represented as a fear structure in memory that contains stimulus (e.g., stimuli associated with the traumatic event, such as features of the perpetrator), response (e.g., fear, physiological reactions, and avoidance), and meaning elements (e.g., dangerous). The authors suggested that the fear structure in PTSD is characterized by

- Particularly strong response elements.
- Unrealistic associations, including benign stimuli and danger- or fear-related stimulus, response, and meaning elements.

- An especially large number of stimulus elements.

According to Foa et al. (1989), the large number of stimulus elements has the effect that many different stimuli can trigger the trauma memory structure, which leads to information about the trauma entering consciousness (intrusive memories) and the strong response elements of the structure being activated (fear, hyperarousal, avoidance). The triggers can include stimuli that are objectively safe, as uncontrollable intensive aversive stimuli break down the discrimination between safety and danger signals (Foa et al., 1992). The large number of stimulus elements makes the fear structure resistant to change. Foa and Rothbaum (1998) also suggested that the fear structure contains a particularly large number of response elements. Foa and Riggs (1993) further proposed that the structure of trauma memories is more fragmented and disorganized than the structure of nontrauma memories (see also Herman, 1992; van der Kolk & Fisler, 1995), which contributes to their resistance to change. According to Foa et al. (1989), the persistence of PTSD can be explained by inadequate activation of the fear network. This hypothesis builds on Foa and Kozak's (1986) theory that activation of the memory is a necessary condition for change. The lack of activation may be due to a range of processes, for example, (1) avoidance strategies and numbing may prevent an adequately long activation of the fear network; (2) the complex network may not be activated entirely because not enough matching cues are present or because the memory is fragmented (Foa & Riggs, 1993); and/or (3) excessively high arousal impedes habituation and processing of new information.

Foa and colleagues further highlighted an important phenomenological feature of intrusive trauma memories: When people with PTSD have memories of the traumatic event, they reexperience the original emotions they had at the time of the event (e.g., Foa & Rothbaum, 1998; see also Bremner, Krystal, Southwick, & Charney, 1995; Brewin, Dalgleish, & Joseph, 1996). This would suggest that these intrusive memories lack the "autonoetic awareness" (the sense or experience of the self in the past) that normally characterizes autobiographical memories (Tulving, 2002). The part of the trauma that is retrieved in the intrusive memory seems to happen in the "here and now." Hackmann, Ehlers, Speckens, and Clark (2004) found that this perceived "nowness" is not restricted to flashback episodes as defined in DSM-IV (American Psychiatric Association, 1994) but also applies to those intrusions listed in criterion B1, "recurrent and distressing recollections of the event."

Ehlers and Clark's (2000) model focuses on this lack of time perspective (perceived "nowness") and the ease with which intrusive memories are triggered. Building on recent research on nontrauma autobiographical memory (Conway, 1997, 2001; Conway & Pleydell-Pearce, 2000) they suggested a deficit in the autobiographical memory for the traumatic event, as did Foa and colleagues and other trauma theorists (e.g., Brewin et al.,

1996; Brewin, 2001). Autobiographical memories are normally organized and elaborated in a way that facilitates intentional retrieval and inhibits cue-driven[1] reexperiencing of an event (e.g., Conway & Pleydell-Pearce, 2000). The intentional recall of an autobiographical event contains both specific information about the event itself and context information. Ehlers and Clark (2000) proposed that trauma memories do not have this level of organization and elaboration. The series of experiences during a traumatic event are thought to be inadequately integrated into their *context* (both within the event and within the context of previous and subsequent experiences or information).[2] This has the effect that the resulting intentional recall is disjointed; that is, although distressing elements are recalled, it may be difficult for the individual to access later information that corrected impressions they had or predictions they made at the time. For example, a man who thought during an assault that he would never see his children again was not able (while recalling this particularly distressing moment) to access the fact that he still lived with his children. He felt overwhelming sadness, as during the event itself. The lack of integration of traumatic moments experienced during the event into a context is also illustrated by Ehlers and Clark's (2000) observation that people with PTSD may have persistent intrusive memories of different parts of the traumatic event that contradict each other in meaning.

Ehlers and Clark (2000) further suggest that poor elaboration of the traumatic experiences during the event leads to poor inhibition of cue-driven retrieval of corresponding elements from the memory. Two additional processes are thought to enhance the probability of cue-driven retrieval: perceptual priming (reduced threshold for perception) for stimuli that occurred at the time of the traumatic event, and strong associative links between these stimuli and between the stimuli and strong affective responses. The three processes are thought to work in conjunction, that is, poor memory organization and elaboration in itself is not sufficient for producing intrusive memories.

The models presented by Foa and colleagues and by Ehlers and Clark suggest that it may be possible to predict chronic PTSD by measuring characteristics of the trauma memories. Two specific hypotheses can be derived from the models:

1. Characteristics of involuntary trauma memories may predict the chronicity of PTSD symptoms. Of particular interest are the *ease of triggering* of intrusive memories by related stimuli, the *lack of time perspective* (perceived *nowness*), and the *lack of context* information.

2. When people with PTSD intentionally recall the trauma, their memories will be *fragmented* and/or *disorganized*. The level of organization may predict chronic PTSD.

In the following, we discuss the empirical results for these hypotheses in turn.

DO TRAUMA MEMORY CHARACTERISTICS PREDICT PTSD?

In the initial aftermath of trauma, intrusive reexperiencing is common. McFarlane (1988) and Shalev (1992) found that the mere presence of intrusions in the initial days after trauma is not a good predictor of subsequent PTSD. However, in line with the first hypothesis, Michael, Ehlers, Halligan, and Clark (2005) found that several characteristics of intrusive memories distinguished between assault survivors with and without PTSD and also predicted subsequent PTSD severity in a prospective longitudinal study. These included: *lack of time perspective* (operationalized by the degree to which the intrusion was experienced as something happening "now"); *lack of context* (operationalized by the degree to which it was experienced as isolated and disconnected from what happened before and afterward); and *distress* caused by the intrusion (see Ehlers & Steil, 1995, for background on this variable). Whether or not participants reported intrusive memories in the first few weeks after the assault explained only 9% of the variance of PTSD severity at 6 months after assault. Among survivors with intrusions, intrusion frequency explained only 8% of the variance of PTSD symptom severity at 6 months. "Nowness," distress, and lack of context explained an additional 43% of the variance. These intrusion characteristics also predicted PTSD severity at 6 months over and above what could be predicted from PTSD diagnostic status at initial assessment. The results on "nowness" as a predictor of chronic PTSD parallel those of a study by Speckens, Ehlers, Hackmann, and Clark (in press) who found that the perceived "here and now" quality of intrusive memories predicted poor response to imaginal exposure to the trauma memory.

Furthermore, Michael et al. (2005) found, in line with Hypothesis 1, that the ease and persistence with which intrusive memories could be triggered by photographs depicting assaults correlated with concurrent and subsequent PTSD severity.

VOLUNTARY RECALL

A series of studies have tested Foa and Riggs's (1993) hypothesis that trauma memories are fragmented and disorganized in PTSD with self-reports, interviews, and objective measures. In the majority of studies using self-report questionnaires and interviews, trauma survivors indeed described their recollection of the traumatic experience to be more fragmented and less clear, to have more gaps, and to follow a less meaningful order than nontrauma memories (Byrne, Hyman, & Scott, 2001; Halligan, Michael, Clark, & Ehlers, 2003; Koss, Figueredo, Bell, Tharan, & Tromp, 1996; Murray, Ehlers, & Mayou, 2002; Tromp, Koss, Figueredo, & Tharan, 1995; van der Kolk & Fisler, 1995). Discrepant results were reported in three studies (Berntsen, Willert, & Rubin, 2003; Porter & Birt, 2001; Rubin, Feldman, & Beckham, 2004). The wording of the questions used to assess fragmentation and the extent to which the studies used clinical or student populations may have contributed to variability. The psychometric properties of the measures used in the studies are in most cases unknown. For example, in the negative study by Berntsen et al. (2003), the fragmentation of explicit trauma recall was assessed with one item, asking "When you recall the traumatic event, do you then think of it as a continuous series of episodes or as some isolated incoherent fragments?" (p. 693), and the negative study by Rubin et al. (2004) used the item "While remembering the event, it comes to me in words or in pictures as a coherent story or episode and not as an isolated fact, observation, or scene" (p. 24). Fragmentation is a complex concept that may be difficult to assess with self-reports, as the questions are very complex and require the respondent to have a high level of introspective ability. A further limitation of all these studies is that it remains unclear whether trauma memories that participants described were retrieved voluntarily or involuntarily.

In the first study using objective measures of trauma fragmentation/ disorganization, Foa and colleagues transcribed the *trauma narratives* given by rape survivors in their first and last imaginal exposure therapy sessions (Foa, Molnar, & Cashman, 1995). The transcriptions were divided into segments that consisted of one thought, action, or speech utterance. These segments were then coded by two blind raters for indicators of fragmentation versus organization. In line with the fragmentation/disorganization hypothesis, the authors found that the narratives from the last session contained significantly more segments that were rated as "organized thoughts" than the pretreatment narratives. Although a total fragmentation score was not reduced over the course of the treatment, a significant correlation between the fragmentation score and the reduction of PTSD symptoms over treatment was found. In a recent study aiming to replicate these results, van Minnen, Wessel, Dijkstra, and Roelofs (2002), did not find an effect of treatment on the number of organized thoughts or the overall fragmentation index. However, the posttreatment narrative contained significantly fewer disorganized thoughts than the pretreatment narratives. In addition, this reduction was significantly related to treatment response.

In three further cross-sectional studies, the Foa et al. (1995) coding scheme (or variants of it) were used to compare trauma survivors with versus without acute stress disorder (Harvey & Bryant, 1999), PTSD (Halligan et al., 2003, Study 1), or intrusive memories (Evans, 2003). As expected, symptomatic participants had more disorganized trauma memories than nonsymptomatic participants. In two prospective longitudinal studies, Murray et al. (2002) and Halligan et al. (2003, Study 2) further found that self-report and objective measures of trauma memory disorganization taken in the initial weeks after the trauma predicted the severity of PTSD symptoms at 6 months. However, change in memory disorganization was not related to change in PTSD symptoms during the follow-up period (Halligan et al., 2003).

Ehring (2004) has recently investigated whether disorganization is specific to trauma memories in PTSD. In line with Foa and Riggs's (1993) hypothesis, trauma narratives were more disorganized than narratives of other very unpleasant life events. Road traffic accident survivors with PTSD showed greater disorganization than those without PTSD. However, contrary to expectation, there was no interaction between PTSD group and narrative type. Participants with PTSD had more disorganized trauma *and* nontrauma narratives than those without PTSD.

Reading level was first used as a measure of trauma memory fragmentation by Amir, Stafford, Freshman, and Foa (1998). In their study, assault survivors gave narratives of their traumatic experiences 2 weeks following the trauma. Narrative fragmentation was operationalized by two reading level indices (Flesch Reading Ease index and Flesch-Kincaid Grade Level). The authors found that low reading levels of trauma narratives predicted PTSD symptom severity at 12 weeks following the assaults. Gray and Lombardo (2001) replicated the relationship between PTSD and low reading level of trauma narratives. However, when scores obtained from tests of verbal intelligence and writing skills were partialed out, the effect of diagnostic group disappeared. In addition, ease of reading was not significantly different between the trauma narrative and two narratives of nontraumatic situations given by the same participant when general cognitive abilities were partialed out.

Low intelligence is a risk factor for PTSD following trauma (McNally & Shin, 1995) and is likely to influence cognitive processing during the trauma (Ehlers & Clark, 2000). Thus it is possible that general cognitive abilities influence the degree of organization with which trauma memories are laid down in memory. The question of whether or not the results obtained with rater assessment of disorganization of trauma narratives are due to differences in verbal intelligence has as yet not been investigated. However, a correlate of intelligence, level of education, does not seem to explain the pattern of results. In the Halligan et al. (2003) studies, level of education was negatively related to PTSD symptom severity, as is to be expected given the relationship between intelligence and PTSD. The correlation between memory disorganization and concurrent and subsequent PTSD severity remained significant when level of education was partialed out.

Overall, the results of the majority of studies using clinical samples supported memory disorganization as one of the factors that contribute to the development of PTSD symptoms. However, disorganization of autobiographical memories in PTSD may not be specific to trauma narratives, possibly reflecting a more general disturbance in autobiographical memory in PTSD (see also the overgeneral recall of autobiographical memories observed in PTSD; e.g., McNally, Lasko, Macklin, & Pitman, 1995). Studies of other populations, such as student or unselected volunteer samples, found less support for the fragmentation/disorganization hypothesis, possibly because of a less strict definition of "trauma."

A closer look at the discrepant findings further suggests that not all indices of fragmentation/disorganization relate equally well to PTSD and recovery. General measures of narrative complexity, such as number of details, do not seem to bear a close relationship to PTSD symptoms (e.g., Porter & Birt, 2001). Aspects of the narrative such as speech fillers or unfinished sentences may also be less useful in assessing memory disorganization, possibly because they mainly reflect general verbal abilities (Halligan et al., 2003; Ehring, 2004). Van der Minnen et al.'s (2002) finding that the change in the number of disorganized segments in the trauma narrative was most closely related to treatment outcome parallels findings from our prospective studies of accident and assault survivors in that the number of disorganized segments had the greatest predictive power (Ehring, 2004; Halligan et al., 2003). Thus the hypothesized disorganization of trauma memories appears to have received more empirical support than has fragmentation.

Some authors have questioned the fragmentation concept on theoretical grounds (Berntsen et al., 2003; McNally, 2003). They argue that fragmentation might simply be an artifact of the method used, as every autobiographical memory encoding is incomplete and the recalled memory therefore fragmented in some way. McNally (2003) argued that instead of postulating special processes for trauma memories, the memory characteristics observed in PTSD could instead by accounted for by well-known processes identified in cognitive psychology, such as attentional narrowing as a consequence of stress (Christianson, 1992; Easterbrook, 1959). However, Ehlers et al. (2002) and Ehlers, Hackmann, and Michael (2004) have argued that attentional narrowing does not explain the content of intrusive trauma memories. Nevertheless, future studies will need to isolate the mechanisms by which memory disorganization contributes to PTSD symptoms.

Further refinements of disorganization measures may be helpful. For example, according to Ehlers and Clark (2000), one would expect memory disorganization to contribute to the easy triggering of reexperiencing symptoms (because of a lack of inhibition of cue-driven retrieval; see earlier discussion). Clinical observations show that people with PTSD tend to reexperience a small number of intrusive memories consisting of brief moments from the event, for example, "seeing headlights coming toward me" or "the perpetrator's eyes staring at me" (Ehlers et al., 2002; Hackmann et al., 2004; van der Kolk & Fisler, 1995). Ehlers et al. (2004) therefore suggested that one would expect mainly those parts of the trauma narrative that correspond to the intrusive memories to show disorganization and to be disjointed from other parts of the trauma memory and that the overall disorganization of the memory would be less relevant in predicting reexperiencing symptoms. Evans (2003) has recently presented data consistent with this hypothesis.

BELIEFS, SCHEMAS, AND APPRAISALS IN PTSD

Foa's theories of anxiety disorders in general, and PTSD in particular (Foa & Kozak, 1986; Foa et al., 1989; Foa & Riggs, 1993; Foa & Rothbaum, 1998), emphasize the close link between fear memories and problematic cognitions. Meaning elements are an essential component of the proposed fear network in memory. For PTSD, Foa and Riggs (1993) specified two schemas involved in chronic PTSD: "I am entirely incompetent" and "The world is entirely dangerous." The authors suggest that what gets encoded during and after the trauma contributes to these schemas. For example, if rape victims think "It is my fault that I am being raped," this will contribute to their schema "I am entirely incompetent"; and if a trauma survivor experiences negative reactions from other people in the aftermath of the event, this will contribute to their schema "The world is entirely dangerous." Foa and Riggs (1993) and Resick and Schnicke (1993) suggested that these trauma-related cognitions may either reflect a confirmation or shattering of previously held beliefs (see also Horowitz, 1976; Janoff-Bulman, 1992; Joseph, Williams, & Yule, 1995; McCann & Pearlman, 1990).

Like Foa and colleagues, Ehlers and Clark (2000) assign a central role to the personal meaning of the traumatic event and its sequelae in the development and maintenance of PTSD. They suggested that persistent PTSD occurs only if individuals process the traumatic experience in a way that produces a sense of a serious current threat. Two key processes are said to lead to a sense of current threat: (1) excessively negative appraisals of the event and/or its sequelae and (2) the characteristics of the trauma memory discussed previously. These processes interact with each other. For example, the disorganization of trauma memories described earlier may contribute to problematic interpretations of the traumatic event. Ehlers et al. (2004) presented case examples illustrating that confusion about the time course of events, problems in accessing important details of the event, and problematic recall stemming from encoding errors at the time of the event may all give rise to problematic appraisals of the trauma, such as "It is my fault," "I should have prevented the event," or "I am going to be attacked again."

The role of beliefs and appraisals of the traumatic event and its aftermath was investigated in a series of cross-sectional (e.g., Clohessy & Ehlers, 1999; Dunmore, Clark, & Ehlers, 1997, 1999; Foa, Ehlers, Clark, Tolin, & Orsillo, 1999; Halligan et al., 2003; Mechanic & Resick, 1993; Resick, Schnicke, & Markway, 1991; Steil & Ehlers, 2000) and prospective longitudinal studies (Andrews, Brewin, & Rose, 2003; Dunmore, Clark, & Ehlers, 2001; Ehlers, Mayou, & Bryant, 1998; Ehring, 2004; Halligan et al., 2003). The results supported the role of problematic beliefs and appraisals in PTSD. The measures consistently distinguished between traumatized people with and without PTSD. Figure 3.1 shows results for the Negative Thoughts about the Self scale of Foa et al.'s (1999) Posttraumatic Cognitions Inventory (PTCI), comparing traumatized people with and without PTSD and people without trauma (who filled out the questionnaire with respect to another very upsetting event). The PTCI showed high specificity and sensitivity in identifying traumatized people with PTSD. Indirect evidence for a possible role of appraisals stems from findings that anger and shame about the trauma predict chronicity of PTSD symptoms (e.g., Andrews, Brewin, Rose, & Kirk, 1999; Foa, Riggs, Massie, & Yarczower, 1995).

Table 3.1 shows a summary of findings from a series of prospective longitudinal studies of motor vehicle accident and assault survivors conducted by our group. Appraisal measures taken in the initial days or weeks after a traumatic event consistently predicted PTSD severity at 6 months or 1 year. In line with the hypothesis that excessively negative appraisals of the trauma and its aftermath maintain PTSD, the cross-sectional studies of Dunmore et al. (1997, 1999) and Halligan et al. (2003, Study 1) found that these appraisals also distinguished between people with persistent PTSD and those who had recovered from PTSD.

"ADDED VALUE" OF MEMORY
AND APPRAISAL MEASURES?

Do the memory and beliefs/appraisal measures described herein improve the prediction of chronic PTSD over and above what can be predicted from trauma severity and other known risk factors? Data from several prospective longitudinal studies suggest that this is the case. For example, Halligan et al. (2003) found that assault characteristics explained 22% of the PTSD symptom variance, whereas memory, processing, and appraisal measures increased prediction accuracy to 71%. Similarly, in a study of children who had experienced a motor vehicle accident (Ehlers, Mayou, & Bryant, 2003), sex and stressor variables explained 14% of the variance, and the accuracy of the prediction increased to 49% when selected variables from Ehlers and Clark's (2000) model were included in the prediction. Further-

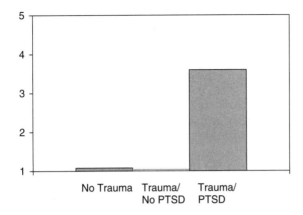

FIGURE 3.1. Results of the Negative Thoughts about the Self scale of the Posttraumatic Cognitions Inventory (Foa et al., 1999).

TABLE 3.1. Summary of Prospective Longitudinal Studies Predicting PTSD at 6 Months or 1 Year from Appraisals of the Trauma or Its Sequelae in the Initial Weeks after Trauma

Type of appraisal investigated/study	Population	Correlation with PTSD severity at follow-up
Negative beliefs about self/the world		
Dunmore et al. (2001)	Assault	.42***
Ehring (2004)	MVA	.66***
Negative interpretations of initial PTSD symptoms		
Ehlers, Mayou, & Bryant (1998)	MVA	.45***
Ehlers, Mayou, & Bryant (2002)	MVA (children)	.35**
Dunmore, Clark, & Ehlers (2001)	Assault	.42***
Halligan, Michael, Clark, & Ehlers (2003)	Assault	.62***
Ehring (2004)	MVA	.50***
Negative interpretation of other people's responses after trauma		
Ehlers, Mayou, & Bryant (2003)	MVA (children)	.41***
Dunmore, Clark, & Ehlers (2001)	Assault	.57***
Perceived permanent change		
Dunmore, Clark, & Ehlers (2001)	Assault	.66***

Note. MVA, motor vehicle accident.
**p < .01; ***p < .001.

more, Ehring (2004) found that the predictive factors identified in Ozer et al.'s (2003) meta-analysis predicted 42% of the variance of PTSD symptom severity, whereas the factors specified in the Ehlers and Clark (2000) model predicted 76% of the variance.

Initial symptom severity is a strong predictor of subsequent PTSD (e.g., Rothbaum et al., 1992). Factors that are hypothesized to maintain PTSD should predict chronic PTSD over and above initial symptom severity. Ehlers and Steil (1995) predicted that negative interpretations of initial PTSD symptoms will motivate trauma survivors to engage in cognitive strategies that are meant to control their symptoms but that maintain the disorder, such as thought suppression or rumination about the event. Interpretations of initial symptoms and the cognitive control strategies should therefore predict PTSD severity at follow-up over and above what can be explained from initial severity. Ehlers, Mayou, and Bryant (1998) and Dunmore et al. (2001) reported empirical results from prospective studies supporting this hypothesis. Further variables in the Dunmore et al. (2001) study that predicted PTSD severity at 6 months over and above PTSD severity at initial assessment were the appraisal that the trauma had permanently changed oneself in a negative way, negative appraisals of one's emotions and mental defeat during the trauma (see also Ehlers, Clark, et al., 1998; Ehlers, Maercker, & Boos, 2000), and negative appraisals of other people's reactions after the event. These data support the role of cognitive factors in the maintenance of PTSD.

CONCLUSION

The results summarized in this chapter suggest that characteristics of the trauma memory and beliefs/appraisals derived from the PTSD models by Foa's group (Foa et al., 1989; Foa & Riggs, 1993; Foa & Rothbaum, 1998) and by Ehlers and Clark (2000) may be useful in predicting who will develop persistent PTSD after a traumatic event. Further work is needed to refine some of the measures used to assess these concepts and to determine the best combination of measures. The prospective longitudinal studies presented in this chapter suggest that maintaining factors play an important part in the prediction of chronic PTSD.

NOTES

1. Cue-driven reexperiencing is the triggering of an aspect of a trauma memory by a stimulus that matches a stimulus that was present at the time of the trauma. Triggering stimuli include low-level physical aspects such as color, sound, movement, shape, and proprioceptive information.

2. A related suggestion is found in Holman and Silver (1998), who observed that temporal disintegration at the time of the trauma—whereby the present moment becomes isolated from the continuity of past and present time—was associated with subsequent distress.

REFERENCES

American Psychiatric Association. (1994). *Diagnostic and statistical manual of mental disorders* (4th ed.). Washington, DC: Author.

Amir, N., Stafford, J., Freshman, M. S., & Foa, E. B. (1998). Relationship between trauma narratives and trauma pathology. *Journal of Traumatic Stress, 11*(2), 385–392.

Andrews, B., Brewin, C. R., & Rose, S. (2003). Gender, social support, and PTSD in victims of violent crime. *Journal of Traumatic Stress, 16*, 421–427.

Andrews, B., Brewin, C. R., Rose, S., & Kirk, M. (1999). Predicting PTSD in victims of violent crime: The role of shame, anger, and blame. *Journal of Abnormal Psychology, 109*, 69–73.

Berntsen, D., Willert, M., & Rubin, D. C. (2003). Splintered memories or vivid landmarks? Qualities and organization of traumatic memories with and without PTSD. *Applied Cognitive Psychology, 17*, 675–693.

Bremner, J. D., Krystal, J. H., Southwick, S. M., & Charney, D. S. (1995). Functional neuroanatomical correlates of the effects of stress on memory. *Journal of Traumatic Stress, 8*, 527–553.

Brewin, C. R. (2001). A cognitive neuroscience account of posttraumatic stress disorder and its treatment. *Behaviour Research and Therapy, 39*, 373–393.

Brewin, C. R., Dalgleish, T., & Joseph, S. (1996). A dual representation theory of post-traumatic stress disorder. *Psychological Review, 103*, 670–686.

Byrne, C. A., Hyman, I. E., Jr., & Scott, K. L. (2001). Comparisons of memories for traumatic events and other experiences. *Applied Cognitive Psychology, 15*, S119–S133.

Christianson, S.-A. (1992). Emotional stress and eyewitness memory: A critical review. *Psychological Bulletin, 112*, 284–309.

Clohessy, S., & Ehlers, A. (1999). PTSD symptoms and coping in ambulance service workers. *British Journal of Clinical Psychology, 38*, 251–266.

Conway, M. A. (1997). What are memories? In M. A. Conway (Ed.), *Recovered memories and false memories* (pp. 1–22). Oxford, UK: Oxford University Press.

Conway, M. A. (2001). Sensory–perceptual episodic memory and its context: Autobiographical memory. *The Royal Society, 356*, 1375–1384.

Conway, M. A., & Pleydell-Pearce, C. W. (2000). The construction of autobiographical memories in the self-memory system. *Psychological Review, 107*, 261–288.

Dunmore, E., Clark, D. M., & Ehlers, A. (1997). Cognitive factors in persistent versus recovered post-traumatic stress disorder after physical or sexual assault: A pilot study. *Behavioural and Cognitive Psychotherapy, 25*, 147–159.

Dunmore, E., Clark, D. M., & Ehlers, A. (1999). Cognitive factors involved in the onset and maintenance of posttraumatic stress disorder after physical or sexual assault. *Behaviour Research and Therapy, 37*, 809–829.

Dunmore, E., Clark, D. M., & Ehlers, A. (2001). A prospective investigation of the role of cognitive factors in persistent posttraumatic stress disorder (PTSD) after physical or sexual assault. *Behaviour Research and Therapy, 39*, 1063–1084.

Easterbrook, J. A. (1959). The effect of emotion on cue utilization and the organization of behavior. *Psychological Review, 66*, 183–201.

Ehlers, A., & Clark, D. M. (2000). A cognitive model of persistent posttraumatic stress disorder. *Behaviour Research and Therapy, 38*, 319–345.

Ehlers, A., Clark, D. M., Dunmore, E., Jaycox, L., Meadows, E., & Foa, E. B. (1998). Predicting response to exposure treatment in PTSD: The role of mental defeat and alienation. *Journal of Traumatic Stress, 11*, 457–471.

Ehlers, A., Hackmann, A., & Michael, T. (2004). Intrusive re-experiencing in post-traumatic stress disorder: Phenomenology, theory, and therapy. *Behaviour Research and Therapy, 12*, 403–415.

Ehlers, A., Hackmann, A., Steil, R., Clohessy, S., Wenninger, K., & Winter, H. (2002). The nature of intrusive memories after trauma: The warning signal hypothesis. *Behaviour Research and Therapy, 40*, 1021–1028.

Ehlers, A., Maercker, A., & Boos, A. (2000). PTSD following political imprisonment: The role of mental defeat, alienation, and permanent change. *Journal of Abnormal Psychology, 109*, 45–55.

Ehlers, A., Mayou, R. A., & Bryant, B. (1998). Psychological predictors of chronic posttraumatic stress disorder after motor vehicle accidents. *Journal of Abnormal Psychology, 107*, 508–519.

Ehlers, A., Mayou, R. A., & Bryant, B. (2003). Cognitive predictors of posttraumatic stress disorder in children: Results of a prospective longitudinal study. *Behaviour Research and Therapy, 41*, 1–10.

Ehlers, A., & Steil, R. (1995). Maintenance of intrusive memories in posttraumatic stress disorder: A cognitive approach. *Behavioural and Cognitive Psychotherapy, 23*, 217–249.

Ehring, T. (2004). *Predictors of posttraumatic stress disorder, phobias and depression after road traffic accidents*. Unpublished doctoral dissertation, King's College, London.

Evans, C. (2003). *Intrusive memories in violent offenders*. Unpublished doctoral dissertation, St. George's Medical School, London.

Foa, E., Ehlers, A., Clark, D. M., Tolin, D. F., & Orsillo, S. M. (1999). The Posttraumatic Cognitions Inventory (PTCI): Development and validation. *Psychological Assessment, 11*, 303–314.

Foa, E. B., & Kozak, M. J. (1986). Emotional processing of fear: Exposure to corrective information. *Psychological Bulletin, 99*, 20–35.

Foa, E. B., Molnar, C., & Cashman, L. (1995). Change in rape narratives during exposure therapy for posttraumatic stress disorder. *Journal of Traumatic Stress, 8*, 675–690.

Foa, E. B., & Riggs, D. S. (1993). Post-traumatic stress disorder in rape victims. In J. M. Oldham, M. B. Riba, & A. Tasman (Eds.), *Annual review of psychiatry* (pp. 273–303). Washington, DC: American Psychiatric Association.

Foa, E. B., Riggs, D. S., Massie, E. D., & Yarczower, M. (1995). The impact of fear activation and anger on the efficacy of exposure treatment for posttraumatic stress disorder. *Behavior Therapy, 26*, 487–499.

Foa, E. B., & Rothbaum, B. O. (1998). *Treating the trauma of rape: Cognitive-behavior therapy for PTSD.* New York: Guilford Press.

Foa, E. B., Steketee, G., & Rothbaum, B. O. (1989). Behavioral/cognitive conceptualizations of post-traumatic stress disorder. *Behavior Therapy, 20,* 155–176.

Foa, E. B., Zinbarg, R., & Rothbaum, B. O. (1992). Uncontrollability and unpredictability in post-traumatic stress disorder: An animal model. *Psychological Bulletin, 112,* 218–238.

Gray, M. J., & Lombardo, T. W. (2001). Complexity of trauma narratives as an index of fragmented memory in PTSD: A critical analysis. *Applied Cognitive Psychology, 15,* S171–S186.

Hackmann, A., Ehlers, A., Speckens, A., & Clark, D. M. (2004). Characteristics and content of intrusive memories in PTSD and their changes with treatment. *Journal of Traumatic Stress, 17,* 231–240.

Halligan, S. L., Michael, T., Clark, D. M., & Ehlers, A. (2003). Posttraumatic stress disorder following assault: The role of cognitive processing, trauma memory, and appraisals. *Journal of Consulting and Clinical Psychology, 71,* 419–431.

Harvey, A. G., & Bryant, R. A. (1999). A qualitative investigation of the organization of traumatic memories. *British Journal of Clinical Psychology, 38,* 401–405.

Herman, J. L. (1992). *Trauma and memory.* New York: Basic Books.

Holman, E. A., & Silver, R. C. (1998). Getting "stuck" in the past: Temporal orientation and coping with trauma. *Journal of Personality and Social Psychology, 74,* 1146–1163.

Horowitz, M. J. (1976). *Stress response syndromes.* New York: Aronson.

Janoff-Bulman, R. (1992). *Shattered assumptions: Toward a new psychology of trauma.* New York: Free Press.

Joseph, S., Williams, R., & Yule, W. (1995). Psychosocial perspectives on post-traumatic stress. *Clinical Psychology Review, 15,* 515–544.

Kessler, R. C., Sonnega, A., Bromet, E., Hughes, M., & Nelson, C. B. (1995). Posttraumatic stress disorder in the National Comorbidity Survey. *Archives of General Psychiatry, 52,* 1048–1060.

Koss, M. P., Figueredo, A. J., Bell, I., Tharan, M., & Tromp, S. (1996). Traumatic memory characteristics: A cross-validated mediational model of response to rape among employed women. *Journal of Abnormal Psychology, 105,* 421–432.

Lang, P. M. (1977). Imagery in therapy: An information processing analysis of fear. *Behavior Therapy, 8,* 862–886.

McCann, I. L., & Pearlman, L. A. (1990). Vicarious traumatization: A framework for understanding the psychological effects of working with victims. *Journal of Traumatic Stress, 3,* 131–149.

McFarlane, A. C. (1988). The phenomenology of posttraumatic stress disorders following a natural disaster. *Journal of Nervous and Mental Disease, 176,* 22–29.

McNally, R. J. (1998). Experimental approaches to cognitive abnormality in post-traumatic stress disorder. *Clinical Psychology Review, 18,* 971–982.

McNally, R. J. (2003). *Remembering trauma.* Cambridge, MA: Harvard University Press.

McNally, R. J., Lasko, N. B., Macklin, M. L., & Pitman, R. K. (1995). Autobiographical memory disturbance in combat-related posttraumatic stress disorder. *Behaviour Research and Therapy, 33,* 619–630.

McNally, R. J., & Shin, L. M. (1995). Association of intelligence with severity of posttraumatic stress disorder symptoms in Vietnam combat veterans. *American Journal of Psychiatry, 152,* 936–938.

Mechanic, M. B., & Resick, P. A. (1993, November). *The Personal Beliefs and Reactions Scale: Assessing rape-related cognitive schemata.* Paper presented at the annual meeting of the International Society for Traumatic Stress Studies, San Antonio, TX.

Michael, T., Ehlers, A., Halligan, S., & Clark, D. M. (2005). Unwanted memories of assault: What intrusion characteristics are associated with PTSD? *Behaviour Research and Therapy, 43,* 613–628.

Murray, J., Ehlers, A., & Mayou, R. A. (2002). Dissociation and posttraumatic stress disorder: Two prospective studies of motor vehicle accident survivors. *British Journal of Psychiatry, 180,* 363–368.

Ozer, E. J., Best, S. R., Lipsey, T. L., & Weiss, D. S. (2003). Predictors of posttraumatic stress disorder and symptoms in adults: A meta-analysis. *Psychological Bulletin, 129,* 52–73.

Porter, S., & Birt, A. R. (2001). Is traumatic memory special? A comparison of traumatic memory characteristics with memory for other emotional life experiences. *Applied Cognitive Psychology, 15,* S101–S117.

Resick, P. A., & Schnicke, M. K. (1993). *Cognitive processing therapy for rape victims.* Newbury Park, CA: Sage.

Resick, P. A., Schnicke, M. K., & Markway, B. G. (1991, November). *The relationship between cognitive content and posttraumatic stress disorder.* Paper presented at the annual meeting of the Association for the Advancement of Behavior Therapy, New York.

Riggs, D. S., Rothbaum, B. O., & Foa, E. B. (1995). A prospective examination of symptoms of posttraumatic stress disorder in victims of nonsexual assault. *Journal of Interpersonal Violence, 10,* 201–214.

Rothbaum, B. O., Foa, E. B., Riggs, D. S., Murdock, T. B., & Walsh, W. (1992). A prospective examination of post-traumatic stress disorder in rape victims. *Journal of Traumatic Stress, 5,* 455–475.

Rubin, D. C., Feldman, M. E., & Beckham, J. C. (2004). Reliving, emotions, and fragmentation in the autobiographical memories of veterans diagnosed with PTSD. *Applied Cognitive Psychology, 18,* 17–35.

Shalev, A. Y. (1992). Posttraumatic stress disorder among injured survivors of a terrorist attack: Predictive value of early intrusion and avoidance symptoms. *Journal of Nervous and Mental Disease, 180,* 505–509.

Speckens, A., Ehlers, A., Hackmann, A., & Clark, D. M. (in press). Changes in intrusive memories associated with imaginal reliving in posttraumatic stress disorder. *Journal of Anxiety Disorders.*

Steil, R., & Ehlers, A. (2000). Dysfunctional meaning of posttraumatic intrusions in chronic PTSD. *Behaviour Research and Therapy, 38,* 537–558.

Tromp, S., Koss, M. P., Figueredo, A. J., & Tharan, M. (1995). Are rape memories different? A comparison of rape, other unpleasant, and pleasant memories among employed women. *Journal of Traumatic Stress, 8,* 607–627.

Tulving, E. (2002). Episodic memory. *Annual Review of Psychology, 53,* 1–25.

van der Kolk, B. A., & Fisler, R. (1995). Dissociation and the fragmentary nature of traumatic memories: Overview and exploratory study. *Journal of Traumatic Stress, 8,* 505–525.

van Minnen, A., Wessel, I., Dijkstra, T., & Roelofs, K. (2002). Changes in PTSD patients' narratives during prolonged exposure therapy: A replication and extension. *Journal of Traumatic Stress, 15,* 255–258.

4

Fearful Imagery and the Anxiety Disorder Spectrum

PETER J. LANG
LISA M. MCTEAGUE
BRUCE N. CUTHBERT

This chapter presents findings from a broad spectrum of anxious patients who participated in studies of physiological reactivity during exposure to fearful imagery. The analytic strategy employed here is novel for research that seeks to relate psychopathology and physiology. Thus it does *not* begin with diagnostic distinctions, symptom measures, or personality question-naires, considering these measures as prima facie definitions of the clinical material, testing whether clinical evaluation predicts differences in physio-logical response patterns. An alternative strategy, pursued here, is to use physiology rather than symptom reports as the predictor variable. Thus we begin with a simple, obligatory reflex—the startle response. The reflex is conceptually interesting in that neuroscience research has demonstrated that its potentiation reliably indexes activation of a neural circuit in the brain (the mammalian defense system) that is normally engaged when or-ganisms confront cues signaling pain or threat to survival. In this analysis, the reflex data (defense system activation) serve as the predictor variable—not the dependent variable. We test the power of the reflex to predict clinical status, as defined by symptom reports, questionnaires, and the diagnostic interview.

In pursuing this strategy, four broad questions are addressed:

1. Does potentiated startle index both fear and anxiety?
2. Do differences in defense system activation—by fearful thoughts and images—predict diagnostic differences along the anxiety spectrum?
3. Do variations in defense system activation predict comorbidity (additional anxiety disorders and depression) in patients with anxiety?
4. Is *negative affect* associated with a less reactive defense response to fearful imagery?

FEAR, POTENTIATED STARTLE, AND THE MAMMALIAN DEFENSE SYSTEM

Our understanding of the brain's defense circuitry comes primarily from neuroscience research with animals—mainly rodents—using relatively simple, classical conditioning procedures. In this work, a nociceptive event (e.g., electric shock) is paired with a previously innocuous light or tone over repeated trials until a connection is formed, such that the animal displays defensive reactions whenever the light or tone appears alone. Employing various neurosurgical, pharmacological, and electrophysiological tools, the links in the neural circuit are traced in the brain, starting from the sensory system, proceeding through the necessary connecting structures, and ending with the autonomic and motoric effector outputs. This research has repeatedly highlighted a small, almond-shaped structure located deep within the temporal lobe—the amygdala—as the center of a defense system mediating the acquisition and orchestrating the expression of conditioned "fear" (Davis, 1992; Gloor, 1960; Gray, 1989; Kapp, Pascoe, & Bixler, 1984; LeDoux, 1987; Sarter & Markowitsch, 1985).

Activation of the defense circuit begins when the lateral and basolateral nuclei of the amygdala receive input that can be relayed from any sensory modality. These nuclei then innervate the amygdala's central nucleus, which in turn projects to a variety of hypothalamic sites, the central gray, facial motor nucleus, and brainstem target areas that initiate a range of defensive behaviors and autonomic reactions that are variously deployed by organisms when under apparent survival threat (see Figure 4.1; cf. Davis, 1992).

These autonomic and somatic patterns have great variety; however, they can be functionally organized into two broad output classes: (1) *defensive immobility* (i.e., freezing, fear bradycardia, and hyperattentiveness; e.g., Campbell, Wood, & McBride, 1997; Kapp, Whalen, Supple, & Pascoe, 1992), in which the organism is vigilant, motorically passive, but primed to respond actively to further stimulation; and (2) *defensive action* (i.e., variations in fight or flight that are more or less direct responses to imminent threat of pain, attack by a predator, etc.). These outputs may be

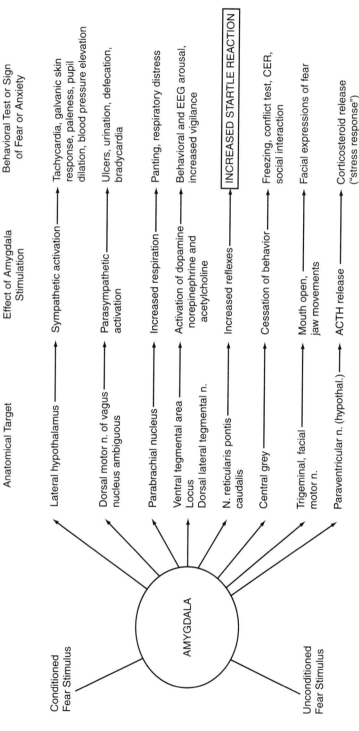

FIGURE 4.1. Schematic diagram showing direct connection between the central nucleus of the amygdala and a variety of hypothalamic and brain stem target areas that may be involved in different animal tests of fear and anxiety. Adapted from Davis (1992). Copyright 1992. Reprinted with permission of Wiley-Liss, Inc., a subsidiary of John Wiley & Sons, Inc.

stages in the normal mammalian defense response, characterized by an initial motor inhibition and an attentional set when threat may be remote and first cued but giving way to action as the signaled event is more imminent. It is apparent, furthermore, that, as representations of simple lights and tones can through aversive association come to activate neural defense circuits in animals, more complex networks of information that characterize human cognition can also come to activate the same defense system. Thus, at the level of human recall and recognition, it is proposed that emotion memory networks are defined by their connections to this primitive motivational circuitry—appetitive or defensive (Lang, 1994). Viewed from this perspective, fear states are defined by defense system activation and its reflexive autonomic and somatic output, whether driven by external threat or internal association. From an evolutionary perspective, human emotions such as fear evolved from preparatory states, evoked by threat cues, in which survival depended on delay or inhibition of overt behavior. In this sense, they derive from the first stage of defense when a threat is encountered, when the organism is immobile and vigilant, autonomically aroused, and primed to respond, but not yet active.

The Startle Reflex and Defense

The obligatory startle reflex—that begins with the eyeblink and that can involve a whole-body flexor response—may be elicited by any abrupt sensory stimulus. In many species, it appears to be a primitive escape response, although in mammals its protective function is less clear. Rodent research has shown, however, that the startle reflex is connected to the defense system and that the reflex is markedly enhanced when the animal is under threat, for example, confronting a conditioned "fear" cue.

Led by Michael Davis (Davis, 2000; Davis & Lang, 2003), researchers have extensively studied the fear conditioning paradigm and its effect on the startle reflex. In this procedure, a startle probe (a brief, abrupt acoustic stimulus) is presented during or shortly after the fear-conditioned cue, and the amplitude of the whole-body reflex is measured through a stability meter under the floor of the cage. As indicated in Figure 4.1, the increment in startle observed under these shock-threat conditions depends on the activation of the amygdala and its direct projections to the pontine center of the normal startle reflex circuit. In this sense, the startle reflex provides a metric for the assessment of defense system activation and, indirectly, the fear state.

Affective Modulation of the Startle Reflex in Humans

It has been demonstrated that reactions to the conditioned shock-fear paradigm are comparable to those found with animals. That is, during extinction, startle probe responses are greater in magnitude (potentiated) when presented during fear-conditioned stimuli than during control stimuli or during the intertrial interval (e.g., Hamm, Greenwald, Bradley, & Lang, 1993). It has also been shown that probe stimuli yield potentiated reflexes when participants are only threatened with shock—with no shocks actually delivered (e.g., Bradley Moulder, & Lang, 2005; Grillon, Ameli, Woods, Merikangas, & Davis, 1991). Furthermore, humans reliably show augmented probe reflex responses when they look at pictures of unpleasant objects or events (Bradley, Codispoti, Cuthbert, & Lang, 2001; Bradley, Codispoti, Sabatinelli, & Lang, 2001) and when they imagine fearful scenarios (Vrana & Lang, 1990; Cuthbert et al., 2003). Furthermore, when confronting images of the phobic object, individuals with phobias show significantly greater startle probe potentiation than nonfearful participants (Hamm, Cuthbert, Globisch, & Vaitl, 1997; Sabatinelli, Bradley, & Lang, 2001). Finally, functional imaging studies of the human brain (e.g., Sabatinelli, Bradley, Fitzsimmons, & Lang, 2005) have shown that the same stimuli that prompt greater potentiated startle in people with snake phobia than in nonfearful participants (e.g., pictures of snakes) also prompt greater activation in the amygdala for those with phobia.

FEARFUL THOUGHTS AND IMAGES: ACTIVATING THE DEFENSE SYSTEM

When prompted by a verbal cue, nearly all human beings directly process the meaning of the stimulus. Furthermore, if the cue refers to an object or event, they retrieve with similar apparent automaticity a memorial image. Leo Tolstoy was said to have tortured his younger brother, telling him that he must *not* think about "white bears." Once prompted, little brother was, of course, unable *not* to have ursine thoughts. Bears kept bobbing up in the conscious stream, white as snow, to the delight of his torturer (see Wegner, Schneider, Carter, & White, 1987). Studies of physiological reactions during imagery suggest that this phenomenon is not wholly cognitive. That is, when participants are told to imagine participating in some action, they experience a subovert activation of the same muscles that would be the motors of the actual behavior (Jacobson, 1931). Similarly, when participants hear text describing fearful situations, they react with a reflex physiology of defense—comparable in pattern to that evoked by actual fearful events.

Measuring Emotional Imagery

Lang and colleagues have carried forward a sustained series of experiments (e.g., Cuthbert et al., 2003; Lang, Levin, Miller, & Kozak, 1983; Miller et al., 1987; Weerts & Lang, 1978; Vrana & Lang, 1990) assessing physiological output during emotional imagery. In this view (Lang, 1977, 1979,

1994), an emotional episode is encoded in memory as an associative network of information units that includes *stimulus* representations (perceptual properties), *meaning* representations (associated semantic information "about" the context), and, most important, *response* representations (the mediators of the behavior, physiology, and expressive language that occurs in an emotional context). It is presumed that the network has neural substrata and that, for emotional imagery, the response component would include activation of motivational systems (appetitive or aversive) and their reflex physiology (Lang, 1994). This view holds that an image can be cued by any external stimulus that matches elements in the network. However, the probability of prompting the entire network depends on the network's associative strength.

As already noted, media—pictures and text—prompt retrieval of episodic emotions in most individuals. For example, the sentence, "The large snake darts forward, fangs protruding, striking my leg in a flash of pain," readily prompts a brief unpleasant image. That is, the verbal cues activate a network of representations that can prompt a transient psychophysiological change. However, if the same verbal cues are presented to an individual with a serious phobia whose snake network has high associative strength, we would anticipate strong activation of the defense system. This would result in change in the facial muscles, increased autonomic arousal, and a strongly potentiated reflex to probe startle stimulation.

Imagery and Anxiety Pathology

That anxiety-disordered patients are fearful, with an associated physiology of defensive arousal, is the syndrome's defining foundation. The veracity of this conception is generally accepted without reservation. Certainly, fear reactions are widely reported by patients, accompanied by reports of "pounding heart," "palpitations," "intense startle," "shortness of breath," "sweaty palms," and "tense muscles." Nevertheless, it is also true that these reports at clinical interviews or on personality questionnaires are rarely accompanied by measurement of the described physiological reactions. Curiously, when psychophysiological studies have been conducted, many anxiety patients appear to have diminished reactions to fear cues.

Summarizing an initial series of imagery studies, Lang (1985) noted that, although nearly all anxiety patients report comparable fearfulness and symptoms of anxious arousal, not all anxiety diagnoses show an accompanying emotional physiology. Basing his interpretation on network theory, Lang proposed that *fearfulness*—defined as a cue-specific defense reaction—actually diminishes along a diagnostic spectrum: specific phobia > social phobia > panic/agoraphobia > generalized anxiety disorder. In this view, patients with specific phobia are the most fearful. This responsiveness is ascribed to the high associative strength (coherence) of the mediating memory networks in the brain, particularly the strong association between neural representations of the cue stimulus (with associated semantic elaborations) and the neural representations that mediate physiological arousal and action. For panic/agoraphobia and generalized anxiety disorder, in contrast, representations of fear cues are embedded in networks of low associative strength, and the activation of defensive reflexes is less reliably related to specific external stimuli or their internal representations. In effect, patients categorized by these diagnoses are persistently apprehensive and distressed, but paradoxically, they appear to be less physiologically fearful.

A series of imagery studies with anxiety patients and fearful volunteers have lent support to this conception (e.g., Lang et al., 1983; Cook, Melamed, Cuthbert, McNeil, & Lang, 1988; McNeil, Vrana, Melamed, Cuthbert, & Lang, 1993). More recently, Cuthbert et al. (2003) studied emotional imagery in more than 100 anxiety patients distributed over four principal diagnoses: specific and social phobia, panic, and posttraumatic stress disorder (PTSD). Extending previous findings based on heart rate and skin conductance, the research assessed blink magnitude to a startle probe administered during imagery. Healthy controls and patients with specific and social phobia all showed significantly larger startle probe responses elicited during fear imagery; in contrast, both patients with PTSD and those with panic disorder with agoraphobia (PDA) failed to show reliable fear potentiation. As previously observed in a smaller sample (Cook et al., 1988), the diagnostic groups did not differ in the extent of self-reported vividness of their imagery, and all reported similarly strong emotional arousal when experiencing fearful images.

Cuthbert and colleagues (2003) noted an inverse relationship over diagnoses between physiological reactivity and self-reported symptomatic distress, negative affect, and the frequency of mood-disorder comorbidity. Furthermore, internal analyses of the group with social phobia showed that even within this diagnosis, as negative affect increased, physiological reactivity decreased. It was suggested that social phobia might be a transition diagnosis (perhaps because it includes both patients with specific performance fears and those with broader social anxiety) on the anxiety spectrum, positioned between the punctuated, reliable reactivity of people with focal phobia and the diffuse and unreliable reactivity of the more chronically anxious (i.e., PDA/PTSD).

STARTLE POTENTIATION DEFINES
AN ANXIETY DISORDER SPECTRUM

The preceding research suggests that semantic cues (about fear situations) engage the defense motive system to varying degrees over the spectrum of anxiety diagnoses. They further suggest that this spectrum reflects differences in fearfulness. Fearfulness is defined here as a characteristic strong, reflexive mobilization in response to threat cues rather than by verbal reports of fear symptoms. Considering the animal model of defense and its support in human basic research, the predictive validity of startle probe potentiation was assessed in a new sample of patients with anxiety disorders who were exposed to fear imagery. This analysis tested the following hypotheses:

1. The incidence of fear-potentiated startle varies significantly over the anxiety spectrum—greater for specific and social phobia than for panic and generalized anxiety disorder (GAD).
2. Fear potentiation is significantly attenuated in those patients showing depressive comorbidity and generalized anxiety symptoms. More broadly, defensive reactions to threat cues are expected to be inversely related to increasing negative affect.

Participants in this research were seen at the University of Florida Fear and Anxiety Disorders Clinic subsequent to clinical referral and newspaper or radio advertisement. Diagnostic interviews were conducted using the Anxiety Disorders Interview Schedule (ADIS-IV; Brown, DiNardo, & Barlow, 1994). The sample comprised 159 participants divided into four principal diagnostic categories[1]: specific phobia (n = 30); social phobia (n = 36); PDA (n = 27); GAD (n = 26). Additionally, a demographically matched, non-treatment-seeking control group (n = 40) that showed no clinically significant anxiety or mood disorder on the ADIS and that was recruited through newspaper advertisements was included. The majority of the sample was European American (78%), approximately 67% of participants were female, and the mean age was 34.4 years (SD = 12.4). Comorbid depression as an additional diagnosis was present in 52% of the patients with anxiety.

Experimental Procedure

After providing informed consent and filling out an anxiety and depression questionnaire battery,[2] participants were then interviewed with the ADIS-IV (Brown et al., 1994). Upon completion of the interview and a short break, the imagery protocol was introduced, and sensors were placed on the participants. Participants were told they would hear a series of tones every several seconds, to relax upon hearing a tone, to breathe out slowly, and to silently repeat the word "one." This secular meditation procedure (Benson, 1975) served as a background task, reducing and stabilizing physiological activity between imagery trials. Participants were told that from time to time in the tone series they would hear a series of imagery scripts. They were to listen carefully to the scripts when presented. At stimulus offset the participant was to vividly imagine the situation described by the sentence—experiencing the scene as an active participant as opposed to an observer. She or he was told to maintain this active imagining until the tone series started again and then to return to silently repeating the word "one." Participants were instructed to keep their eyes closed throughout the entire session.

Twenty-four imagery sentence prompts were constructed to correspond to 12 pleasant, unpleasant, and neutral content categories. The sentences were 18–20 words long, written to communicate affective meaning within the first 3 to 4 words. The sentences were digitized into 6-second audio files and presented over headphones. Participants rated their emotional experience during imagery on the dimensions of affective valence, emotional arousal, and dominance/in control (the Self-Assessment Manikin [SAM]; Lang, 1980). The data for the six threat/fear sentences (attacking animals, attacking humans, social performance) are considered in the following analyses.

Imagery trials were embedded in the tone-relaxation series. Thus several tones preceded the presentation of an image text (listening), followed by an imagery period, and then a return to relaxation (Figure 4.2). Acoustic startle probes consisting of a 50-millisecond presentation, 95-decibel burst of white noise with instantaneous rise time were administered occasionally during the relaxation period, during the first or second 6 seconds of imagery, or during both imagery periods.

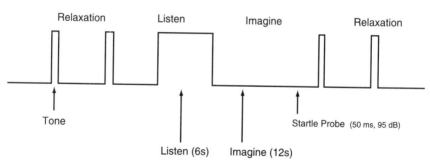

Animal Threat *"I recoil as the large dog strains forward, snarling with teeth bared, and leaps out at me."*

Human Threat *"Alone in an alley my heart pounds in fear as, knives out, laughing with menace, the street gang surrounds me."*

Social Threat *"My heart pounds in the suddenly silent room; everyone is watching me, waiting to hear what I will say."*

FIGURE 4.2. Trial structure and sample scenes. *Top:* A single trial consisted of initial tone-cued relaxation periods, then listening to a script, followed by imagery, and finally a tone-cued return to relaxation. Startle probes were presented 3–10.5 seconds into the imagery period and during intertrial intervals. *Bottom:* Exemplar scripts depicting scenes of threat.

As in other research with humans (e.g., Bradley, Codispoti, Cuthbert, et al., 2001), the eyeblink component of the startle reflex was measured based on the action of the orbicularis occuli muscle, scored as the maximum tension increase deviated from the onset level. Trials with clear artifacts were rejected, whereas trials with no responses were scored as zero magnitude blinks.

Differences in the Patient Reports of Experienced Emotion

There were no group differences in the rated unpleasantness of the threat imagery experiences. All diagnostic groups, including controls, found them similarly unpleasant (SAM; Lang, 1980). However, the rated intensity or arousal during threatening imagery differed significantly across diagnostic groups, $F(4, 156) = 5.25$, $p < .01$. As illustrated in Figure 4.3, patients with social phobia, PDA, and GAD rated fearful scenes to be significantly *more* arousing than either controls or those with specific phobia (each respective comparison, $p < .05$). The patients with PDA, GAD, and social anxiety reported feeling less dominant and "in control" during threatening imagery than did those with social phobia, PDA, or GAD.

Startle Potentiation Discriminates among Diagnoses

Under nonchallenge conditions (either for an initial startle series during a resting baseline or for probes during the intertrial intervals), there were no significant differences among diagnostic groups in startle reactivity (both F values n.s.). However, as expected, diagnostic differences emerged when participants were presented with the threatening texts, $F(4, 158) = 2.63$, $p < .05$. As shown in Figure 4.4, larger startle blinks were elicited during imagery by those with specific phobia than by controls ($p < .05$) or people with PDA ($p < .05$) and GAD ($p < .05$). Patients with social phobia also showed larger blinks than those with PDA ($p < .05$) and GAD ($p = .08$). Similar to previous findings (Cuthbert et al., 2003), patients with PDA showed attenuated defensive reactivity during threatening or fearful imagery compared with those with specific and social phobia. This new sample of patients with GAD also showed less defensive responding than those with the more "fearful" disorders. Considering patients with specific and social phobias to be predominantly "fearful" and those with PDA and GAD predominantly "anxious," the mean difference in the probe startle magnitude between these combined groups is significant, $F(1, 117) = 8.07$, $p < .01$.

Overall, the analysis of groups defined by principal diagnosis shows an inverse relationship over the anxiety spectrum between the degree of defensive reactivity (startle potentiation) and self-report of emotional distress. That is, potentiation during fearful imagery is *least* for the diagnostic groups

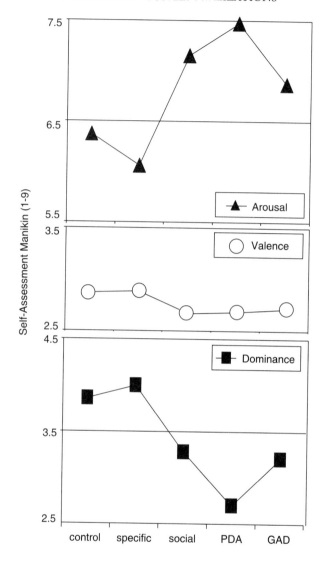

FIGURE 4.3. Evaluative judgment by principal anxiety diagnosis of arousal (*top*), pleasure (*middle*), and dominance (*bottom*).

that, during imagined fear, report the greatest emotional arousal (PDA and GAD). Interestingly, anxiety comorbidity (interview-based, DSM-IV) is also inversely related to startle potentiation, showing an increasing incidence across the spectrum, $F(3, 118) = 6.23, p < .001$, from specific phobia to GAD. Furthermore, patients with specific phobia reported the least syndromal depression, followed by those with social phobia, PDA, and GAD. Thus there is a consistent increase in reports of distress (negative affect) across the anxi-

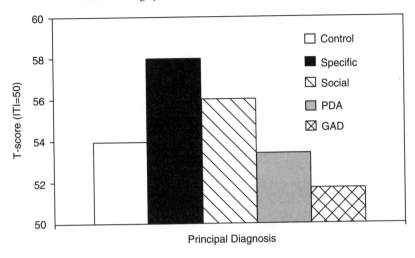

FIGURE 4.4. Mean startle blink magnitude when imagining threatening scenes by principal anxiety diagnosis.

ety-disorder spectrum that, paradoxically, covaries with a systematic decrease in potentiated startle.

High- and Low-Threat Responders

In the following analyses, the entire patient sample was divided into two groups, based on high or low defensive activation during the fear challenge. The aim was to determine whether the physiological response alone would reliably predict differences in diagnosis and, independent of diagnosis, whether physiological reactivity predicted differences in symptom severity. A median split on blink magnitude during fear imagery defined a group high in reactivity to threat ($n = 60$) and a group that did not react strongly to threat ($n = 59$), $F(1, 117) = 106.4$, $p < .0001$.[3] Interestingly, the low-threat responders responded to fear images with reflexes similar to those obtained during the intertrial or relaxation period; that is, low responders did not show normal potentiation. Figure 4.5 depicts the percentage of low-threat responders in each diagnostic group, illustrating that individuals with specific (33%) and social phobia (39%) were less likely than those with PDA (59%) and GAD (73%) to be characterized as low responders (group difference, $\chi^2 = 11.68$, $p < .01$).

Threat Startle Responder Status Predicts Measures of Generalized Anxiety

Figure 4.6 includes four graphs. The upper left graph (a) is the comparison of blink magnitude by high- and low-threat responder status, $F(1,$

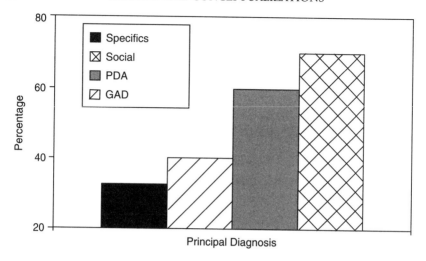

FIGURE 4.5. Percentage of each principal anxiety-disorders group that includes low-threat or low-defensive responders.

117) = 106.4, p .0001. Graph (b) shows the comparison of trait anxiety for high- and low-threat responders, which depicts the opposite pattern to that shown in graph (a). That is, those who showed larger blink magnitude during threat (i.e., high threat/defensive responders) reported *less* trait anxiety (State–Trait Anxiety Inventory [STAI]; Spielberger, Gorsuch, Lushene, Vagg, & Jacobs, 1983), $F(1, 112) = 6.01$, $p < .05$. A similar result was obtained predicting anxious distress from the General Distress–Anxious Symptoms subscale of the Mood and Anxiety Symptom Questionnaire (MASQ; Watson et al., 1995). Patients who showed larger blink magnitude again (c) reported *less* symptomatology of anxious mood, $F(1, 110) = 4.73$, $p < .05$. Last, results shown in graph (d) show startle probe prediction of self-reported symptoms of physiological activation as indexed by the Anxious Arousal scale of the MASQ. Again, it is a paradoxical pattern—patients who demonstrate the least defensive physiology report the *most* symptoms of physiological hyperarousal, $F(1, 114) = 2.71$, $p = .05$. In short, those with the most robust defensive reactivity reported significantly *less* anxious distress on all measures.

Predicting Depression from Responder Status

The same pattern depicted for generalized anxiety emerged for multiple indices of depression. Thus low-threat responders were *more* likely to have a diagnosis of comorbid depression as determined from the ADIS-IV administration, $\chi^2 = 3.95$, $p < .05$. Low-threat responders had higher levels of

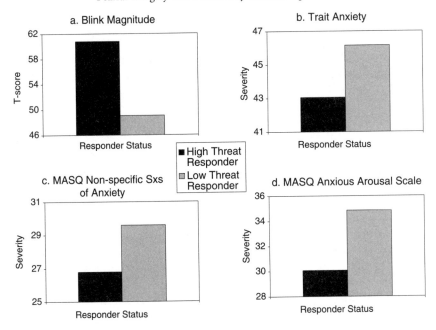

FIGURE 4.6. Predicting generalized anxiety from low- and high-threat responder status reveals that those with the most robust defensive reactivity reported *less* generalized, anxious distress. (a) Comparison of blink magnitude by high- and low-responder status. (b) Comparison of trait anxiety for high and low responders. (c) Predicting general, anxious distress from the MASQ (i.e., General Distress–Anxious Symptoms subscale) from high- and low-threat-responder status. (d) Predicting self-reported symptoms of physiological arousal (i.e., Anxious Arousal scale of the MASQ) from high- and low-threat-responder status.

cognitive and somatic symptoms of depression (Beck Depression Inventory [BDI]; Beck, Steer, & Brown, 1996), $F(1, 118) = 4.00$, $p < .05$, as well as increased anhedonia (MASQ Anhedonia subscale), $F(1, 112) = 3.33$, $p < .05$. In summary, those with the most reliable defensive reactivity reported significantly fewer depressive symptoms.

Threat Responder Status Predicts Symptom Severity within Diagnosis

It is expected that those diagnosed with specific phobia, the quintessential "fear" disorder, would show a significant positive relationship between threat potentiation and measures of phobic symptom severity. And, in fact, high-threat responders reported more specific phobias at interview (ADIS-IV; Brown et al., 1994) and had higher mean Fear Survey Schedule (FSS) scores (Wolpe & Lang, 1964). However, as over two-thirds of those with specific phobia were high responders, there were not enough low responders for meaningful analysis. Among those with social phobia, however, high ($n = 51$) and low ($n = 49$) responders were more balanced, and analysis could proceed. Consistent with the assumption that social phobia is predominantly a "fear" disorder, high defensive responding was associated with greater social fearfulness rated on the FSS ($p < .05$) and more reported symptoms on the Avoidant Personality scale of the Structured Clinical Interview for DSM-IV Axis II Personality Disorders (SCID-II) screener (First, Gibbon, Spitzer, Williams, & Benjamin, 1997) ($p < .05$).

In contrast, the relationship between startle potentiation and severity was reversed for PDA and GAD. Thus low-responding patients with PDA reported more symptoms than high-threat responders on the Anxiety Sensitivity Index (ASI; Reiss & McNally, 1985) ($p < .01$) and revealed more agoraphobic apprehension ($p < .01$) and avoidance ($p < .01$) on the ADIS-IV (Brown et al., 1994). Similarly, low responders with GAD endorsed greater interference of generalized anxiety symptoms, more excessive worry, and poorer control of worry, as rated on the ADIS-IV (all $p < 05$). In summary, high-threat responders with social phobia displayed greater diagnosis-specific symptom severity, whereas high-defensive responders with principal PDA or GAD showed less diagnosis-specific symptom severity. These data suggest that heightened defensive reactivity is associated with phobic or fearful avoidance but that defense reflexes are attenuated in diagnoses characterized by generalized anxiety, worry, and anxious apprehension.

Negative Affect

Generalized anxiety and depression appear to make individual contributions to the attenuation of startle potentiation. This was evident when the patient sample was divided into fear disorders (specific and social) and anxious disorders (GAD and PDA), and further into subgroups with or without comorbid depression. In a 2×2 analysis of variance with fearfulness versus anxiety and presence/absence of depression as two independent variables predicting blink magnitude during threat imagery, a main effect for the fearful/anxious distinction emerged, $F(1, 112) = 7.37$, $p < .01$). Patients with circumscribed fear as opposed to generalized anxiety, irrespective of depression status, demonstrated augmented blink response. Looking next at the nondepressed and depressed groups revealed reduced startle reactivity in those with comorbid depression, main effect, $F(1, 112) = 6.98$, $p < .01$. Follow-up comparisons showed that the main effect of startle attenuation with comorbid depression is reliable for both fearful ($p < .01$) and anxious disorders ($p < .01$). Interestingly, in comparing both depressed groups, the fearful-depressed group still exhibited greater startle potentiation than the anxious-depressed group ($p < .05$) suggesting that the principal presenting problem, phobia or anxiety, and presence or absence of comorbid depression separately modulate physiological reactivity.[4]

DISCUSSION AND CONCLUSIONS

The results affirm the value of the probe startle reflex in discriminating among anxiety diagnoses and in defining the predicted anxiety spectrum. The data are consistent with previous research that emphasized autonomic responses and support the view that associative connections between semantic processes and the brain's defense motive system are attenuated in disorders characterized by more generalized anxiety. These new data suggest, furthermore, that the deficit is a general response to semantic fear cues, that is, it is not specific to contents with specific clinical relevance (as highlighted in previous research; Cook et al., 1988; Cuthbert et al., 2003). The fear scenes analyzed here describe events that most people find fearful. In fact, these same threat contents have been shown to prompt significant potentiated blink reflex responses in healthy control participants—markedly larger than those that occur during neutral or less arousing affective imagery (McTeague, Bradley, & Lang, 2002). In brief, it appears that reactivity to threats of all types is greater in specific phobia than in nonphobic controls. But surprisingly, this defense reaction to threat imagery is markedly attenuated in patients with PDA and effectively absent in those with GAD relative to normal participants.

The anxiety spectrum defined here by the probe startle response is similar to a spectrum based on comorbidity noted by other investigators. For example, in a sample of 968 patients, Brown, Campbell, Lehman, Grisham, & Mancil (2001) determined that principal anxiety disorders differed significantly in the incidence of additional anxiety diagnoses. Patients with PDA and GAD showed the highest risk for an additional anxiety disorder; 47% and 52%, respectively. Conversely, those with specific (27%) and social (26%) phobias showed significantly reduced risk. Rates of additional mood disorders differed similarly across the anxiety spectrum. Principal PDA (33%) and GAD (36%) were associated with increased risk, whereas specific phobia (10%) showed a significantly reduced risk of comorbid mood disorders.

When patients with anxiety were divided into those responding with relatively stronger or weaker reflex to threat, attenuated potentiation was strongly associated with interview and questionnaire responses defined as increases in both comorbid generalized anxiety and depression. These results suggest an additive effect of anxiety and depression, supporting Clark and Watson's (1991) concept of *negative affect*. It would appear that potentiated startle could be a physiological marker for this concept. Paradoxically, however, increased negative affect is associated with a lessening of specific fear reactivity.

When high- and low-startle responders are analyzed within diagnostic groups, it is clear that some diagnoses can be characterized as "fearful," following the animal model of conditioned defense activation, whereas others are not fearful in this sense and are perhaps better described as "anxious." Thus, for the fearful disorders specific phobia and social phobia, high-threat responders are patients displaying the greatest symptom severity at interview and on questionnaires. In contrast, for the anxiety disorders PDA and GAD, high-threat responders show significantly less symptom severity. In effect, high-responding anxious patients have a "healthier" (more normal) reflexive response to rational fear cues and report less anxiety.

The results highlight the marked discordance in "anxious" patients between actual physiological reactivity and verbal report of fear and fearful physiology. That is, the patients reporting their experience of threat imagery to be the most emotionally arousing (e.g., those with PDA) were nevertheless significantly less likely to be physiological responders. In the analysis of the entire patient sample, it was the low-startle responders who reported the most physiological symptoms (e.g., on the Anxious Arousal scale of the MASQ and the Anxiety Sensitivity Index).

Future Directions for the Research

It is not clear what mechanism, cognitive or neurophysiological, can fully account for these data. The startle reflex is an obligatory response, and although it can be modulated by foreground factors, intentional suppression has not been demonstrated. Alternatively, patients with high negative affect might somehow disattend to the evocative texts—contrive *not* to think about fearful white bears. The notion of strategic cognitive avoidance of fearful information is replete in the clinical literature (e.g., Hayes, Strosahl, & Wilson, 1999) but seriously lacking in empirical support. An opposite finding is often the result of research. For example, increases (not decreases) in self-reported distress and intrusive thoughts have been reported in a wide array of thought-suppression studies (e.g., see Wenzlaff & Wegner, 2000, for a review). Furthermore, paradoxical increases in autonomic arousal have been demonstrated during purposeful emotional suppression: Gross and Levenson (1993, 1997) showed that deliberate restriction of facial expressivity (i.e., expressive suppression) during negative films resulted in less self-reported negative emotionality but heightened—not reduced—sympathetic responses. Finally, most studies of anxiety patients suggest that, rather than showing disattention to unpleasant cues, the attention of anxious participants is drawn to, even automatically "captured" by, negative stimulation (Mathews & MacLeod, 1994).

There is similarly no obvious physiological theory to adequately explain the phenomenon. One possibility is that negative affect defines a state something like "learned helplessness," as described in animal research: After extended experience with unpredictable and uncontrollable shock, animal participants become nonreactive, with no apparent capacity to respond to further challenges (e.g., Dwivedi, Mondal, Payappagoudar, & Rizavi, 2005; Dwivedi, Mondal, Shukla, Rizavi, & Lyons, 2004; Moreau, Scherschlicht, Jenck, & Martin, 1995). This state is characterized by biochemical changes that alter autonomic and central neural responses and that could result in a compromised defense circuit in the brain, reducing startle potentiation. For research with human participants, considering the broad bodily changes implied by the helplessness model, it will be important to examine defensive startle attenuation in the context of other tasks. Now that modulatory effects of text imagery have been firmly established, it will be important to examine anxiety spectral effects on the reflex using other tasks, for example, in response to external cues—other media, unpleasant pictures (e.g., Bradley, Codispoti, Cuthbert, & Lang, 2001; Bradley, Codispoti, Sabatinelli, & Lang, 2001), or threat of shock (e.g., Bradley Moulder, & Lang, 2005; Grillon et al., 1991).

In conclusion, these findings demonstrate that a simple reflex measure can reliably define an anxiety disorder spectrum, discriminating predominantly fearful disorders from disorders characterized by generalized anxiety and depression. The data also suggest that attenuated fear-potentiated startle may represent a physiological marker for negative affect, broadening this concept and linking it to a deficit in defense system activation. Finally, the predictive power of this methodology is sufficiently robust that it could be considered a practical supplement to questionnaire and interview evaluations in determining diagnosis, developing treatment plans, and monitoring patient progress.

ACKNOWLEDGMENTS

This work was supported in part by National Institute of Mental Health (NIMH) Grant Nos. MH37757 and P50-MH52384, an NIMH Behavioral Science grant to the Center for the Study of Emotion and Attention (CSEA), University of Florida, Gainesville, Florida. Many thanks to various members of the NIMH Center for the Study of Emotion and Attention for their assistance, especially Cyd Strauss, Marie-Claude Laplante, and Margaret Bradley.

NOTES

1. PTSD and OCD samples are also being collected, but at the time of writing, they were not yet of sufficient size for inclusion in this chapter.

2. The questionnaire battery included the Beck Depression Inventory (BDI; Beck et al., 1996), the State–Trait Anxiety Inventory (STAI; Spielberger et al.,

1983), the Anxiety Sensitivity Index (Reiss & McNally, 1985), the Mood and Anxiety Symptom Questionnaire (MASQ) subscales to assess the tripartite structure of negative affect (i.e., General Distress–Mixed Symptoms of anxiety and depression [MASQ GDM], General Distress–Anxious Symptoms [MASQ GDA], General Distress–Depressed Symptoms [MASQ GDD], Anxious Arousal [AA], and Anhedonic Depression [AD]; Watson & Clark, 1991).

3. Startle blinks were referenced to the distribution of reflexes obtained during nonimagery, intertrial intervals.

4. The evaluation interview included a systematic inquiry into medication use. In a subsequent comparison of patients who were taking psychotropic drugs for their presenting problems (e.g., selective serotonin reuptake inhibitors, monoamine oxidase inhibitors, benzodiazepines) with those who were not, no difference in blink magnitude during threat imagery was found, $F(1, 117) = 1.37$, n.s. This result was the same when those on and off medication are compared *within* principal diagnoses (all comparisons n.s.).

REFERENCES

Beck, A. T., Steer, R. A., & Brown, G. K. (1996). *Manual for the Beck Depression Inventory—Second edition*. San Antonio, TX: Psychological Corporation.

Benson, H. (1975). *The relaxation response*. New York: Morrow.

Bradley, M. M., Codispoti, M., Cuthbert, B. N., & Lang, P. J. (2001). Emotion and motivation: I. Defensive and appetitive reactions in picture processing. *Emotion, 1*, 276–298.

Bradley, M. M., Codispoti, M., Sabatinelli, D., & Lang, P. J. (2001). Emotion and motivation: II. Sex differences in picture processing. *Emotion, 1*, 300–319.

Bradley, M. M., Moulder, B., & Lang, P. J. (2005). When good things go bad: The reflex physiology of defense. *Psychological Science, 16*, 468–473.

Brown, T. A., Campbell, L. A., Lehman, C. L., Grisham, J. R., & Mancil, R. B. (2001). Current and lifetime comorbidity of the DSM-IV anxiety and mood disorders in a large clinical sample. *Journal of Abnormal Psychology, 110*, 585–599.

Brown, T. A., DiNardo, P. A., & Barlow, D. H. (1994). *The Anxiety Disorder Interview Schedule for DSM-IV*. Albany: State University of New York, Center for Stress and Anxiety Disorders.

Campbell, B. A., Wood, G., & McBride, T. (1997). Origins of orienting and defensive responses: An evolutionary perspective. In P. J. Lang, R. F. Simons, & M. T. Balaban (Eds.), *Attention and orienting: Sensory and motivational processes* (pp. 41–67). Mahwah, NJ: Erlbaum.

Clark, L. A., & Watson, D. (1991). Tripartite model of anxiety and depression: Psychometric evidence and taxonomic implications. *Journal of Abnormal Psychology, 100*, 316–336.

Cook, E. W., III, Melamed, B. G., Cuthbert, B. N., McNeil, D. W., & Lang, P. J. (1988). Emotional imagery and the differential diagnosis of anxiety. *Journal of Consulting and Clinical Psychology, 56*, 734–740.

Cuthbert, B. N., Lang, P. J., Strauss, C., Drobes, D., Patrick, C. J., & Bradley, M. M. (2003). The psychophysiology of anxiety disorder: Fear memory imagery. *Psychophysiology, 40,* 407–422.

Davis, M. (1992). The role of the amygdala in conditioned fear. In J. Aggleton (Ed.), *The amygdala: Neurobiological aspects of emotion, memory, and mental dysfunction* (pp. 255–305). New York: Wiley-Liss.

Davis, M. (2000). The role of the amygdala in conditioned and unconditioned fear and anxiety. In J. P. Aggleton (Ed.), *The amygdala* (Vol. 2., pp. 213–287). Oxford, UK: Oxford University Press.

Davis, M., & Lang, P. J. (2003). Emotion. In M. Gallagher & R. J. Nelson (Eds.), *Handbook of psychology: Vol. 3. Biological psychology* (pp. 405–439). New York: Wiley.

Dwivedi, Y., Mondal, A. C., Payappagoudar, G. V., & Rizavi, H. S. (2005). Differential regulation of serotonin (5HT)2A receptor mRNA and protein levels after single and repeated stress in rat brain: Role in learned helplessness behavior. *Neuropharmacology, 48,* 204–214.

Dwivedi, Y., Mondal, A. C., Shukla, P. K., Rizavi, H. S., & Lyons, J. (2004). Altered protein kinase A in brain of learned helpless rats: Effects of acute and repeated stress. *Biological Psychiatry, 56,* 30–40.

First, M. B., Gibbon, M., Spitzer, R. L., Williams, J. B., & Benjamin, L. S. (1997). *User's Guide for the Structured Clinical Interview for DSM-IV Axis II Personality Disorders (SCID-II).* Washington, DC: American Psychiatric Press.

Gloor, P. (1960). Amygdala. In J. Field (Ed.), *Handbook of physiology: Section 1. Neurophysiology* (pp. 1395–1420). Washington, DC: American Physiological Society.

Gray, T. S. (1989). Autonomic neuropeptide connections of the amygdala. In Y. Tache, J. E. Morley, & M. R. Brown (Eds.), *Neuropeptides and stress* (pp. 92–106). New York: Springer.

Grillon, C., Ameli, R., Woods, S. W., Merikangas, K., & Davis, M. (1991). Fear-potentiated startle in humans: Effects of anticipatory anxiety on the acoustic blink reflex. *Psychophysiology, 28,* 588–595.

Gross, J. J., & Levenson, R. W. (1993). Emotional suppression: Physiology, self-report, and expressive behavior. *Journal of Personality and Social Psychology, 64,* 970–986.

Gross, J. J., & Levenson, R. W. (1997). Hiding feelings: The acute effects of inhibiting negative and positive emotion. *Journal of Abnormal Psychology, 106,* 95–103.

Hamm, A. O., Cuthbert, B. N., Globisch, J., & Vaitl, D. (1997). Fear and startle reflex: Blink modulation and autonomic response patterns in animal and mutilation fearful subjects. *Psychophysiology, 34,* 97–107.

Hamm, A. O., Greenwald, M. K., Bradley, M. M., & Lang, P. J. (1993). Emotional learning, hedonic change, and the startle probe. *Journal of Abnormal Psychology, 102*(3), 453–465.

Hayes, S. C., Strosahl, K. D., & Wilson, K. G. (1999). *Acceptance and commitment therapy.* New York: Guilford Press.

Jacobson, E. (1931). Electrical measurements of neuromuscular states during mental activities: V. Variation of specific muscles contracting during imagination. *American Journal of Physiology, 96,* 115–121.

Kapp, B. S., Pascoe, J. P., & Bixler, M. A. (1984). The amygdala: A neuroanatomical systems approach to its contribution to aversive conditioning. In N. Butters & L. S. Squire (Eds.), *The neuropsychology of memory* (pp. 473–488). New York: Guilford Press.

Kapp, B. S., Whalen, P. J., Supple, W. F., & Pascoe, J. P. (1992). Amygdaloid contributions to conditioned arousal and sensory information processing. In J. P. Aggleton (Ed.), *The amygdala: Neurobiological aspects of emotion, memory, and mental dysfunction* (pp. 229–254). New York: Wiley-Liss.

Lang, P. J. (1977). Imagery in therapy: An information processing analysis of fear. *Behavior Therapy, 8*, 862–886.

Lang, P. J. (1979). A bio-informational theory of emotional imagery. *Psychophysiology, 16*, 495–512.

Lang, P. J. (1980). Behavioral treatment and bio-behavioral assessment: Computer applications. In J. B. Sidowski, J. H. Johnson, & T. A. Williams (Eds.), *Technology in mental health care delivery systems* (pp. 119–137). Norwood, NJ: Ablex Publishing.

Lang, P. J. (1985). The cognitive psychophysiology of emotion: Fear and anxiety. In A. H. Tuma & J. D. Maser (Eds.), *Anxiety and the anxiety disorders* (pp. 131–170). Hillsdale, NJ: Erlbaum.

Lang, P. J. (1994). The motivational organization of emotion: Affect-reflex connections. In S. VanGoozen, N. E. Van de Poll, & J. A. Sergeant (Eds.), *Emotions: Essays on emotion theory* (pp. 61–93). Hillsdale, NJ: Erlbaum.

Lang, P. J., Levin, D. N., Miller, G. A., & Kozak, M. J. (1983). Fear imagery and the psychophysiology of emotion: The problem of affective response integration. *Journal of Abnormal Psychology, 92*, 276–306.

LeDoux, J. E. (1987). Emotion. In V. B. Mountcastle, F. Plum, & St. R. Geiger (Eds.), *Handbook of physiology. Section I: The nervous system* (Vol. 5, pp. 419–459). Bethesda, MD: American Psychological Association.

Mathews, A., & MacLeod, C. (1994). Cognitive approaches to emotion and emotional disorders. *Annual Review of Psychology, 45*, 25–50.

McNeil, D. W., Vrana, S. R., Melamed, B. G., Cuthbert, B. N., & Lang, P. J. (1993). Emotional imagery in simple and social phobia: Fear versus anxiety. *Journal of Abnormal Psychology, 102*, 212–225.

McTeague, L. M., Bradley, M. M., & Lang, P. J. (2002). Creating a mental image: Is a picture worth a thousand words? *Psychophysiology, 39*(Suppl. 1), S57.

Miller, G. A., Levin, D. N., Kozak, M. J., Cook, E. W., III, McLean, A., Jr., & Lang, P. J. (1987). Individual differences in imagery and the psychophysiology of emotion. *Cognition and Emotion, 1*, 367–390.

Moreau, J. L., Scherschlicht, R., Jenck, F., & Martin, J. R. (1995). Chronic mild stress induced anhedonia model of depression; sleep abnormalities and curative effects of electroshock treatment. *Behavioral Pharmacology, 6*, 682–687.

Reiss, S., & McNally, R. J. (1985). Expectancy model of fear. In S. Reiss & R. R. Bootzin (Eds.), *Theoretical issues in behavior therapy* (pp. 107–121). San Diego, CA: Academic Press.

Sabatinelli, D., Bradley, M. M., Fitzsimmons, J. R., & Lang, P. J. (2005). Parallel amygdala and inferotemporal activation reflect emotional intensity and fear relevance. *NeuroImage, 24*, 1265–1270.

Sarter, M., & Markowitsch, H. J. (1985). Involvement of the amygdala in learning and memory: A critical review, with emphasis on anatomical relations. *Behavioral Neuroscience, 99*, 342–380.

Spielberger, C. D., Gorsuch, R. L., Lushene, P. R., Vagg, P. R., & Jacobs, G. A. (1983). *Manual for the State–Trait Anxiety Inventory (STAI)*. Palo Alto, CA: Consulting Psychologists Press.

Vrana, S. R., & Lang, P. J. (1990). Fear imagery and the startle probe reflex. *Journal of Abnormal Psychology, 99*, 181–189.

Watson, D., Clark, L. A., & Weber, K. (1991). *The Mood and Anxiety Symptom Questionnaire*. Unpublished manuscript, University of Iowa, Iowa City.

Watson, D., Weber, K., Assenheimer, J. S., Clark, L. A., Strauss, M. E., & McCormick, R. A. (1995). Testing a tripartite model: I. Evaluating the convergent and discriminant validity of anxiety and depression subscales. *Journal of Abnormal Psychology, 104*, 3–14.

Weerts, T. C., & Lang, P. J. (1978). Psychophysiology of fear imagery: Differences between focal phobia and social performance anxiety. *Journal of Consulting and Clinical Psychology, 46*, 1157–1159.

Wegner, D. M., Schneider, D. J., Carter, S. R., & White, T. L. (1987). Paradoxical effects of thought suppression. *Journal of Personality and Social Psychology, 53*, 5–13.

Wenzlaff, R. M., & Wegner, D. M. (2000). Thought suppression. *Annual Review of Psychology, 51*, 59–91.

Wolpe, J., & Lang, P. J. (1964). A fear survey schedule for use in behavior therapy. *Behavior Research Therapy, 2*, 27–30.

5

Emotional Processing Theory and the Recollection of Forgotten Trauma

RICHARD J. MCNALLY

In the fall of 1991, the Society for Research in Psychopathology held its annual meeting on the campus of Harvard University. Edna Foa was one of the featured speakers. After her presentation, we wandered around the campus, talking about all sorts of things, as usual. The conversation drifted to the sociology of science, and I made passing reference to "the Index." Edna asked, "What's that?" I replied, "The Social Sciences Citation Index—a measure of the impact an investigator's work has had on the field" (see Simonton, 1988, pp. 84–94). She still had no idea what I was talking about. So we went into the Widener Library and consulted the bulky volume for the year 1990. Each annual volume lists the number of times that an author's publications have been cited by other scholars during that year. Opening the book, I turned to the page for "Foa, E. B." Following her name were columns of fine print, listing all the articles that had appeared in 1990 that had cited her work. "*That*," I said to Edna, "is impact."

Many of Edna's publications have been widely cited, but one stands out above all the rest: "Emotional Processing of Fear: Exposure to Corrective Information," cowritten with Michael Kozak and published in *Psychological Bulletin* in 1986. Figure 5.1 graphically depicts its impact over the years.

Building on the insights of Lang (1977, 1979) and Rachman (1980), Foa and Kozak (1986) sought to integrate findings from clinical psychology,

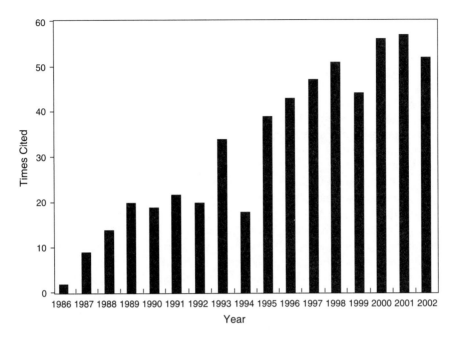

FIGURE 5.1. The frequency with which Foa and Kozak's (1986) article has been cited in the scientific literature as a function of year.

psychophysiology, and cognitive psychology in a framework for understanding pathological fear and its treatment. But concepts integral to their framework—*cognitive avoidance, meaning propositions,* and *emotional processing* (see Foa, Huppert, & Cahill, Chapter 1, this volume)—have broader relevance. More specifically, they have implications for the most contentious controversy to afflict our field in decades: the debate over the reality of recovered memories of childhood sexual abuse (CSA; McNally, 2003a). In this chapter, I use concepts from emotional processing theory to organize presentation of recent work by our group regarding cognitive functioning in people reporting recovered memories of trauma (McNally, 2003b; McNally, Clancy, & Barrett, 2004).

Our research on this topic began after I had interviewed several women who had responded to a newspaper advertisement soliciting volunteers for a neuroimaging study on recollection of memories of CSA (Shin et al., 1999). Although each claimed to have been sexually abused as a child, none had memories of abuse. All had inferred their (presumably repressed) memories of abuse from diverse indicators (e.g., depressed mood, nightmares, inexplicable uneasiness in the presence of a stepfather). Lacking explicit autobiographical memories of trauma, these women were unsuitable for the neuroimaging study. But they sparked our interest in recruiting and researching participants who believed they harbored repressed memories of CSA.

Our first series of studies comprised four groups of women: (1) those who believed they suffered from inaccessible memories of CSA (repressed-memory group); (2) those who never forgot their CSA (continuous-memory group); (3) those who reported having recalled memories of CSA that they had not thought about in many years (recovered-memory group), and (4) those who reported never having been exposed to CSA (control group).

These studies revealed that participants who reported recovered and (especially) repressed memories of CSA tend to endorse more symptoms of emotional distress than do participants who report never having forgotten their abuse or those who report never having been abused (McNally, Clancy, Schacter, & Pitman, 2000a). Participants with repressed and recovered memories, however, did not exhibit selective processing of threat cues in the emotional Stroop paradigm (McNally, Clancy, Schacter, & Pitman, 2000b), unlike patients with posttraumatic stress disorder (PTSD; McNally, Kaspi, Riemann, & Zeitlin, 1990). Although participants in the recovered-memory group were not prone to believe they had experienced unusual childhood events (e.g., getting stuck in a tree) after having visualized them during guided imagery (Clancy, McNally, & Schacter, 1999), they did exhibit heightened false-memory effects in a paradigm devised by Deese (1959) and revived and modified by Roediger and McDermott (1995). In the Deese–Roediger–McDermott (DRM) paradigm, participants are exposed to words sharing a common theme (e.g., *candy, sour, bitter, sugar*) that converge on a nonpresented word that captures the gist of the list (*sweet*). Using a version of this paradigm, we found that participants in the recovered-memory group were more likely than those in the control, repressed-memory, and continuous-memory groups to "recognize" gist words that had not, in fact, been presented (Clancy, Schacter, McNally, & Pitman, 2000).

COGNITIVE AVOIDANCE AND DIRECTED FORGETTING OF TRAUMA CUES

But most relevant to emotional processing theory are studies on cognitive avoidance and its purported role in forgetting trauma. No one disputes that CSA survivors try to avoid thinking about their abuse. Whether motivation to forget translates into ability to do so is an empirical question. Certainly the putative ability to engage in cognitive avoidance has figured prominently in theories of repressed or dissociated memories of CSA. For example, Terr (1991) asserted that children can blunt the emotional impact of sexual abuse by dissociating their attention during episodes of molestation. Such cognitive avoidance purportedly makes it difficult for abuse survivors to remember their CSA except under special circumstances years later. In fact, some trauma theorists believe that the worse the abuse, the less likely the survivor will be able to remember it. As Spiegel (1997) put it, "the nature of traumatic dissociative amnesia is such that it is not subject to the same rules of ordinary forgetting: it is more, rather than less, common after repeated episodes; involves strong affect; and is resistant to retrieval through salient cues" (p. 6).

We have conducted experiments designed to test for mechanisms that ought to be operative if people can forget and then recover memories of CSA. Researchers have used two directed-forgetting methods to investigate cognitive avoidance in the laboratory (McNally, 2005). In the item method, participants are shown a series of words on a computer screen. Shortly after each word's appearance, instructions inform the participant either to remember or to forget the previous word. They are later asked to recall all words, regardless of initial instruction. Most often, participants recall more "remember" words than "forget" words—an effect usually attributed to attentional disengagement following "forget" instructions.

In our first directed-forgetting experiment (McNally, Metzger, Lasko, Clancy, & Pitman, 1998), we tested three groups of women. One group had CSA-related PTSD, another had experienced CSA but did not have PTSD, and a third group had neither experienced CSA nor had PTSD. Each participant saw a series of words on a computer screen. Each word appeared for 2 seconds before being replaced by a cue that instructed the person either to remember (RRRR) or to forget (FFFF) the word she had just seen. Words either were related to trauma (e.g., *incest, abused*), were positive (e.g., *elation, affection*), or were neutral (e.g., *lamp, stairs*). Immediately after this encoding phase, participants were asked to write down as many words as they could remember, irrespective of whether the word had been followed by "remember" or "forget" instructions. The cognitive avoidance (or dissociative or avoidant encoding) hypothesis implies that abuse survivors with PTSD should recall few trauma-related "remember" words relative to positive and neutral "remember" words and relative to psychiatrically healthy CSA survivors and control participants who presumably lack the motivation (and skill) to expel trauma-related material from awareness.

The results were exactly the opposite of these predictions. CSA survivors with PTSD exhibited memory deficits, to be sure, but for positive and neutral words they were supposed to remember. They did not exhibit the predicted skill in disengaging attention from trauma words, thereby impairing later recollection of them. Indeed, these participants remembered the trauma words all too well, including those they had been instructed to forget. Rather than exhibiting superior cognitive avoidance skills, CSA survivors with PTSD exhibited a breakdown in the ability to avoid and forget. CSA survivors without PTSD were indistinguishable from control participants. Both groups recalled "remember" words more often than "forget" words, regardless of the valence of the word.

The psychiatrically impaired survivors in this study had PTSD. Accordingly, this group may not have been especially suitable for testing the hypothesis that CSA survivors possess superior cognitive avoidance capabilities. In our next experiment, we replicated the aforementioned procedure, testing women who reported either repressed memories of CSA, recovered memories of CSA, or no history of CSA (McNally, Clancy, & Schacter, 2001). If anyone should exhibit superior ability to disengage attention from trauma cues and limit subsequent recall of them, it should be individuals who report having forgotten their abuse for years (recovered-memory group) or who believe they still cannot remember it (repressed-memory group).

But as it turns out, neither of these groups exhibited impaired recall of trauma words. Indeed, they exhibited normal directed-forgetting performance, recalling "remember" words more often than "forget" words, regardless of valence. Taken together, these two studies indicated that none of the groups reporting CSA exhibited superior ability to disengage attention from threat words, thereby impairing subsequent recall. To be sure, these directed-forgetting experiments concern mere trauma words, not autobiographical memories of abuse. But if survivors possess skills for forgetting memories of abuse, one would expect that being able to forget mere words would be easy.

In our next experiment, we used the list method to test for enhanced directed forgetting of trauma cues (McNally, Clancy, Barrett, & Parker, 2004). In the list method, participants are shown a series of words; halfway through the list, they are told to forget all the words they have seen so far. After viewing the remaining items, they are asked to recall all words, regardless of whether they were from the first or second half of the list. Most often, participants exhibit a recall deficit for words from the block they were told to forget—an effect attributed to retrieval inhibition of encoded, but inaccessible, words.

In this study, we tested men and women who reported either repressed, recovered, or continuous memories of CSA or no history of CSA. Participants saw a series of words that were either trauma-related or positive, and they rated the emotional significance of each word. Halfway through the first block of words, the experimenter told the participant that the words shown so far were just for practice and that these words could be forgotten. The second block of intermixed trauma and positive words then appeared, and the individual continued to rate the emotionality of each word. Participants then received a surprise recall test for all words, including those from the first block that they had been told to forget. Contrary to prediction, the repressed- and recovered-memory groups did not exhibit deficits in the ability to recall trauma words from the first block. Indeed, all four groups exhibited a directed-forgetting effect, as evinced by greater recall of words from the second block than from the first block. Moreover, there was a main effect of valence: All groups recalled trauma words more often than positive words.

However, DePrince and Freyd (2004) have argued that our experiments provide inadequate tests of the hypothesis of superior forgetting skills in dissociative CSA survivors. They claim that these survivors coped with abuse by disengaging their attention during molestation episodes. Accordingly, an appropriate test would require participants to perform the directed-forgetting task under divided rather than selective attention conditions. Testing college students, some with reported abuse histories, DePrince and Freyd (2004) found that those scoring high on a dissociation questionnaire exhibited impaired recall of trauma words encoded under divided, but not selective, attention conditions relative to students scoring low on dissociation.

In our most recent experiment, we replicated DePrince and Freyd's procedure with adults who reported either recovered memories of CSA, continuous memories of CSA, or no history of CSA (McNally, Ristuccia, & Perlman, 2005). Participants saw four blocks of intermixed trauma and neutral words on a computer screen. Two blocks were encoded under selective attention conditions, and two were encoded under divided attention conditions. Under selective attention, each word appeared in black letters against a white background. Under divided attention, words changed colors from red to blue (and vice versa). For example, the word *molested* might appear in blue letters for the first second of the 6-second presentation time, switch to red letters for the next 2 seconds, and then back to blue letters for the final 3 seconds. Participants' attention was divided because they had to press the space bar whenever a word changed color while simultaneously trying to encode it. Finally, one selective attention block and one divided attention block were followed by "forget" instructions, and one selective attention and one divided attention block were followed by "remember" instructions. After all blocks had been presented, participants attempted to recall words from all blocks.

Although a memory deficit for trauma words encoded during divided attention was expected in the recovered-memory group, all three groups recalled trauma words far more often than neutral words, regardless of instructions and regardless of encoding condition. The memorability of trauma-related material was so striking that it overrode all other variables.

In summary, although most CSA survivors are motivated to avoid thinking about their abuse, we have found no evidence of their enhanced ability to do so—at least in the cognitive psychology laboratory.

MEANING PROPOSITIONS AND THE
TRANSFORMATION OF MEMORY

Foa and Kozak (1986) stressed the importance of meaning propositions in the emotional processing of fear. Patholytic changes in the meaning of stimuli and responses were awarded considerable significance. However, the reverse can also occur, as we have learned in our research on recovered memories of sexual abuse.

In an interview study of 27 adults (17 women) who reported recovering memories of CSA after many years of not having thought about their abuse, we found evidence of meaning changing in pathogenic directions (Clancy & McNally, in press). On average, they reported having been nonviolently molested (e.g., fondled) when they were about 8 years old. Approximately 21 years later, they encountered reminders that prompted recollection of these long-forgotten events. Although 93% remembered experiencing the abuse as confusing, upsetting, and disgusting, only two remembered having experienced intense fear. Indeed, only two said that they had understood it as sexual at the time.

However, after having remembered these long-forgotten events, they regarded them as more traumatizing in retrospect, now that they understood them as sexual abuse. In fact, 100% reported that the abuse had had multiple adverse effects on their lives, and no fewer than seven qualified for a current diagnosis of abuse-related PTSD, delayed onset. That is, the retrospective reappraisal—change in meaning—managed to convert a forgotten memory of an adverse childhood experience into a PTSD-inducing event.

EMOTIONAL PROCESSING
OF "FALSE MEMORIES" OF TRAUMA

Although our research group has been studying recovered memories of sexual abuse for the past several years, we have often found it difficult to determine whether the recollected events were true or false. Corroboration has been tough to come by. Accordingly, we have been studying individuals whose memories we suspect are probably false: those who report having been abducted by space aliens (Clancy, McNally, Schacter, Lenzenweger, & Pitman, 2002; McNally, Lasko, et al., 2004). The typical "abductee" experiences a terrifying episode of sleep paralysis (discussed later), misinterpreted as an alien encounter, and then contacts a mental health professional who "helps" the abductee recover detailed (and presumably false) memories of being sexually probed by aliens on spaceships and so forth.

In one experiment (McNally, Lasko, et al., 2004), we tested whether people who report alien abduction exhibit the psychophysiological reactivity typical of PTSD patients who recollect their traumatic events in the laboratory (Orr, Metzger, & Pitman, 2002). Using a script-driven imagery protocol (Lang, Levin, Miller, & Kozak, 1983), we asked 10 abductees to provide material for five autobiographical memory scripts: two related to traumatic alien encounters, one related to another extremely stressful experience, one related to a very positive experience, and one concerning a neutral experience. Using this material, we created 30-second audiotaped scripts for presentation in the psychophysiology laboratory. Control participants, who denied ever having been abducted by space aliens, heard the scripts of the abductees. If processing "false" emotional memories is functionally akin to processing genuine emotional memories, psychophysiological reactivity to abduction scripts and stressful scripts should provoke greater heart rate, skin conductance, and electromyographic activity in the abductee group than in the control group. This is precisely what happened. Accordingly, belief that one has been traumatized—whether the belief is true or false—seems to drive a physiological reaction hitherto attributed to traumatic conditioning experiences that have occurred.

The physiological data are fully concordant with the view that these individuals genuinely believed they had been abducted. Our psychiatric interviews uncovered no evidence of major mental illness (e.g., schizophrenia). What, then, is going on? What are the ingredients for a space-alien abductee? Our work with this population suggests the following recipe (Clancy et al., 2002; McNally & Clancy, 2005; McNally, Lasko, et al., 2004). First, the typical abductee endorses a wide range of "New Age"-like beliefs, including astral projection, past lives, and alien visitation. Second, thanks to Hollywood, all are acquainted with the standard abduction narrative. The person is whisked out of the bedroom window at night and transported to a spaceship, where little gray beings perform various medical and sexual procedures on the abductee. Third, they score high on a questionnaire measure of Absorption, a trait related to fantasy proneness and rich imaginative capabilities. Fourth, they experience episodes of sleep paralysis, accompanied by hypnopompic hallucinations of figures in the bedroom, lights flashing, sounds buzzing, tingling sensations coursing through the body, and feelings of levitating off one's bed. These harmless events occur when people awaken from rapid eye movement (REM) sleep—the stage of sleep when we do most of our dreaming and during which we are entirely paralyzed. The person awakens before the paralysis has waned and experiences terror at the temporary inability to move. The hallucinations occur as remnants of REM mentation intrude into wakefulness—dreaming with one's eyes open, so to speak. Fifth, most seek mental health professionals specializing in hypnotic memory recovery who interpret the sleep paralysis episode as an alien encounter and then "help" the person recall the blocked memories of what had happened next (e.g., being medically probed on a spaceship). By the time we have assessed these abductees in our research program, they have fully embraced the social role

of alien abductee, and most resist the aforementioned mundane explanation for their abduction memories.[1] In fact, although our abductees described their sleep paralysis episodes and subsequent recovery of abduction
memories as terrifying, all stated that they were ultimately glad to have
been abducted. They noted how their alien encounters deepened their
spiritual appreciation of the universe, confirming that wise beings exist
"out there" who care for us and the fate of the Earth.

Max Weber (1919/1946) famously proclaimed that secular science
produces "disenchantment of the world" (p. 155), robbing it of its mystery
and its meaning by expelling the gods. The entire space-alien-abductee phenomenon represents an effort to reenchant the world.

CONCLUSION

Foa and Kozak's (1986) emotional processing theory was developed to provide a framework for elucidating the mechanisms underlying pathological
fear and its treatment. But, as evident from the studies cited in this chapter,
the conceptual reach of their theory extends far beyond behavior therapy
for phobia and related disorders. Indeed, its relevance spans issues ranging
from reports of repressed memories of sexual abuse to reports of abduction
by space aliens. Whether emotional processing theory turns out to be correct in all its details matters less than the heuristic impact it has had on our
field.

ACKNOWLEDGMENT

Research cited in this chapter is supported by National Institute of Mental Health
Grant No. MH61268 awarded Richard J. McNally.

NOTE

1. Not all traumatologists buy this explanation for alien abduction accounts.
In a public discussion of our research on the Traumatic Stress electronic mailing list,
one social worker hypothesized that our participants had actually been molested by
members of a Satanic cult who, in turn, used mind-control programming to convince them that they had been molested by space aliens (P. Spinal-Robinson, personal communication, July 31, 2004). Of course, others may argue that cult victims
have actually been molested by space aliens who, in turn, have used mind-control
programming to convince them that they had been molested by Satanists. Such are
the complexities of science.

REFERENCES

Clancy, S. A., & McNally, R. J. (in press). Recovered memories of childhood sexual abuse: Forgetting as a consequence of voluntary suppression. *Scientific Review of Mental Health Practice.*

Clancy, S. A., McNally, R. J., & Schacter, D. L. (1999). Effects of guided imagery on memory distortion in women reporting recovered memories of sexual abuse. *Journal of Traumatic Stress, 12,* 559–569.

Clancy, S. A., McNally, R. J., Schacter, D. L., Lenzenweger, M. F., & Pitman, R. K. (2002). Memory distortion in people reporting abduction by aliens. *Journal of Abnormal Psychology, 111,* 455–461.

Clancy, S. A., Schacter, D. L., McNally, R. J., & Pitman, R. K. (2000). False recognition in women reporting recovered memories of sexual abuse. *Psychological Science, 11,* 26–31.

Deese, J. (1959). On the prediction of occurrence of particular verbal intrusions in immediate recall. *Journal of Experimental Psychology, 58,* 17–22.

DePrince, A. P., & Freyd, J. J. (2004). Forgetting trauma stimuli. *Psychological Science, 15,* 488–492.

Foa, E. B., & Kozak, M. J. (1986). Emotional processing of fear: Exposure to corrective information. *Psychological Bulletin, 99,* 20–35.

Lang, P. J. (1977). Imagery in therapy: An information processing analysis of fear. *Behavior Therapy, 8,* 862–886.

Lang, P. J. (1979). A bio-informational theory of emotional imagery. *Psychophysiology, 16,* 495–512.

Lang, P. J., Levin, D. N., Miller, G. A., & Kozak, M. J. (1983). Fear behavior, fear imagery, and the psychophysiology of emotion: The problem of affective-response integration. *Journal of Abnormal Psychology, 92,* 276–306.

McNally, R. J. (2003a). *Remembering trauma.* Cambridge, MA: Belknap Press/Harvard University Press.

McNally, R. J. (2003b). Recovering memories of trauma: A view from the laboratory. *Current Directions in Psychological Science, 12,* 32–35.

McNally, R. J. (2005). Directed forgetting tasks in clinical research. In A. Wenzel & D. C. Rubin (Eds.), *Cognitive methods and their application to clinical research* (pp. 197–212). Washington, DC: American Psychological Association Press.

McNally, R. J., & Clancy, S. A. (2005). Sleep paralysis, sexual abuse, and space alien abduction. *Transcultural Psychiatry, 42,* 113–122.

McNally, R. J., Clancy, S. A., & Barrett, H. M. (2004). Forgetting trauma? In D. Reisberg & P. Hertel (Eds.), *Memory and emotion* (pp. 129–154). Oxford, UK: Oxford University Press.

McNally, R. J., Clancy, S. A., Barrett, H. M., & Parker, H. A. (2004). Inhibiting retrieval of trauma cues in adults reporting histories of childhood sexual abuse. *Cognition and Emotion, 18,* 479–493.

McNally, R. J., Clancy, S. A., & Schacter, D. L. (2001). Directed forgetting of trauma cues in adults reporting repressed or recovered memories of childhood sexual abuse. *Journal of Abnormal Psychology, 110,* 151–156.

McNally, R. J., Clancy, S. A., Schacter, D. L., & Pitman, R. K. (2000a). Personality profiles, dissociation, and absorption in women reporting repressed, recovered, or continuous memories of childhood sexual abuse. *Journal of Consulting and Clinical Psychology, 68*, 1033–1037.

McNally, R. J., Clancy, S. A., Schacter, D. L., & Pitman, R. K. (2000b). Cognitive processing of trauma cues in adults reporting repressed, recovered, or continuous memories of childhood sexual abuse. *Journal of Abnormal Psychology, 109*, 355–359.

McNally, R. J., Kaspi, S. P., Riemann, B. C., & Zeitlin, S. B. (1990). Selective processing of threat cues in posttraumatic stress disorder. *Journal of Abnormal Psychology, 99*, 398–402.

McNally, R. J., Lasko, N. B., Clancy, S. A., Macklin, M. L., Pitman, R. K., & Orr, S. P. (2004). Psychophysiological responding during script-driven imagery in people reporting abduction by space aliens. *Psychological Science, 15*, 493–497.

McNally, R. J., Metzger, L. J., Lasko, N. B., Clancy, S. A., & Pitman, R. K. (1998). Directed forgetting of trauma cues in adult survivors of childhood sexual abuse with and without posttraumatic stress disorder. *Journal of Abnormal Psychology, 107*, 596–601.

McNally, R. J., Ristuccia, C. S., & Perlman, C. A. (2005). Forgetting trauma cues in adults reporting continuous or recovered memories of childhood sexual abuse. *Psychological Science, 16*, 336–340.

Orr, S. P., Metzger, L. J., & Pitman, R. K. (2002). Psychophysiology of post-traumatic stress disorder. *Psychiatric Clinics of North America, 25*, 271–293.

Rachman, S. (1980). Emotional processing. *Behaviour Research and Therapy, 18*, 51–60.

Roediger, H. L., III, & McDermott, K. B. (1995). Creating false memories: Remembering words not presented in lists. *Journal of Experimental Psychology: Learning, Memory, and Cognition, 21*, 803–814.

Shin, L. M., McNally, R. J., Kosslyn, S. M., Thompson, W. L., Rauch, S. L., Alpert, N. M., et al. (1999). Regional cerebral blood flow during script-driven imagery in childhood sexual abuse-related PTSD: A PET investigation. *American Journal of Psychiatry, 156*, 575–584.

Simonton, D. K. (1988). *Scientific genius: A psychology of science*. Cambridge, UK: Cambridge University Press.

Spiegel, D. (1997). Foreword. In D. Spiegel (Ed.), *Repressed memories* (pp. 5–11). Washington, DC: American Psychiatric Press.

Terr, L. C. (1991). Childhood trauma: An outline and overview. *American Journal of Psychiatry, 148*, 10–20.

Weber, M. (1946). Science as a vocation. In H. H. Gerth & C. W. Mills (Eds. & Trans.), *From Max Weber: Essays in sociology* (pp. 129–156). New York: Oxford University Press. (Original work published 1919)

PART II

Assessment of and Treatments for Pathological Anxiety

6

Assessment Strategies in the Anxiety Disorders

DAVID RIGGS
TERENCE M. KEANE

Anxiety is defined as an "apprehensive anticipation of future danger or misfortune accompanied by a feeling of dysphoria or somatic symptoms of tension," (American Psychiatric Association, 2000, p. 820). Closely related to anxiety is the basic emotion of fear. However, theorists have argued that fear and anxiety are distinct (Antony & Barlow, 1996; Lang, McTeague, & Cuthbert, Chapter 4, this volume). Anxiety is seen as anticipatory in that it is focused on upcoming events that are seen as uncontrollable, unpredictable, and potentially dangerous. This anticipation leads to worry and negative affect. In contrast, fear is focused on the present situation and represents an alarm reaction to danger perceived in the immediate environment. Thus a person confronted with a large growling dog may become fearful but will experience anxiety in anticipation of a visit with a friend who owns a large dog.

Lang (1971) conceptualized the related states of fear and anxiety as incorporating responses in each of three channels: cognitive, behavioral, and physiological. Responses in the cognitive realm include anticipation of negative outcomes, biases in information processing, and anxious beliefs. In the behavioral arena, responses include avoidance, distractions, compulsive rituals, and other behaviors that function to increase perceived safety. Physiological responses include a variety of reactions that are consistent with increased autonomic arousal, such as dizziness, increased heart rate and respiration, and sweating. Empirical studies suggest that the three response channels described by Lang (1971) are not always highly correlated; therefore, it is important to assess reactions in each of the three areas.

Assessment of anxiety and fear should incorporate multiple issues. These include such things as diagnostic features, severity of symptoms, medical conditions that may cause or exacerbate the anxiety symptoms, and the course of the symptoms. Additional areas that may need to be assessed include skills deficits that may contribute to the problem or limit treatment options, family history of anxiety and other mental health problems, and treatment history and preferences (Antony, 2001).

A variety of assessment methods are available for collecting information related to fear and anxiety. The choice of method(s) used will depend on the goals of the assessment and the resources available to complete the assessment. Diagnostic interviews are available for the anxiety disorders in general and for many of the specific disorders included in the DSM-IV (American Psychiatric Association, 1994). Standardized, semistructured diagnostic interviews such as the Structured Clinical Interview for DSM-IV (SCID; First, Spitzer, Gibbon, & Williams, 1996) and the Anxiety Disorders Interview Schedule for DSM-IV (ADIS-IV; Brown, Di Nardo, & Barlow, 1994) represent an excellent means for assessing diagnostic criteria and thus providing a differential diagnosis. Similarly, disorder-specific interviews have been developed to evaluate symptoms of a particular disorder. However, these interviews can be time-consuming and require extensive training. Self-report instruments that focus the assessment on symptoms of a specific disorder or on characteristics of anxiety or fear that transcend specific diagnoses are available. These instruments are generally less time-intensive to administer than a diagnostic interview, but they also allow less flexibility. In addition to these assessment techniques, anxiety and fear may be evaluated using behavioral assessments such as the behavioral approach test, in which a person is asked to confront a feared situation or stimulus, and self-monitoring of specific aspects of anxiety, such as the frequency of compulsive rituals. Similarly, the physiological component of anxiety and fear may be assessed by measuring indices of physiological reactivity, such as heart rate and skin conductance. In this chapter we discuss the assessment of patients by diagnosis, focusing on posttraumatic stress disorder (PTSD), social phobia (SP), obsessive–compulsive disorder (OCD), and panic disorder (PD).

POSTTRAUMATIC STRESS DISORDER

PTSD was initially conceptualized by the diagnostic manuals in mental health as a relatively rare condition owing to a belief that traumatic events such as war, sexual assault, violence, and disasters constituted events beyond the usual experiences of humans. The development of specific, measurable diagnostic criteria for PTSD led to diagnostic interviews, psychological tests and questionnaires, and ultimately to the conduct of epidemiological studies. Therein, we learned that exposure to traumatic events was indeed common in the general population of the United States (e.g., 61% of men and 51% of women; Kessler et al., 1995) and that PTSD was among the most common of all disorders, with approximately 11% of women and 5% of men developing this condition at some time in their lives. Thus what was previously considered a relatively low prevalence condition in America was found to be among the most common of all mental health conditions, surpassed only by alcohol abuse, depression, and social phobia. The assessment and treatment of PTSD is, therefore, a major concern for the public health of all Americans.

For many people, exposure to a traumatic event results in extreme emotional reactions in the short term, but fortunately most people do recover. However, a significant minority of those exposed do eventually develop PTSD. The development of appropriate assessment measures to be used in the clinical setting was among the very first goals of clinical researchers attempting to improve the treatment of those with PTSD. In the 25 years since the inception of the diagnostic category, clinical researchers have developed many outstanding measures of PTSD suitable for use in every clinical setting, in research laboratories, and in epidemiological field studies (see Keane & Barlow, 2002; Keane, Weathers, & Foa, 2000). Although the progress is excellent for adults, more work remains in the field of assessment of adolescents and children. This section focuses on the assessment of PTSD in adults.

Assessment Issues

Features of PTSD

PTSD is characterized by high levels of anxiety, depression, and related symptomatology. The diagnostic criteria include exposure to a traumatic event, with attendant intense emotional reactions. The expression of symptoms includes experiences that recapitulate the traumatic event, such as nightmares, flashbacks, and preoccupation with the event and/or sensory cues associated with the traumatic event itself. Typically these reliving experiences incorporate some or all of the memory of the traumatic event; when reliving the traumatic event, the individual feels anxiety, fear, horror, anger, or other strong emotions associated with the event.

In addition to reliving experiences, the diagnostic criteria also include avoidance and withdrawal. The avoidance may take the form of behavioral avoidance of people and places associated with the traumatic event or of emotional or cognitive avoidance. For some people, the emotional reactions to cues associated with the traumatic event are so strong and distressing that their lives become increasingly restricted. This restriction can be emotional, as in the case of emotional numbing, or social, in that individuals may become significantly withdrawn from family and friends.

Other symptoms that constitute the diagnostic picture for PTSD are viewed as hyperarousal and can include concentration and memory impairment, insomnia, irritability and anger, hypervigilance, and exaggerated startle responses. PTSD is often comorbid with alcohol and drug abuse, depression, social anxiety disorder, and panic.

Differential Diagnosis

PTSD is most often seen as a disorder that combines features of the mood disorders, other anxiety disorders, dissociative disorders, and the personality disorders. For this reason, a thorough and complete history that focuses on exposure to the most high-frequency traumatic events is key to accurate diagnosis. Past child abuse and neglect are now commonly assessed in diagnostic interviews, but exposure to natural disasters, industrial and moving vehicle accidents, and domestic and community violence are less frequently assessed. Sexual assault and rape are commonly assessed among women, but less so among men. When violence within the family is involved or if the aftermath of sexual assault is troubling an individual, people may be reluctant to openly communicate these experiences. The shame or humiliation commonly associated with these events highlights the importance of early screening for these life experiences. Missing the exposure component will increase the likelihood that an inaccurate diagnosis will ensue.

It is clear that PTSD is one disorder that frequently follows exposure to a traumatic event, but it is not the only one. Depression, phobia, panic, substance abuse, and adjustment disorder are frequent outcomes as well. The prevalence of dissociative disorders following exposure to traumatic events is not known at the moment, but they are likely frequent sequelae.

Assessment Strategies

Structured Diagnostic Interviews

Clinician-administered structured diagnostic interviews are valuable tools for assessing PTSD (Keane et al., 1996). Whereas it is standard practice in clinical research settings to employ structured diagnostic interviews, the use of these types of interviews in the clinical setting is less common, with perhaps the single exception of clinical forensic practice (Keane, 1995; Keane, Buckley, & Miller, 2003). Several structured interviews are available that were developed for the assessment of PTSD either as modules of comprehensive diagnostic assessment tools or as independent PTSD measures. These are described next.

Structured Clinical Interview for DSM-IV (SCID-IV). The SCID-IV (First et al., 1997) is designed to assess a broad range of psychiatric conditions on Axis I and Axis II. It is divided into separate modules corresponding to DSM-IV (American Psychiatric Association, 1994) diagnostic criteria, with each module providing the interviewer with specific prompts and follow-up inquiries intended to be read verbatim to respondents. The SCID is intended for use only by clinicians and highly trained interviewers.

Although the administration of the full SCID-IV can be time-consuming, the modular structure allows clinicians to limit their assessment to conditions that are frequently comorbid with PTSD. Within the context of a trauma clinic, it is recommended that the anxiety disorders, affective disorders, and substance use disorder modules be given. Administration of the psychotic screen will also help to rule out conditions that require a different set of interventions (Keane & Barlow, 2002).

The SCID–PTSD module is considered psychometrically sound. Keane et al. (1998) examined the interrater reliability of the SCID by asking a second interviewer to listen to audiotapes of an initial interview. They found a kappa of .68 and agreement across "lifetime," "current," and "never" levels of PTSD of 78%. Similarly, in a sample of patients who were reinterviewed within a week by a different clinician, they found a kappa of .66 and diagnostic agreement of 78%. The SCID–PTSD module also yielded substantial sensitivity (.81) and specificity (.98) and a robust kappa (.82) in one clinical sample against a composite PTSD diagnosis (Kulka et al., 1988), indicating good diagnostic utility.

Clinician-Administered PTSD Scale (CAPS). Developed by the National Center for PTSD (Blake et al., 1990), the CAPS is currently the most widely used structured interview for diagnosing and measuring the severity of PTSD (Weathers, Keane, & Davidson, 2001). The CAPS assesses all DSM-IV (American Psychiatric Association, 1994) diagnostic criteria for PTSD, including Criteria A (exposure), B–D (core symptom clusters), E (chronology), and F (functional impairment), as well as associated symptoms of guilt and dissociation. The CAPS also promotes uniform administration and scoring through carefully phrased prompt questions and explicit rating scale anchors with clear behavioral referents.

Weathers et al. (2001) extensively reviewed the psychometric studies conducted on the CAPS. Weathers, Ruscio, and Keane (1999) examined the reliability and validity data of the CAPS across five samples of male Vietnam veterans collected at the National Center for PTSD. Robust estimates were found for interrater reliability over a 2–3 day interval for each of the three symptom clusters (.86–.87 for frequency, .86–.92 for intensity, and .88–.91 for severity) and all 17 symptoms (.91 for total frequency, .91 for total intensity, and .92 for total severity). Test–retest reliability for a

CAPS-based PTSD diagnosis was also high (kappa = .89 in one sample and 1.00 in a second sample). Thus the data indicate that trained and calibrated raters can achieve a high degree of consistency in using the CAPS to rate PTSD symptom severity and diagnose PTSD. Weathers et al. (1999) also found high internal consistency across all 17 items in a research sample (alphas of .93 for frequency and .94 for intensity and severity) and a clinical sample (alphas of .85 for frequency, .86 for intensity, and .87 for severity), supporting its use in research and clinical settings.

Strong evidence for validity of the CAPS was also provided by Weathers et al. (1999), who found that the CAPS total severity score correlated highly with other measures of PTSD (Mississippi Scale = .91, MMPI–PTSD Scale = .77, the number of PTSD symptoms endorsed on the SCID = .89, and the PTSD Checklist = .94; Weathers, Litz, Herman, Huska, & Keane, 1993).

The CAPS has now been used successfully in a wide variety of trauma populations (e.g., combat veterans and survivors of rape, crime, motor vehicle accidents, incest, the Holocaust, torture, and cancer), has served as the primary diagnostic or outcome measure in more than 200 empirical studies on PTSD, and has been translated into at least 12 languages (Weathers et al., 2001). Thus the existing data strongly support its continued use in both clinical and research settings.

PTSD Symptom Scale—Interview (PSS-I). Developed by Foa, Riggs, Dancu, and Rothbaum (1993), the PSS-I is a structured interview designed to assess symptoms of PTSD in individuals with a known trauma history. Using a Likert scale, interviewers rate the severity of 17 symptoms corresponding to the DSM criteria for PTSD. The PSS-I was originally tested in a sample of women with a history of rape and nonsexual assault (Foa et al., 1993) and was found to have strong psychometric properties. Foa and colleagues reported high internal consistency (Cronbach alphas = .85 for full scale, .65–.71 for subscales), test–retest reliability over a 1-month period (.80), and interrater agreement for a PTSD diagnosis (kappa = .91, 95% agreement). With respect to validity, the PSS-I was significantly correlated with other measures of traumatic stress (e.g., .69, Impact of Event Scale Intrusion score, Horowitz, Wilner & Alvarez, 1979; and .67, Rape Aftermath Symptom Test [RAST] total score, Kilpatrick, 1988) and demonstrated good diagnostic utility when compared with a SCID–PTSD diagnosis (sensitivity = .88, specificity = .96). The PSS-I appears to possess many strong features that warrant its use in clinical and research settings, especially with sexual-assault survivors.

Structured Interview for PTSD (SIP). Originally developed by Davidson, Smith, and Kudler (1989), the SIP is designed to diagnose PTSD and to measure symptom severity. It includes 17 items focused on the DSM-IV

(American Psychiatric Association, 1994) criteria for PTSD, as well as two items focused on survivor and behavior guilt. Each item is rated by the interviewer on a Likert scale. There are initial probe questions and follow-up questions to promote a more thorough understanding of the respondent's symptom experiences. The SIP takes 10–30 minutes to administer depending on the level of symptomatology present.

Psychometric data for the SIP is good. In a sample of combat veterans, Davidson et al. (1989) reported high interrater reliability (.97–.99) on total SIP scores and perfect agreement on the presence or absence of PTSD across raters. High alpha coefficients have also been reported (.94 for the veteran sample; Davidson et al., 1989, and .80 for PTSD patients enrolled in a clinical trial; Davidson, Malik, & Travers, 1997). In the veteran sample, test–retest reliability for the total SIP score was .71 over a 2-week period. With respect to validity, the SIP was significantly correlated with other measures of PTSD, but not with measures of combat exposure (.49–.67; Davidson et al., 1989, 1997). Davidson et al. (1989) compared the SIP scores of current and remitted SCID-defined PTSD cases and reported good sensitivity (.96) and specificity (.80) against the SCID. The SIP correctly classified 94% of cases relative to a structured clinical interview (Davidson et al., 1997). Overall, the SIP appears to be a sound instrument.

Self-Report PTSD Questionnaires

Numerous self-report measures have been developed as a method for obtaining information on PTSD. For the most part, self-report measures are used as continuous measures of PTSD to reflect symptom severity, but in several cases specific cutoff scores have been developed to provide a diagnosis of PTSD. These measures are generally more time- and cost-efficient than structured interviews and can be especially valuable when used as screens for PTSD. The data also support the use of self-report questionnaires alone in clinical and research settings when it is not feasible or practical to administer a structured interview. Many of the measures can be used interchangeably, as the findings appear to be robust for the minor variations in methods and approaches involved. In selecting a particular instrument, the clinician is encouraged to examine the data for that instrument for the population on which it is to be employed.

Impact of Event Scale—Revised (IES-R). Developed by Horowitz et al. (1979), the IES is one of the most widely used self-report measures to assess psychological responses to a traumatic stressor. Since the publication of DSM-IV (American Psychiatric Association, 1994), a revised 22-item version of the scale (IES-R; Weiss & Marmar, 1997) was developed that includes items on hyperarousal symptoms and flashback experiences to more closely parallel DSM-IV criteria for PTSD. To complete the measure, respondents who have experienced a traumatic event rate on a Likert scale "how distressed or bothered" they were by each symptom during the preceding week. It takes approximately 10 minutes to complete.

Although much data existed on the psychometric properties of the original IES, data on the psychometric properties of the revised IES-R are preliminary in nature. In two studies that incorporated four samples of emergency workers and earthquake survivors, Weiss and Marmar (1997) reported satisfactory internal consistency for each of the subscales (alphas = .87–.92 for Intrusion, .84–.86 for Avoidance, and .79–.90 for Hyperarousal). Test–retest reliability data from two samples yielded a range of reliability coefficients for the subscales (Intrusion = .57–.94, Avoidance = .51–.89, Hyperarousal = .59–.92). They suggest that the shorter interval between assessments and the greater recency of the traumatic event for one sample contributed to higher coefficients of stability for that sample.

Convergent and discriminant validity data are not yet available for the IES-R. Many questions were raised about the validity of the original scale, in part because it did not assess all DSM criteria for PTSD (see Weathers, Keane, King, & King, 1996). Although it now more closely parallels DSM-IV (American Psychiatric Association, 1994), some consider the items measuring numbing to be limited (Foa, Cashman, Jaycox, & Perry, 1997). Additional studies with the revised instrument are needed to establish its reliability and validity and ensure its continued use in clinics and research settings.

Mississippi Scale for Combat-Related PTSD. Developed by Keane, Caddell, and Taylor (1988), the 35-item Mississippi Scale is widely used to assess combat-related PTSD symptoms. The scale items were selected from an initial pool of 200 items generated by experts to closely match the DSM-III (American Psychiatric Association, 1980) criteria for the disorder. The Mississippi Scale has been updated and now assesses the presence of symptoms reflecting the DSM-IV (American Psychiatric Association, 1994) criteria for PTSD and several associated features. Respondents are asked to rate, on a Likert scale, the severity of symptoms over the time period occurring "since the event." The Mississippi Scale yields a continuous score of symptom severity, as well as diagnostic information. It is available in several languages and takes 10–15 minutes to administer.

The Mississippi Scale has excellent psychometric properties. In Vietnam-era veterans seeking treatment, Keane et al. (1988) reported high internal consistency (alpha = .94) and test–retest reliability (.97) over a 1-week time interval. In a subsequent validation study, the authors found substantial sensitivity (.93) and specificity (.89) with a cutoff of 107, and an overall hit rate of 90% when the scale was used to differentiate between a group with PTSD and two comparison groups without PTSD. These findings suggest that the Mississippi Scale is a valuable self-report tool in settings in which assessment of combat-related PTSD is needed.

Posttraumatic Diagnostic Scale (PDS). Developed by Foa et al. (1997), the PDS is a 49-item scale designed to measure DSM-IV (American Psychiatric Association, 1994) PTSD criteria and symptom severity. The PDS reviews trauma exposure and identifies the most distressing trauma. It also assesses Criterion A2 (physical threat or helplessness), Criteria B–D (intensity and frequency of all 17 symptoms), and Criterion F (functional impairment). This scale has been used with several populations, including combat veterans, accident victims, and sexual- and nonsexual-assault survivors. The PDS can be administered in 10–15 minutes.

The psychometric properties of the PDS were evaluated among 264 volunteers recruited from several PTSD treatment centers, as well as from non-treatment-seeking populations at high risk for trauma (Foa et al., 1997). Investigators reported high internal consistency for the PTSD total score (alpha = .92) and subscales (alphas = .78–.84) and satisfactory test–retest reliability coefficients for the total PDS score and for the symptom cluster scores (.77–.85). With regard to validity, the PDS total score correlated highly with other scales that measure traumatic responses (IES Intrusion = .80 and Avoidance = .66; RAST = .81). In addition, the measure yielded good sensitivity (.89) and specificity (.75) and high levels of diagnostic agreement with a SCID diagnosis (kappa = .65, 82% agreement). Based on these data, the PDS is an effective and efficient screening tool for PTSD.

PTSD Checklist (PCL). Developed by researchers at the National Center for PTSD (Weathers et al., 1993), the PCL is a 17-item self-report measure of PTSD. Different scoring procedures may be used to yield either a continuous measure of PTSD symptom severity or a dichotomous indicator of diagnostic status. Furthermore, dichotomous scoring methods include either an overall cutoff score or a symptom cluster scoring approach. Respondents are asked to rate, on a Likert scale, "how much each problem has bothered them" during the previous month. The time frame can be adjusted as needed to suit the goals of the assessment. The PCL has been used extensively in both research and clinical settings and takes 5–10 minutes to administer. If needed, a 17-item Life Events Checklist, developed as a companion to the CAPS and aimed at identifying exposure to potentially traumatic experiences and establishing Criterion A for the diagnosis, can be used with the PCL.

The PCL was originally validated in a sample of Vietnam and Persian Gulf War veterans and found to have strong psychometric properties (Weathers et al., 1993). Keen, Kutter, Niles, and Krinsley (2004) examined the psychometric properties of the updated PCL in veterans with both combat- and non-combat-related traumas and found evidence for high internal consistency (alpha = .96 for all 17 symptoms). Test–retest reliability measurement is robust (.96) over a 2–3 day interval, and other investigators have documented adequate test–retest reliability of this measure over a 2-week time frame (Ruggiero, Del Ben, Scotti, & Rabalais, 2003).

With respect to validity, Keen et al. (2004) found that the scale was highly correlated with other measures of PTSD, including the Mississippi Scale (.90) and CAPS (total symptom severity = .79). Using a cutoff score of 60, slightly higher than that used by Weathers et al. (1993), Keen et al. (2004) also found that the PCL had a sensitivity of .56, a specificity of .92, and overall efficiency of .84 when compared with the CAPS, indicating good diagnostic power.

Summary

The recent advances in the assessment of PTSD suggest that the state of the art is nothing short of excellent (Wilson & Keane, 2004). Yet much more work remains to be done. Assessment methods for evaluating adolescents and children are emerging and will soon be used more comprehensively in clinical and research settings. Many of the assessment tools under development are now being translated into other languages, and their cultural sensitivity and appropriateness are being assessed. With traumatic events showing no signs of abatement, future emphases on the study of cultural influences in the assessment of PTSD are warranted (Keane, Weathers, & Kaloupek, 1996).

PANIC DISORDER

PD is characterized by the presence of repeated and unexpected panic attacks and related fear of further attacks, fear of the consequences of the attacks (e.g., having a heart attack, going crazy), or changes in behavior to reduce the likelihood or severity of an attack (e.g., avoiding situations, not going out alone). When these behavioral changes center on the avoidance of numerous situations in which panic attacks might occur or in which it would be difficult to escape or get help should an attack occur, the person may be diagnosed with agoraphobia along with the PD. Prevalence estimates for PD range between 1.5 and 3.5% of the population, and symptoms of panic tend to be chronic, with some waxing and waning over time (American Psychiatric Association, 1994).

Assessment Issues

Features of PD

When assessing PD it is important to document the nature of the panic attacks, including determining how frequently they occur, in what situations they occur, at what times of day they occur, the specific symptoms that are experienced, and what thoughts accompany the attacks (e.g., "I am going to die"; "oh, no, not another one"). These features include aspects of each

of Lang's three channels of anxiety: physiological arousal, cognitive evaluation, and behavioral avoidance. Physiological symptoms of panic attacks
include increased heart rate, respiration, and perspiration. The patient may
also experience dizziness, nausea, and tingling in the extremities as a result
of physiological arousal. Identifying what reactions a particular person has
and which ones contribute to increased distress can be important for
understanding the nature of the attacks and planning treatment (McCabe,
2001).

In addition to the physiological symptoms of the panic attacks, a complete assessment includes the cognitive evaluation that the person makes of
these reactions. PD is typically related to catastrophic thoughts related to
the panic symptoms or to their consequences, beliefs about issues related to
control, and information processing biases (for a review see Khawaja &
Oei, 1998). Accurately identifying these cognitive distortions and biases is
important for developing an effective treatment plan. Similarly important
for treatment planning and outcome evaluation is the identification of
avoided situations that may become goals for exposure exercises and also
measures of progress through treatment. Critical to this process is the identification of subtle avoidance strategies (e.g., always being accompanied by
a trusted person, avoiding heavy jackets) and other safety behaviors (e.g.,
always carrying medication, distraction). These behaviors, though not as
impairing as agoraphobic avoidance, serve to maintain the panic symptoms
and may interfere with treatment if they are not targeted.

Differential Diagnosis

When assessing persons for panic disorder, it is important to keep in mind
that panic attacks are not specific to PD. Panic attacks, or symptoms that
mimic panic attacks, may also occur with other anxiety disorders, some
medical conditions, and the use of certain drugs and other substances.
When endeavoring to make a differential diagnosis of PD, it is important
first to have the patient complete a medical evaluation to rule out the possibility that the panic symptoms are caused by a medical condition (e.g.,
hyperthyroidism). Also, the use of cocaine, caffeine, and other substances
may lead to elevated arousal and symptoms that mimic panic, as can withdrawal from other substances, such as alcohol. Prior to diagnosing PD, it is
necessary to rule out the possibility that the symptoms are caused by the
use or withdrawal of substances.

Differentiating PD from other anxiety disorders (once medical and
substance use issues have been ruled out) requires careful assessment of the
nature and characteristics of the panic attacks. One important characteristic that can serve to differentiate PD from other disorders that may include
panic attacks is the determination of whether or not the panic attacks are
cued by a particular situation or stimulus. In PD, panic attacks are typically
uncued. That is, they seem to happen "out of the blue," without warning

and without an evident trigger. In contrast, panic symptoms associated with other anxiety disorders such as SP and PTSD typically occur in response to specific cues in the environment or to specific thoughts. Thus someone with SP will have panic attacks only in social situations, and persons with PTSD will panic only when reminded of their traumas.

Not everyone with PD will describe his or her panic attacks as uncued. Some individuals, particularly those who have lived with panic for a period of time, will identify certain internal sensations (e.g., an increased heart rate, shortness of breath, dizziness) as triggers for their panic attacks. Typically, it is thought that these individuals have come to recognize early stages of anxious arousal that precipitate full panic attacks. To confirm that the attacks were at one time uncued, it may be necessary to assess the person's experience of his or her first few attacks.

Another means of differentiating panic attacks associated with PD from those related to other disorders is to identify the focus of the person's fears during the attacks. Most individuals with PD report that they fear the attacks or the consequences of the attack rather than the consequences of the situation in which the attack occurs. Thus people with PD, SP, and PTSD may all report that they fear being at a party, but the focus of these fears will be different. Patients with PD might report fearing the physical or psychological consequences of the panic attack (e.g., heart attack, losing control, having someone notice their panic), whereas patients with SP might fear doing or saying something embarrassing, and persons with PTSD may fear an attack from someone at the party. Similarly, although patients with PD and patients with other anxiety disorders may avoid similar situations, the reasons that they avoid these situations will be different.

Assessment Strategies

A variety of assessment tools have been developed to evaluate PD symptoms and related characteristics, and many of them have developed cutoff scores that indicate a high likelihood of meeting a PD diagnosis. However, the semistructured clinical interviews, such as the SCID (First et al., 1996) and the ADIS (Brown et al., 1994), remain the "gold standard" for obtaining the needed information to accurately diagnose PD and the other anxiety disorders. Because of the overlap in symptoms across the anxiety disorders, these interviews that probe for symptoms of all the anxiety disorders provide the best means of making an accurate differential diagnosis.

Self-report instruments have been designed to assess many of the core features of PD. For example, a number of scales measure sensitivity to physiological arousal, including the Anxiety Sensitivity Index (ASI; Peterson & Reiss, 1993), the Body Sensations Interpretation Questionnaire (Clark et al., 1997), the Anxiety Sensitivity Profile (Taylor & Cox, 1998), and the Body Sensations Questionnaire (BSQ; Chambless, Caputo, Bright, & Gallagher,

1984). Each of these measures asks the respondents to indicate the level of fear or distress that they would experience in response to specific physiological sensations. Similarly, self-report instruments have been designed to assess cognitive distortions that are characteristic of PD. These instruments include the Agoraphobic Cognitions Questionnaire (AgCQ; Chambless et al., 1984) and the Catastrophic Cognitions Questionnaire (Khawaja, Oei, & Baglioni, 1994). Others, such as the Body Vigilance Scale (BVS; Schmidt, Lerew, & Trakowski, 1997), measure cognitive biases such as attention to bodily sensations. Agoraphobic avoidance may also be measured using self-report instruments. The Mobility Inventory for Agoraphobia (Chambless, Caputo, Jasin, Gracely, & Williams, 1985) and the Panic and Agoraphobia Scale (PAS; Bandelow, 1999) offer measures of the severity of agoraphobic avoidance. Similarly, the Texas Safety Maneuver Scale (TSMS; Kamphuis & Telch, 1998) can be used to examine more subtle forms of avoidance.

Behavioral assessment techniques, in particular self-monitoring of panic attacks and avoidance behaviors, can prove quite valuable when assessing PD patients. Self-monitoring with panic diaries (e.g., Barlow & Craske, 2000; De Beurs, Chambless, & Goldstein, 1997) can provide very useful information regarding the frequency, severity, and specificity of symptoms of panic attack. The diaries can also provide information regarding in what situations the panic attacks occur and whether they follow any pattern (e.g., more likely to occur in the morning). This information can be used to guide treatment, to evaluate the impact of specific interventions (e.g., exposure exercises, cognitive restructuring), and to assess treatment gains.

SOCIAL PHOBIA

SP is a disorder characterized by significant and persistent fear in social and/or performance situations in which scrutiny or embarrassment could occur. SP is typically chronic, and it may lead to significant impairment, but often those who suffer with SP do not seek treatment (Magee, Eaton, Wittchen, McGonagle, & Kessler, 1996). Social situations are typically avoided, and exposure to such situations almost always results in intense feelings of fear that may include panic attacks. It is also common that persons with social phobia will present with substantial anticipatory anxiety about upcoming social events. When avoidance is not possible, persons with social phobia may try to endure the situation despite their distress, and often they will employ strategic behaviors to manage their fear. SP is one of the most common anxiety disorders, with lifetime prevalence rates of about 13% (Kessler et al., 1994). The disorder tends to persist without treatment, but in some cases symptoms appear to remit over time or fluctuate as a function of external demands (e.g., having to speak in public for a new job, moving to a new school, etc.)

Assessment Issues

Features of SP

Assessment of SP should detail the situations that the patient fears and/or avoids, the intensity of the patient's fear, and an examination of safety behaviors that the patient might use to endure social situations when they cannot be avoided entirely. With regard to the situations that elicit fear, almost any situation that includes social interaction or performance demands may become a source of anxiety for the patient with SP. For each patient, it is important to determine which specific situations produce fear and which do not. For some patients, most social situations will elicit fear, but for about one-third of them, the fears are limited to public speaking (Kessler, Stein, & Berglund, 1998).

Differential Diagnosis

The most likely complication to arise in diagnosing SP is differentiating this disorder from other anxiety disorders. Although fear and avoidance of social situations defines SP, it may also be present in other anxiety disorders, including PD, OCD, and PTSD. As discussed earlier, one means of differentiating these disorders is to identify the focus of the fear. Patients with SP tend to focus their fear on the possibility that they will do or say something that will cause others to judge them negatively. In contrast, OCD patients may fear social situations because they may become contaminated with germs, and PTSD patients may fear that someone might attack them. When patients with SP must remain in social situations, they sometimes engage in strategic behaviors to reduce or manage their fear (e.g., placing their hands in their pockets to avoid trembling). Because these behaviors serve to reduce distress, they may appear similar to compulsive rituals seen in OCD; however, the goal of the behavior is to reduce the chance of negative social judgments rather than avoiding germs, as might be the case in OCD.

Assessment Strategies

As with other anxiety disorders, a comprehensive assessment of social phobia will include a clinical interview, clinician and patient ratings of the patient's symptoms, and behavioral assessments. These different strategies may be emphasized or deemphasized depending on the goal of the assessment. As discussed earlier, semistructured clinical interviews provide the best means to differentially diagnose SP, but these interviews may fail to capture all of the information needed to develop a treatment plan or to assess progress through treatment.

A number of clinician rating scales and self-report instruments have been developed to measure various aspects of SP. For example, the Liebowitz Social Anxiety Scale (LSAS; Liebowitz, 1987) and the Brief Social Phobia Scale (Davidson et al., 1991) are both clinician-rated scales that provide estimates of fear and avoidance across a range of social and evaluative situations. Similarly, the Social Interaction Anxiety Scale (SIAS; Mattick & Clarke, 1998) and the Social Phobia and Anxiety Inventory (SPAI; Turner, Beidel, & Dancu, 1996) are self-report instruments that provide estimates of fear related to a range of social situations. Other self-report instruments are designed to assess fear of specific types of situations, such as the Self-Statements during Public Speaking Scale (SSPS; Hofmann & DiBartolo, 2000) that measures fear of public speaking and the Social Phobia Scale (SPS; Mattick & Clarke, 1998) that assesses fear of being scrutinized.

Several methods have been suggested to evaluate maladaptive cognitions related to social situations owing to the extent to which they are implicated in social phobia. These include thought listing (in which the client writes down his or her thoughts), articulated thoughts (in which the client speaks aloud his or her thoughts while completing a social task), and structured measures to assess specific thoughts (Orsillo & Hammond, 2001). Recently, researchers, and to a lesser extent clinicians, are beginning to use paradigms developed in experimental cognitive psychology, such as the modified Stroop task and the visual dot probe, to assess attentional and interpretational bias associated with social situations.

Behavioral assessment techniques that can be useful in evaluating SP include behavioral approach tests, in which the patient with SP is asked to participate in a social interaction while subjective, objective, and possibly physiological assessments are made. Self-monitoring of fear-producing situations, cognitions, distress, and avoidance and safety behaviors are also valuable assessment tools. Finally, it is important to remember that the assessment process itself could be a fear-eliciting situation for the patient. This may make the evaluation more difficult, but it also provides an opportunity to observe the patient in a social situation and may provide valuable information about the patient.

OBSESSIVE–COMPULSIVE DISORDER

OCD is characterized by the presence of (1) recurrent intrusive and distressing thoughts, images, or urges and (2) repetitive and/or ritualized behaviors or thoughts that function to reduce (at least temporarily) the distress that results from the obsessions (American Psychiatric Association,

1994). Patients with OCD may also exhibit avoidance of stimuli that increase obsessional thoughts. It is estimated that OCD affects approximately 2.5% of the U.S. population at some point in their lifetimes (Karno, Golding, Sorenson, & Burnam, 1988; Rasmussen & Eisen, 1992; Sasson et al., 1997). If untreated, OCD is typically a chronic disorder. Over time, the symptoms may wax and wane in severity, but they rarely remit without treatment.

Among patients with OCD, it is more common for a person to have at least one other psychiatric disorder than to complain of OCD alone (Sasson et al., 1997; Tukel, Polat, Ozdemir, Aksut, & Turksoy, 2002). As many as two-thirds of patients with OCD are also diagnosed with depression (Crino & Andrews, 1996; Rasmussen & Eisen, 1992; Sasson et al., 1997; Tukel et al., 2002). Other common diagnoses are simple phobia, social phobia, dysthymia, and substance use disorders, occurring in 10–20% of samples of obsessive-compulsive patients (Crino & Andrews, 1996; Mayerovitch et al., 2003; Rasmussen & Eisen, 1992; Sasson et al., 1997; Tukel et al., 2002).

Assessment Issues

Features of OCD

Many OCD classification schemes differentiate among patients based on the topography of the ritualistic activity (i.e., compulsions), probably because it is relatively easy to observe overt compulsions. However, it is important to remember that topographically similar compulsions may be associated with different obsessions. Therefore, it is important to identify obsessions, as well to fully understand the manifestation of the disorder. The predominant ritual may be used to classify an individual with OCD (e.g., as a washer, a checker, a repeater), but because typical presentation includes multiple forms of rituals, it is more appropriate to classify symptoms rather than individuals. Thus a patient may be described as having washing and repeating rituals.

Ritualistic washing is the most common compulsion and may involve patients washing themselves and/or cleaning their environment. Typically, cleaning rituals are performed to decrease discomfort associated with obsessional fears about germs or diseases. Another common compulsion is repetitive checking. Patients typically check to assure themselves that a feared catastrophe will not, or has not, happened. Patients may check any number of things, but some of the most common are checking to make sure that doors are locked, faucets and electrical appliances are off or unplugged, that one has not lost important possessions (e.g., keys, wallet), or that one has not hit a pedestrian while driving.

Other rituals such as repeating, ordering, and counting are less commonly reported predominant compulsions. Like checking, these rituals may serve to prevent disasters, but often the mechanism through which they operate is more superstitious or magical. However, many people with these compulsions complete them to reduce distress or to make things "feel right" rather than to prevent a disaster. When assessing OCD, it is important to remember that repeating and counting and checking (in the form of reviewing) may manifest as mental rituals with little or no observable behavior.

Hoarding, a class of OCD that involves accumulating excessive amounts of material, is atypical in that many hoarders engage in little compulsive activity. Instead, hoarding may best be characterized as avoidant, with the patient avoiding the act of discarding things (e.g., newspapers, string) for fear of not having them in the future. However, some hoarders do compulsively accumulate certain materials (e.g., subscribing to multiple newspapers, downloading excessive amounts of information from the Internet, buying many "copies" of an item). Over time, avoidance of discarding can result in overwhelming accumulations, even in the absence of active gathering rituals. A diagnosis of OCD is complicated when the hoarded material is "collectible" or potentially valuable. In these cases, the diagnosis relies more on the distress associated with the loss or failure to obtain the object or on the impairment resulting from the collection and associated activities (e.g., oven filled with comic books, failure to go to work in order to tend to collection).

Differential Diagnosis

Diagnosing OCD is complicated by the frequent presence of other mental disorders and also because many of the symptoms of OCD overlap or closely resemble the symptoms of other disorders. For example, many people with depression experience ruminations that may appear obsessive but that do not warrant a diagnosis of OCD. Similar ruminations or worry can be seen in patients with generalized anxiety disorder (GAD). PTSD is also characterized by intrusive, unwanted distressing thoughts and/or images. The primary distinctions between obsessions and the intrusive thoughts associated with other disorders have to do with the content of the thought and/or the patient's reaction to the thoughts. For example, the intrusive thoughts associated with PTSD typically focus on recollections of a past trauma, whereas obsessions in OCD are almost always focused on some event that might happen in the future. Depressive ruminations are typically congruent with the person's mood, and rarely does the person try to suppress them. In contrast, people with OCD go to great lengths to try to eliminate their obsessions.

Like patients with OCD, individuals with PTSD may also develop repetitive behaviors or routines that serve to reduce perceived risk and that may appear similar to compulsive rituals. For example, a person with PTSD might check the doors and windows repeatedly to reduce the risk of an intruder entering. Patients with OCD will experience dramatic increases in distress if their rituals are interrupted. In contrast, individuals with PTSD rarely experience such distress.

Avoidance behaviors, common across the anxiety disorders, can complicate the diagnostic picture as well. As discussed previously, the key to deciding which diagnosis is most appropriate is determining the meaning of the fear, that is, what exactly is being avoided. For example, a person with SP and one with OCD may both avoid social situations, but the individual with SP is fearful of social scrutiny, whereas the person with OCD may fear contracting an illness through shaking hands.

Diagnostic complications also arise with disorders such as hypochondriasis and body dysmorphic disorder (BDD), in which individuals manifest worries that they have a physical malady (illness in the case of hypochondriasis and a physical defect in BDD). Some people with OCD may have similar fears about their physical health (particularly in the case of contamination fears) or appearance. In the case of OCD, these are often accompanied by checking rituals and seeking reassurance from others to reduce distress. People with BDD or hypochondriasis may report similar rituals (e.g., repeatedly seeking consultation from physicians). When additional obsessions or compulsions are present that are not directly related to the physical concern, a diagnosis of OCD is probably warranted (Riggs & Foa, 1993); however, differentiating between OCD and these two disorders is often difficult.

Ritualized and repetitive motor behaviors may occur in Tourette's disorder and related tic disorders. In most cases, differentiating these disorders relies on determining the function of the behaviors. In OCD, the rituals function to lessen the distress associated with the obsession. In contrast, in tic disorders, the behaviors do not reduce distress but are generally perceived as involuntary and unintentional. This task is complicated by the fact that a subgroup of patients with OCD also suffer from a tic disorder.

In some cases, obsessive beliefs are held so strongly that they appear delusional, raising the possibility that a person should be diagnosed with delusional disorder or schizophrenia. Typically, obsessions of delusional intensity are almost always accompanied by rituals, but such rituals are usually absent in patients with delusional disorder. Like schizophrenic delusions, obsessions seen in OCD may be rather bizarre; however, even with bizarre obsessions of delusional intensity, patients with OCD rarely manifest other symptoms of schizophrenia.

Assessment Strategies

A number of assessment instruments have been developed to diagnose and/or measure the severity of OCD. These instruments vary in form (i.e., interview vs. self-report) and focus (i.e., documenting symptoms vs. identifying treatment targets). One of the most commonly used instruments is the Yale–Brown Obsessive Compulsive Scale (Y-BOCS). The Y-BOCS is a clinician-rated measure that provides an estimate of symptom severity. The Y-BOCS also includes an extensive checklist that provides information about the content of the obsessions and compulsions that can be quite useful clinically.

Several self-report instruments designed to assess OCD symptom severity have been developed. These include the Obsessive–Compulsive Inventory (OCI; Foa, Kozak, Salkovskis, Coles, & Amir, 1998), the Maudsley Obsessive–Compulsive Inventory (MOCI; Hodgson & Rachman, 1977), and the Padua Inventory (PI; Sanavino, 1988). Two additional measures are more focused. The Obsessive Thoughts Questionnaire (Cottraux, 1989) assesses obsessional fears, and the Compulsive Activity Checklist (Freund, Steketee, & Foa, 1987) evaluates impairment due to compulsive rituals.

Several additional self-report instruments are designed to assess cognitive factors associated with the disorder rather than OCD symptoms. These include the Frost Indecisiveness Scale (Frost & Shows, 1993) that measures decision-making difficulties. The Thought–Action Fusion Scale (Shafran, Thordarson, & Rachman, 1996) measures the tendency of respondents to (1) believe that thinking something makes it more likely to happen and (2) believe that thinking about an unacceptable action is equivalent to carrying out that action. Two additional scales, the Responsibility Attitudes Scale and the Responsibility Interpretations Questionnaire (Salkovskis et al., 2000), were designed to measure beliefs about responsibility that are thought to be related to OCD.

As with the other anxiety disorders, behavioral assessments can be a valuable component of a comprehensive evaluation. Self-monitoring of obsessions and rituals can provide vital information about situations that trigger obsessions, as well as a clearer understanding of the functional relationship between the obsessions and compulsions. Clinicians who conduct careful behavioral observations of patients with OCD will often discover numerous subtle rituals and avoidance behaviors that the patient does not report verbally. Often these behaviors are so subtle or carried out so automatically that the patient does not even recognize that they are part of the disorder.

SUMMARY

Advances in the assessment of anxiety disorders are unparalleled in all of psychopathology. Since the development of the more specific set of diagnostic criteria that characterized DSM-III (American Psychiatric Association, 1980) researchers in the anxiety disorders concentrated significant effort to ensure the ready availability of reliable, sensitive, and specific measures of each of the conditions. At this time, the effort appears to have been successful. In each of the major anxiety disorders, clinicians and researchers possess numerous options to consider when assessing the diagnostic criteria and other relevant dimensions of the anxiety disorders. Future work will focus increasingly on refining these measures, making them more portable for ease in application, and assessing their generalizability across countries, cultures, languages, and age groups. Through such efforts to enhance assessment of anxiety disorders, it is clear that treatment access will improve, as will treatment outcomes.

REFERENCES

American Psychiatric Association. (1980). *Diagnostic and statistical manual of mental disorders* (3rd ed.). Washington, DC: Author.

American Psychiatric Association. (1994). *Diagnostic and statistical manual of mental disorders* (4th ed.). Washington, DC: Author.

American Psychiatric Association. (2000). *Diagnostic and statistical manual of mental disorders* (4th ed., text rev.). Washington, DC: Author.

Antony, M. M. (2001). Assessment of anxiety and the anxiety disorders: An overview. In M. M. Antony, S. M. Orsillo, & L. Roemer (Eds.), *Practitioner's guide to empirically based measures of anxiety* (pp. 9–17). New York: Kluwer Academic/Plenum Publishers.

Antony, M. M., & Barlow, D. H. (1996). Emotion theory as a framework for explaining panic attacks and panic disorder. In R. M. Rapee (Ed.), *Current controversies in the anxiety disorders* (pp. 55–76). New York: Guilford Press.

Bandelow, B. (1999). *Panic and Agoraphobia Scale (PAS) manual.* Seattle, WA: Hogrefe & Huber.

Barlow, D. H., & Craske, M. G. (2000). *Mastery of your Anxiety and Panic—III (Client Workbook).* San Antonio, TX: Psychological Corporation.

Blake, D. D., Keane, T. M., Wine, P. R., Mora, C., Taylor, K. L., et al. (1990). Prevalence of PTSD symptoms in combat veterans seeking medical treatment. *Journal of Traumatic Stress, 3*(1), 15–27.

Brown, T. A., DiNardo, P., & Barlow, D. H. (1994). *Anxiety Disorders Interview Schedule for DSM-IV.* San Antonio, TX: Psychological Corporation.

Chambless, D. L., Caputo, G. C., Bright, P., & Gallagher, R. (1984). Assessment of fear of fear in agoraphobics: The Body Sensations Questionnaire and the Agoraphobic Cognitions Questionnaire. *Journal of Consulting and Clinical Psychology, 52*, 1090–1097.

Chambless, D. L., Caputo, G. C., Jasin, S. E., Gracely, E. J., & Willaims, C. (1985). The Mobility Inventory for Agoraphobia. *Behaviour Research and Therapy, 23*, 35–44.

Clark, D. M., Salkovskis, P. M., Ost, L. G., Breitholtz, E., Koehler, K. A., Westling, B. E., et al. (1997). Misinterpretation of body sensations in panic disorder. *Journal of Consulting and Clinical Psychology, 65*, 203–213.

Cottraux, J. (1989). Behavioural psychotherapy for obsessive–compulsive disorder. *International Review of Psychiatry, 1*(3), 227–234.

Crino, R. D., & Andrews, G. (1996). Obsessive–compulsive disorder and Axis I comorbidity. *Journal of Anxiety Disorders, 10*(1), 37–46.

Davidson, J. R., Book, S. W., Colkert, J. T., Tupler, L. A., et al. (1997). Assessment of a new self-rating scale for posttraumatic stress disorder. *Psychological Medicine, 27*(1), 153–160.

Davidson, J. R., Malik, M. L., & Sutherland, S. N. (1997). Response characteristics to antidepressants and placebo in post-traumatic stress disorder. *International Clinical Psychopharmacology, 12*(6), 291–296.

Davidson, J. R. T., Potts, N. L. S., Richichi, E. A., Ford, S. M., Krishnan, R. R., Smith, R. D., & Wilson, W. (1991). The Brief Social Phobia Scale. *Journal of Clinical Psychiatry, 52*, 48–51.

Davidson, J., Smith, R., & Kudler, H. (1989). Validity and reliability of the DSM-III criteria for posttraumatic stress disorder: Experience with a structured interview. *Journal of Nervous and Mental Disease, 177*(6), 336–341.

de Beurs, E., Chambless, D. L., & Goldstein, A. J. (1997). Measurement of disorder: A multicenter trial. *Journal of the American Academy of Child and Adolescent Psychiatry, 31*(1), 45–49.

First, M. B., Spitzer, R. L., Gibbon, M., & Williams, J. B. (1996). *Structured Clinical Interview for DSM-IV Axis I Disorders—Patient Edition (SCID-I/P, version 2.0).* New York: New York State Psychiatric Institute, Biometrics Research Department.

First, M. B., Spitzer, R. L., Gibbon, M., & Williams, J. B. (1997). *Structured Clinical Interview for DSM-IV Axis I Disorders (SCID-I), Clinician Version.* Washington, DC: American Psychiatric Press.

Foa, E. B., Cashman, L., Jaycox, L., & Perry, K. (1997). The validation of a self-report measure of posttraumatic stress disorder: The Posttraumatic Diagnostic Scale. *Psychological Assessment, 9*, 445–451.

Foa, E. B., Kozak, M. J., Salkovskis, P. M., Coles, M. E., & Amir, N. (1998). The validation of a new obsessive–compulsive disorder scale: The Obsessive–Compulsive Inventory. *Psychological Assessment, 10*(3), 206–214.

Foa, E. B., Riggs, D. S., Dancu, C. V., & Rothbaum, B. O. (1993). Reliability and validity of a brief instrument for assessing post-traumatic stress disorder. *Journal of Traumatic Stress, 6*, 459–474.

Freund, B., Steketee, G. S., & Foa, E. B. (1987). Compulsive Activity Checklist (CAC): Psychometric analysis with obsessive–compulsive disorder. *Behavioral Assessment, 9*(1), 67–79.

Frost, R. O., & Shows, D. L. (1993). The nature and measurement of compulsive indecisiveness. *Behaviour Research and Therapy, 31*, 683–692.

Hodgson, R., & Rachman, S. (1977). Obsessional compulsive complaints. *Behaviour Research and Therapy, 15*, 389–395.

Hofmann, S. G., & DiBartolo, P. M. (2000). An instrument to assess self-statements during public speaking: Scale development and preliminary psychometric properties. *Behavior Therapy, 31*, 499–515.

Horowitz, M. J., Wilner, N., & Alvarez, W. (1979). Impact of Event Scale: A measure of subjective stress. *Psychosomatic Medicine, 41*, 209–218.

Kamphuis, J. H., & Telch, M. J. (1998). Assessment of strategies to manage or avoid perceived threats among panic disorder patients: The Texas Safety Maneuver Scale (TSMS). *Clinical Psychology and Psychotherapy, 5,* 177–186.

Karno, M., Golding, J. M., Sorenson, S. B., & Burnam, M. A. (1988). The epidemiology of obsessive–compulsive disorder in five U.S. communities. *Archives of General Psychiatry, 45*(12), 1094–1099.

Keane, T. M. (1995). Guidelines for the forensic psychological assessment of posttraumatic stress disorder claimants. In R. I. Simon (Ed.), *Posttraumatic stress disorder in litigation: Guidelines for forensic assessment* (pp. 99–115). Washington, DC: American Psychiatric Press, Inc.

Keane, T. M., & Barlow, D. H. (2002). Posttraumatic stress disorder. In D. H. Barlow, *Anxiety and its disorders: The nature and treatment of anxiety and panic* (2nd ed., pp. 418–453). New York: Guilford Press.

Keane, T. M., Buckley, T., & Miller, M. (2003). Guidelines for the forensic psychological assessment of posttraumatic stress disorder claimants. In R. I. Simon (Ed.), *Posttraumatic stress disorder in litigation: Guidelines for forensic assessment* (2nd ed., pp. 119–140). Washington, DC: American Psychiatric Association Press.

Keane, T. M., Caddell, J. M., & Taylor, K. L. (1988). Mississippi Scale for Combat-Related Posttraumatic Stress Disorder: Three studies in reliability and validity. *Journal of Consulting and Clinical Psychology, 56,* 85–90.

Keane, T. M., Kaloupik, D. G., & Weathers, F. W. (1996). Ethnocultural considerations in the assessment of PTSD. In M. J. Friedman & A. J. Marsella (Eds.), *Ethnocultural aspects of posttraumatic stress disorder: Issues, research, and clinical applications* (pp. 183–205). Washington, DC: American Psychological Association.

Keane, T. M., Kolb, L. C., Kaloupek, D. G., Orr, S. P., Blanchard, E. B., Thomas, R. G., et al. (1998). Utility of psychophysiology measurement in the diagnosis of posttraumatic stress disorder: Results from a department of Veteran's Affairs cooperative study. *Journal of Consulting and Clinical Psychology, 66*(6), 914–923.

Keane, T. M., Weathers, F. W., & Foa, E. B. (2000). Diagnosis and assessment. In T. M. Keane & E. B. Foa (Eds.), *Effective treatments for PTSD: Practice guidelines from the International Society for Traumatic Stress Studies* (pp. 18–36). New York: Guilford Press.

Keen, S. M., Kutter, C. J., Niles, B. L., & Krinsley, K. E. (2005). Psychometric properties of the PTSD Checklist. Manuscript submitted for publication. *Journal of Traumatic Stress.*

Kessler, R. C. (1994). The National Comorbidity Survey of the United States. *International Review of Psychiatry, 6*(4), 365–376.

Kessler, R. C., Sonnega, A., Bromet, E., Hughes, M., et al. (1995). Posttraumatic stress disorder in the National Comorbidity Survey. *Archives of General Psychiatry, 52*(12), 1048–1060.

Kessler, R. C., Stein, M. B., & Berglund, P. A. (1998). Social phobia subtypes in the National Comorbidity Survey. *American Journal of Psychiatry, 155,* 613–619.

Khawaja, N. G., & Oei, T. P. S. (1998). Catastrophic cognitions in panic disorder with and without agoraphobia. *Clinical Psychology Review, 18,* 341–365.

Khawaja, N. G., Oei, T. P. S., & Baglioni, A. J. (1994). Modification of the Catastrophic Cognitions Questionnaire (CCQ-M) for normals and patients: Exploratory and LISREL analyses. *Journal of Psychopathology and Behavioral Assessment, 16,* 325–342.

Kilpatrick, D. (1988). *Rape Aftermath Symptom Test.* Oxford: Pergamon Press.

Kulka, R. A., Schlenger, W. E., Fairbank, J. A., Hough, R. L., Jordon, B. K., Marmar, C. R., & Weiss, D. S. (1988). *Contractual report of findings from the National Vietnam Veterans Readjustment Study: Executive summary, description of findings, and technical appendices.* New York: Brunner/Mazel.

Lang, P. J. (1971). The application of psychophysiological methods to the study of psychotherapy and behavior modification. In A. E. Bergin & S. L. Garfield (Eds.), *Handbook of psychotherapy and behavior change* (pp. 75–125). New York: Wiley.

Liebowitz, M. R. (1987). Social phobia. *Modern Problems in Pharmacopsychiatry, 22,* 141–173.

Magee, W. J., Eaton, W. W., Wittchen, H. U., McGonagle, K. A., & Kessler, R. C. (1996). Agoraphobia, simple phobia, and social phobia in the National Comorbidity Survey. *Archives of General Psychiatry, 53,* 159–168.

Mattick, R. P., & Clarke, J. C. (1998). Development and validation of measures of social phobia scrutiny fear and social interaction anxiety. *Behaviour Research and Therapy, 36,* 455–470.

Mayerovitch, J. I., du Fort, G. G., Kakuma, R., Bland, R. C., Newman, S. C., & Pinard, G. (2003). Treatment seeking for obsessive–compulsive disorder: Role of obsessive–compulsive disorder symptoms and comorbid psychiatric diagnoses. *Comprehensive Psychiatry, 44*(2), 162–168.

McCabe, R. E. (2001). Panic disorder and agoraphobia: A brief overview and guide to assessment. In M. M. Antony, S. M. Orsillo, & L. Roemer (Eds.), *Practitioner's guide to empirically based measures of anxiety* (pp. 87–94). New York: Kluwer Academic/Plenum Publishers.

Orsillo, S. M., & Hammond, C. (2001). Social phobia: A brief overview and guide to assessment. In M. M. Antony, S. M. Orsillo, & L. Roemer (Eds.), *Practitioner's guide to empirically based measures of anxiety* (pp. 159–164). New York: Kluwer Academic/Plenum Publishers.

Peterson, R. A., & Reiss, S. (1993). *Anxiety Sensitivity Index—Revised test manual.* Worthington, OH: IDS.

Rasmussen, S. A., & Eisen, J. L. (1992). The epidemiology and differential diagnosis of obsessive–compulsive disorder. *Journal of Clinical Psychiatry, 53*(Suppl.), 4–10.

Riggs, D. S., & Foa, E. B. (1993). Obsessive–compulsive disorder. In D. H. Barlow (Ed.), *Clinical handbook of psychological disorders: A step-by-step treatment manual* (2nd ed., pp. 189–239). New York: Guilford Press.

Ruggiero, K. J., Del Ben, K., Scotti, J. R., & Rabalais, A. E. (2003). Psychometric properties of the PTSD Checklist—Civilian Version. *Journal of Traumatic Stress, 16,* 495–502.

Salkovskis, P. M., Wroe, A. L., Gledhill, A., Morrison, N., Forrester, E., Richards, C., et al. (2000). Responsibility attitudes and interpretations are characteristic of obsessive–compulsive disorder. *Behaviour Research and Therapy, 38,* 347–372.

Sanavio, E. (1988). Obsessions and compulsions: The Padua Inventory. *Behaviour Research and Therapy, 26,* 169–177.

Sasson, Y., Zohar, J., Chopra, M., Lustig, M., Iancu, I., & Hendler, T. (1997). Epidemiology of obsessive–compulsive disorder: A world view. *Journal of Clinical Psychiatry, 58*(12), 7–10.

Schmidt, N. B., Lerew, D. R., & Trakowski, J. H. (1997). Body vigilance in panic disorder: Evaluating attention to bodily perturbations. *Journal of Consulting and Clinical Psychology, 65,* 214–220.

Shafran, R., Thordarson, D. S., & Rachman, S. (1996). Thought–action fusion in obsessive compulsive disorder. *Journal of Anxiety Disorders, 10,* 379–391.

Taylor, S., & Cox, B. J. (1998). An expanded Anxiety Sensitivity Index: Evidence for a hierarchic structure in a clinical sample. *Journal of Anxiety Disorders, 12,* 463–483.

Tukel, R., Polat, A., Ozdemir, O., Aksut, D., & Turksoy, N. (2002). Comorbid conditions in obsessive–compulsive disorder. *Comprehensive Psychiatry, 43,* 204–209.

Turner, S. M., Beidel, D. C., & Dancu, C. V. (1996). *SPAI: Social Phobia and Anxiety Inventory.* North Tonawanda, NY: Multi-Health Systems.

Weathers, F. W., Keane, T. M., & Davidson, J. R. T. (2001). The Clinician-Administered PTSD Scale (CAPS): A review of the first ten years of research. *Depression and Anxiety, 13,* 132–156.

Weathers, F. W., Keane, T. M., King, L. A., & King, D. W. (1996). Psychometric theory in the development of posttraumatic stress disorder assessment tools. In J. P. Wilson & T.M. Keane (Eds.), *Assessing psychological trauma and PTSD* (pp. 98–135). New York: Guilford Press.

Weathers, F. W., Litz, B. T., Herman, D. S., Huska, J. A., & Keane, T. M. (1993, October). *The PTSD Checklist (PCL): Reliability, validity, and diagnostic utility.* Poster presented at the annual meeting of the International Society for Traumatic Stress Studies, San Antonio, TX.

Weathers, F. W., Ruscio, A. M., & Keane, T. M. (1999). Psychometric properties of nine scoring rules for the Clinician-Administered PTSD Scale (CAPS). *Psychological Assessment, 11,* 124–133.

Weiss, D., & Marmar, C. (1997). The Impact of Event Scale—Revised. In J. P. Wilson & T. M. Keane (Eds.), *Assessing psychological trauma and PTSD* (pp. 399–411). New York: Guilford Press.

Wilson, J., & Keane, T. M. (2004). *Assessing psychological trauma and PTSD* (2nd ed.). New York: Guilford Press.

7

Social Phobia

Then, Now, the Future

JONATHAN R. T. DAVIDSON

Social phobia (SP; also referred to as social anxiety disorder [SAD]) is the most common anxiety disorder in the United States (Kessler et al., 1994) and is responsible for a great deal of morbidity, increased health utilization, and general failure of affected individuals to fulfill their potential (Katzelnick et al., 2001). Social phobia as seen and studied today is more complex than when it was first introduced into DSM-III. Then it corresponded much more closely to performance anxiety, with examples being given of fear of speaking, of performing in public, of using public restrooms, of eating in public, and of writing in the presence of others. DSM-III went on to say that "generally an individual has only one social phobia." It goes without saying that today we would disagree with this statement. Avoidant personality disorder was seen as a separate concern, and the term "generalized social phobia" was not in use. Most of the drug treatment research at that time involved studying the use of beta-blockers, which showed modest benefit at best and are of limited value for our current conceptualization of social phobia (Sutherland & Davidson, 1995). Principles and techniques of psychosocial treatment were at a rudimentary stage. The field has moved on considerably, and most of this chapter focuses on treating the more commonly seen and clinically disabling generalized form of social phobia (GSP).

In managing SP, the following important goals can be identified: (1) reduction of fear, (2) correction of maladaptive cognitive patterns, (3) reduction of avoidance, (4) reduction of physiological arousal, (5) reduction of any comorbid disorders that may be present, (6) restoration of daily function, and (7) improvement in quality of life.

There are two broad treatment approaches, both of which possess well-established efficacy in SP: cognitive-behavioral therapy (CBT) and pharmacotherapy. Two principal approaches for treating SP are described, as well as an ongoing collaboration between the Duke University group, which I lead, and the University of Pennsylvania group, led by Edna Foa. Foa's unique contributions to social phobia research are identified.

PSYCHOSOCIAL APPROACHES
TO THE TREATMENT OF SP

Of the available psychosocial treatments, exposure-based procedures, cognitive restructuring techniques, social skills training, and interpersonal therapy have all been studied, with CBT having received the most attention.

A number of reviews have compared the effect of treatment over time relative to various types of control intervention. In the first analysis, Feske and Chambless (1995) compared the effects of cognitive restructuring and exposure. Their review focused on the question of whether additional cognitive restructuring enhanced exposure. Exposure, both alone and combined with cognitive restructuring, produced equal pre- to posttreatment effect sizes, as well as treatment adherence.

In a subsequent review, Taylor (1996) found that social skills training, cognitive restructuring, exposure, and combined treatment were all superior to a wait-list control condition over short-term treatment. However, further gains were noted with longer follow-up. Of interest, although combination treatment produced a significantly greater effect size than the wait-list control condition immediately posttreatment, the difference had lessened at 3 months' follow-up.

Gould, Buckminster, Pollack, Otto, and Yap (1997) undertook a meta-analysis of published studies and found that treatments that included exposure, whether administered alone or in combination with cognitive restructuring, produced the greatest treatment effect. Cognitive treatment and social skills training, when given alone, were less effective.

In a more recent meta-analysis, Federoff and Taylor (2001) compared different forms of psychosocial treatment. All were moderately effective, without any difference between treatments and without any greater effect being noted when they were combined, similar to the analysis of Feske and Chambless (1995). The authors argued for enhanced, modified forms of CBT in order to improve efficacy, pointing out that older forms of CBT were, surprisingly, not as effective in the short term as pharmacotherapy. Clark et al. (2003), Clark and Wells (1995), and Huppert, Roth, and Foa (2003) have further enhanced the content and delivery of CBT in SP, as described later.

The question has sometimes arisen as to whether CBT administered in a group format is more effective than when given individually. From the preceding reviews (Gould et al., 1997; Federoff & Taylor, 2001), it does not appear that one has any advantage over the other. One significant problem is that group treatment is difficult to schedule; also, many patients with SAD find group treatment difficult to accept. Furthermore, one recent report (Stangier, Heidenreich, Peitz, et al., 2003) found that cognitive-behavioral group therapy was inferior to the individual form, although both were superior to the wait-list control condition. On the other hand, at least compared with pharmacotherapy, CBGT enjoys a substantial cost advantage, whereas individual CBT showed less difference (Gould et al., 1997).

Interpretation of the preceding meta-analyses should be tempered by the fact that sample sizes were relatively small and thus underpowered to detect differences between CBT and medication.

Interpersonal therapy has been well established as an effective treatment for depression. Lipsitz, Markowitz, Cherry, and Fyer (1999) suggested that it could also benefit SP. However, this was a small study, and, although 78% responded to treatment, much further evaluation of this treatment is clearly necessary.

CONCERNING CBT FOR SP:
ADDITIONAL CONSIDERATIONS

Given that CBT is clearly effective and that exposure appears to be perhaps of greatest importance, what are the outstanding questions? As with pharmacotherapy (described in the next section), not everyone responds adequately to CBT, and even those judged to be "responders" often show significant residual pathology. Could there be certain subtypes of SP, or certain aspects of it, that are more resistant to CBT? For example, there is evidence (Davidson, Foa, Connor, & Churchill, 2002) that CBT is no more effective than placebo for treating the hyperhidrosis found in SP, an often troublesome aspect of the illness. Also, remission rates are low from both CBT and pharmacotherapy. Thus further refinements and modifications of CBT might still generate greater improvement. There also is a subtype of social phobia that appears not to respond well to CBT; namely, the tendency to react to situations with anger. These patients are more likely to drop out of therapy early (Zaider & Heimberg, 2003) . Could CBT be modified in order to enhance its effectiveness in those who have difficulties regulating anger?

Comorbidity with other Axis I disorders is often found in SP (Kessler et al., 1994). In particular, other anxiety disorders, depression, and alcohol abuse/dependence frequently co-occur. In a follow-up study by Heimberg, those who had SP with a mood disorder were not as well at the end of treatment, even though CBT had been of benefit (Zaider & Heimberg, 2003). Similarly, studies by Chambless, Tran, and Glass (1997) found that those with depression and SP were less likely to improve on social skills and social anxiety after a course of CBT.

One study exists with a population of alcohol abusers with social anxiety problems (Randall et al., 2001), which showed no advantage to incorporating CBT in addressing social anxiety, as well as standard CBT for alcoholism. As discussed later, it is possible that, in some situations in which comorbidity is present, sequencing of treatments produces a better effect than the simultaneous initiation of both.

On the question of response to CBT in nongeneralized social phobia (NGSP), limited data are available. Two studies (Hope, Heimberg, & Bruch, 1995; Brown, Heimberg, & Juster, 1995) suggest that NGSP responds to CBT perhaps more rapidly and to a shorter course of treatment than is the case for GSP (Hope et al., 1995).

Two other important challenges include (1) application of CBT early in the course of GSP (e.g., in childhood or late teenage years, before many of the chronic maladaptive and comorbid problems have set in), and (2) more widespread dissemination of CBT (e.g., via Internet, hand-held computer, community-based peer-led programs).

PHARMACOTHERAPY FOR SAD: EVIDENCE FOR EFFICACY

Selective Serotonin Reuptake Inhibitors and Serotonin–Norepinephrine Reuptake Inhibitors

Several published placebo-controlled trials have evaluated selective serotonin reuptake inhibitor (SSRI) and serotonin–norepinephrine reuptake inhibitor (SNRI) treatments. Two studies with fluvoxamine have shown response rates of 46 and 43% versus 7 and 23%, respectively, on placebo (van Vliet, den Boer, Westenberg, 1994; Steini, Fyer, Davidson, Pollack, & Witte, 1999). With sertraline, response rates are 50 and 53% relative to 9 and 29%, respectively, on placebo (Katzelnick et al., 1995; van Ameringen et al., 2001). Three trials with paroxetine have shown efficacy rates of 55, 70, and 66% on drug, versus 24, 8, and 32%, respectively, on placebo (Stein et al., 1998; Allgulander, 1999; Baldwin, Bobes, Stein, Scharwaechter, & Faure, 1999). Two published studies of fluoxetine have failed to show efficacy relative to placebo (Kobak, Greist, Jefferson, & Katzelnick, 2002; Clark et al., 2003). A study with the SNRI drug venlafaxine-XR has shown superior effect over placebo (Liebowitz, Allgulander, Mangano, & Costa, 2003).

Benzodiazepines

Good benefit has been demonstrated with two benzodiazepine drugs, clonazepam and bromazepam, relative to placebo, and modest benefits were noted with alprazolam. In the study by Davidson et al. (1993), 78% responded to clonazepam versus 20% on placebo, and in the study by Versiani, Nardi, Figueira, and Marques (1997), the response rate to bromazepam was 82% compared with 20% on placebo. In the study by Gelernter et al. (1991), 38% responded to alprazolam compared with 20% on placebo. The rapid onset of action noted with clonazepam and the generally very high response rates noted for clonazepam and bromazepam might suggest that benzodiazepines could be the first-choice treatment in pharmacotherapy of SP. Although their effectiveness is unquestioned, limitations of benzodiazepines include their limited range of efficacy for some comorbid Axis I disorders (e.g., depression, PTSD), as well as the fact that some individuals are likely to misuse benzodiazepines or to experience discontinuation problems. Nonetheless, they are important options, both for uncomplicated SP and for those who do not respond to antidepressant drugs or those who require augmentation of preexisting pharmacotherapy.

Monoamine Oxidase Inhibitors

The monoamine oxidase inhibitors (MAOIs) were the first drugs to be studied systematically in SP, with four studies each of phenelzine and moclobemide and three for brofaromine. Rates of response to phenelzine were 69, 64, 65, and 85%, versus rates of response to placebo of 20, 23, 33, and 15%, respectively (Gelernter et al., 1991; Liebowitz et al., 1992; Heimberg et al., 1998; Versiani et al., 1992). With moclobemide, response rates were 65, 38, 17, and 47%, versus response rates to placebo of 15, 15, 33, and 13%, respectively (Versiani et al., 1992; Noyes et al., 1997; Schneier et al., 1998; International Multicenter Clinical Trial Group [IMCTG], 1997). With brofaromine, response rates in three studies were 50, 78, and 26% versus rates of 19, 23, and 0%, respectively, for placebo (Lott et al., 1997; Fahlen, 1995; van Vliet, Westenberg, & den Boer, 1992).

Although MAOIs such as phenelzine are highly effective, if not the most effective of all pharmacotherapies for SP, their use is severely restricted because of toxicity and intolerance of their many side effects. The reversible and selective inhibitors of MAO type A (RIMA), such as moclobemide and brofaromine, have offered much more promise of greater safety and greater acceptability. However, their overall performance has been disappointing, and neither of these RIMA drugs is available in the United States.

Other Drugs

Two anticonvulsant drugs, gabapentin and pregabalin, whose actions are mediated through the alpha-2 delta calcium channel, are both more effective than placebo in SP. Response rates for gabapentin were 38% versus

17% on placebo (Pande et al., 1999), whereas with pregabalin at 600 mg per day, the response rate was 43% compared with 22% in the placebo group (Pande et al., 2004).

The atypical antipsychotic drug olanzapine has been shown superior to placebo in GSP (Barnett, Kramer, Casat, Connor, & Davidson, 2002). Atypical neuroleptics, although carrying concerns about weight gain and alterations in glucose metabolism, may be a useful option for more severely affected and treatment-resistant patients with SP.

Drugs with Limited Benefit

The anxiolytic drug buspirone, a serotonin $(5\text{-}HT)_{1A}$ partial agonist, was found to be ineffective in a placebo-controlled trial (van Vliet, den Boer, Westenberg, & Pian, 1997). A $5\text{-}HT_3$ antagonist, ondansetron, showed statistically significant benefits greater than placebo, although their magnitude was of very little relevance (Davidson et al., 1997). Thus, merely because a drug has "serotonergic" agonist or antagonist properties, we cannot conclude ipso facto that it will be useful in SP.

The beta-blocker drug atenolol is ineffective in generalized social anxiety (Liebowitz et al., 1992; Turner, Beidel, & Jacob, 1995). There is evidence, however, that beta blockers may be more useful for NGSP (Liebowitz et al., 1992), thus they may have a limited place in the management of social anxiety when characterized by autonomic symptoms such as palpitations and tremor in a public speaking or performance setting. Sutherland and Davidson (1995) have reviewed the pre-DSM-III literature, suggesting modest benefit for beta blockers in performance anxiety.

Effect Sizes

A review by Hidalgo, Barnett, and Davidson (2001) noted the following effect sizes (adjusted for sample size) for each group of drugs. The strongest effect size was for benzodiazepines (1.12), followed by phenelzine (0.97), SSRIs (0.68), anticonvulsants (0.46), RIMA drugs (0.41), and buspirone and beta blockers 0.14.

RELAPSE RATES FOLLOWING DISCONTINUATION OF PHARMACOTHERAPY

In one trial of clonazepam, patients received open-label treatment for approximately 6 months, then were randomized to receive either continued clonazepam or placebo for 6 more months. There was a statistically significant difference in favor of clonazepam maintenance, which appeared to have a relapse-preventing effect (Connor et al., 1998). Stein, Versiani, Hair, and Kumar (2002) studied the use of paroxetine for relapse prevention over 24 weeks. After 2 months, groups were randomized to either continue on the drug or to receive a placebo. Among those remaining on the drug, only 14% relapsed, compared with 39% in the group that took placebo.

In a study with sertraline conducted over a 44-week period, those who remained on the drug showed a relapse rate of only 4%, as compared with 36% among those switched to a placebo after 20 weeks of treatment with sertraline (Walker et al., 2000).

Thus it can be said that for both SSRI and benzodiazepine treatment, continuation to 6 months and beyond is associated with a significantly lower relapse rate as compared with discontinuation. The object of pharmacotherapy, as with psychosocial treatment, is to achieve the fullest possible response (i.e., remission) and, in the case of pharmacotherapy, to continue treatment for a minimum of 12 months in those with a long-standing history of GSP.

PHARMACOTHERAPY OF SP: FURTHER CHALLENGES

As with CBT, present-day pharmacotherapy has its shortcomings, and there is room for improvement. Five predictors of nonresponse to SSRIs, benzodiazepines, or MAOIs have been identified. These are (1) more severe symptoms; (2) excessive use of alcohol; (3) family history of social phobia; (4) passive-dependent and borderline personality disorders; and (5) high systolic blood pressure and heart rate (Davidson, 1998). The last mentioned is of particular interest, because Gelernter and colleagues (Gelernter, Page, Stein, & Woods, 2004) have shown that the gene that encodes the norepinephrine (and dopamine) transporter protein is a likely physiological and positional candidate influencing SP risk. Based on the finding that high basal sympathetic arousal predicts poorer response to SSRIs, other therapeutic approaches (e.g., CBT, noradrenergic drugs) might be preferred in this subgroup.

COMPARISONS OF PHARMACOTHERAPY AND PSYCHOSOCIAL TREATMENT

Given the reasonable yet limited response to each treatment approach alone, could there be a case for combining or possibly sequencing the two treatment approaches? The literature is scanty. The earliest studies to compare drug and psychosocial treatment failed to generate any meaningful results. Unfortunately, the two drugs involved, buspirone and propranolol, are of no real benefit for GSP; therefore, very little can be concluded from these small-scale trials (Clark & Agras, 1991; Falloon, Lloyd, & Halpin, 1981).

More recently, a comparative study evaluated clonazepam and CBT, finding equal benefit from both treatments. Among the completer sample, but not in the lost observation carried forward analysis, clonazepam was associated with significantly greater improvement on fear of negative evaluation (Otto et al., 2000).

A primary care study has compared sertraline with brief CBT, specifically adapted for use in the primary care setting. Each treatment was also combined, and a placebo was utilized as control (Blomhoff et al., 2001). Sertraline, whether given alone or with CBT, was superior to placebo, but CBT with placebo was not superior to placebo alone in the short term. However, at 6 months' follow-up, neither group who received sertraline fared as well as did those who had received CBT without sertraline. The authors concluded that, for CBT to be fully effective, relatively severe levels of social anxiety were necessary, and the early administration of a drug could perhaps undermine the effect of CBT by rapidly lowering symptoms. Thus, once the drug is taken away, relapse is more likely, perhaps because appropriate learning of new behaviors, social skill sets, and interpretation biases has not taken place. This would not be expected to happen if CBT alone had produced major gains in the beginning. Although we have not found a similar outcome in our study (described later) at 1-year follow-up, neither did we see any kind of enhancement from simultaneous administration of both treatments. Nonetheless, these findings raise the question as to how drug treatment and CBT might be best combined and under what circumstances.

We should also keep in mind the fact that SSRI drugs and CBT may in fact be working in opposite (i.e., antagonistic) ways, at least in depression (Goldapple et al., 2004), and not inconceivably also in social phobia and other forms of anxiety. Should this be the case, then potentiation is perhaps unlikely under conditions of simultaneous initiation, and at best there would be equivalence relative to each treatment alone. We do not know whether, in some cases, there would be diminution of effect for CBT; our results do not show this to be the case.

Let us consider the neurobiological mechanisms of CBT and of SSRI drugs such as paroxetine in depression. CBT works uniquely in brain regions related to self-focus (medial frontal, anterior cingulate, and orbitofrontal cortex), whereas paroxetine works initially in regions that subserve vegetative, autonomic, and circadian activities (ventral subgenual cingulate, anterior insula, hypothalamus, and brain stem). Both treatments ultimately produce a resetting of function in brain regions subserving attention, cognitive function, and memory enhancement/consolidation (i.e., dorsolateral prefrontal and inferior parietal cortex and posterior cingulate cortex). However, they do this in opposite ways. Thus CBT reduces metabolic activity in cortex while increasing it in the hippocampus; paroxetine, on the other hand, enhances cortical and reduces hippocampal activity. The two treatments thus may be engaging in a form of neurobiological tug-of-war. Therefore, perhaps a case could be made for sequencing the treatments (e.g., drug first, followed by CBT), with greatest benefit to be found, speculatively, in those who are only partial responders to the drug. We have found this to be the case in an unpublished collaborative study between Foa, Rothbaum and Davidson in PTSD, and it bears study in SP. Perhaps, where depression is comorbid with SP, this approach has particular appeal.

An alternative view of the relationship of CBT and medication to neurobiology has been put forward by Furmark et al. (2002). These authors note that CBT and citalopram reduced blood flow in the amygdalar-hippocampal regions, suggesting a common site of action. Moreover, the degree of attenuation predicted lasting improvement at 1 year. According to this model, each treatment could enhance the effect of the other, suggesting a possible potentiating effect from combined therapy over monotherapy.

RECENT DEVELOPMENTS: CONTRIBUTIONS OF THE PENN GROUP

In their seminal and widely quoted 1986 paper, Foa and Kozak presented a coherent system for understanding emotional processing of fear and the importance of exposure to corrective information. Their adumbration of emotional processing theory holds the presence of fear structures that serve as blueprints for response to danger, in which the following three representations occur: (1) information about the stimulus, (2) the response, and (3) an interpreted meaning of the two. Pathological fear structures are held to underlie anxiety, in which the representations do not correspond to reality. Successful psychosocial treatment activates abnormal elements in the structure and then presents new (reality-based and adaptive) information to replace the older, maladaptive fear structure. Foa and Kozak (1986) argued that both exposure and cognitive therapy are aimed at modifying dysfunctional cognitions that maintain symptoms of social phobia and that both therapeutic approaches involve confrontation of avoided social situations. As noted earlier, however, exposure appears to be the most effective component of CBT for social phobia and affects not only anxiety and avoidance but also cognitive dysfunction. As a rule, psychosocial treatment for anxiety in general, and social phobia in particular, typically includes both exposure and cognitive therapy.

Foa and her colleagues have modified the content and delivery of CBT for social phobia, which, along with education, exposure, and cognitive restructuring, was enriched by the addition of social skills training (SST). This modified form of CBT, which the authors refer to as comprehensive

CBT (CCBT), was developed because of the recognition that social skills deficits are often a critical element underlying negative beliefs, as well as being an effect of same, and thus can occupy an etiological role (Foa, Franklin, & Kozak, 2001). In this regard, Foa differs from the views held by Clark and Wells (1995) and Rapee and Heimberg (1997), who see poor social skills as being mainly a consequence of the safety behaviors that occur in SP. Thus, Foa and her colleagues (Franklin, Jaycox, & Foa, 1999; Franklin et al., 2001) include SST as an important element in the treatment package for CCBT. One study (Herbert et al., in preparation) has shown that CCBT is superior to CBT. The large collaborative study by Davidson, Foa and colleagues (2004) at Duke and Penn has now demonstrated that CCBT works as effectively as an antidepressant drug and is superior to placebo in the treatment of GSP. This two-site collaborative study tested the efficacy of four types of treatment versus placebo. The specific hypotheses were as follows:

1. To compare the immediate effects at 14 weeks of fluoxetine, CCBT, placebo, combined CCBT/fluoxetine, and combined CCBT/placebo.
2. To evaluate the maintenance of therapeutic gains for the different treatments by following responders for 88 weeks after discontinuing CCBT and fluoxetine.
3. To demonstrate that each treatment is transportable, that is, that CCBT can be successfully implemented in a center with primary allegiance to pharmacotherapy and that fluoxetine can likewise be successfully implemented at a center that specializes in CBT.
4. To investigate mechanisms of therapeutic change by examining the relationship between cognitive distortions and social skills deficits and the extent to which changes in these variables mediate reductions in symptoms by the different treatments.
5. To explore predictors of treatment response.

We took care to standardize treatment delivery. Initial training in CBGT was facilitated by R. G. Heimberg, and we taped the group sessions for viewing by cognitive therapists at each site. Similarly, for medication sessions, treatment was given according to a manual developed for the study, and a senior psychopharmacologist listened to the tapes to rate treatment adherence. We held regular conference calls between sites, as well as supervisory conference calls to maintain treatment delivery standards.

All patients had to fulfill DSM-IV (American Psychiatric Association, 1994) criteria for GSAD without any other primary Axis I disorder. Fluoxetine was initiated at 10 mg per day, and the dose was increased up to a possible maximum 60 mg according to tolerability and response. CCBT was administered once a week for 14 weeks. CBT was given according to the manual developed for the study. Blinded independent raters were used for the primary measure, which was a combination of the Clinical Global Improvement Scale and the Brief Social Phobia Scale.

Results of the study have been presented elsewhere (Davidson et al., 2004).

Overall, we have successfully conducted a two-site study of the treatment of GSP. Each site was able to demonstrate superior efficacy of both pharmacotherapy and CBT over placebo, indicating that implementation of treatments was achieved successfully at both centers. We concluded that participants with both GSP and depression are more challenging to treat and that further work is required for us to better understand how this population can be treated optimally. We also believe that sequential administration of medication followed by CBT might help enhance the effects of treatment, as opposed to initiating both simultaneously. This conclusion is reinforced by a recent positive experience with a controlled trial of an SSRI and prolonged exposure in PTSD (Rothbaum et al., 2004). (Rothbaum, B.O., Foa, E.B., Davidson, J.R.T., Cahill, S., Connor, K.M., & Astin, M. Augmentation of sertraline with prolonged exposure in the treatment of PTSD, submitted June 2004).

Specifically, with respect to SP and depression, Foa and her colleagues have subsequently further modified CCBT so that it can be applied to patients with and without comorbid depression. The depression modules contain two core efficacious techniques, behavioral activation and cognitive therapy (Martell, Addis, & Jacobson, 2001). The goal of this treatment is to increase activities that are pleasurable and/or associated with mastery, while simultaneously decreasing activities that are associated with negative feelings. Pilot data have been collected from a series of patients with SP and major depression or dysthymia that show very encouraging reduction of social anxiety and depression. Thus CCBT, in response to both emerging empirical data and modification of theory, has been adapted. Both individualized format and a modularized form of delivery are now available (Clark, 2001). In the latest modification of CCBT, Foa and her colleagues have incorporated techniques to eliminate the safety behaviors that often sustain the disorder, as well as encouraging outward focus (Clark & Wells, 1995; Huppert, Roth, & Foa, 2003). It is precisely by such modifications that we may be able to advance CBT from a treatment that merely improves to one that leads more people into full remission. Such a challenge, of course, must also be met with pharmacotherapy.

Foa and colleagues have elaborated on the potential cognitive mechanisms involved in the maintenance of SP. They have provided some of the foundation of the biases in interpretation that exist in SP. Specifically, they have demonstrated the exaggerated estimations of probability and cost of negative outcomes related to social interactions (Foa, Franklin, Perry, & Herbert, 1996; Amir, Foa, & Coles, 1998; Gilboa-Schectman, Franklin, &

Foa, 2000). They showed, moreover, that successful treatment of GSP with CBT is associated with reduced probability and cost estimates in mildly negative social situations (Foa et al., 1996) and that changes in cost estimates were more predictive than change in probability biases with respect to lowered social anxiety symptoms, a finding that has recently been independently supported (Uren, Szabo, & Lovibond, 2004). Foa's group was also the first to compare patients with GSP treated with CCBT with those who were untreated, along with nonanxious controls. By the end of treatment, the group with CCBT was similar to the nonanxious control group, and lower than the untreated patient group. Thus CCBT does reduce negative interpretative bias (Franklin, Huppert, Langner, Leiberg & Foa, submitted).

Edna Foa and her colleagues have also innovated the use of imaginal exposure as a therapeutic procedure in GSP, particularly when the predicted outcome is difficult to demonstrate (such as an audience's evaluation of a performance) or when the individual is unwilling to engage in direct exposure (Huppert, Roth, & Foa, 2003).

ACKNOWLEDGMENTS

I am grateful to Jonathan Huppert, PhD, and Frank Keefe, PhD, as well as to grant support (No. R10MH49339) from the National Institute of Mental Health to Jonathan R. T. Davidson.

REFERENCES

Allgulander, C. (1999). Paroxetine in social anxiety disorder: A randomized placebo-controlled study. *Acta Psychiatrica Scandinavica, 100*, 193–198.

American Psychiatric Association (1994). *Diagnostic and statistical manual of mental disorders* (4th ed.). Washington, DC: Author.

Amir, N., Foa, E. B., & Coles, M. E. (1998). Negative interpretation bias in social phobia. *Behavior Research and Therapy, 36*, 959–970.

Baldwin, D., Bobes, J., Stein, D. J., Scharwaechter, I., & Faure, M. (1999). Paroxetine in social phobia/social anxiety disorder: Randomized, double-blind, placebo-controlled study. *British Journal of Psychiatry, 175*, 120–126.

Barnett, S. D., Kramer, M. L., Casat, C. D., Connor, K. M., & Davidson, J. R. T. (2002). Efficacy of olanzapine in social anxiety disorder: A pilot study. *Journal of Psychopharmacology, 16*, 365–368.

Blomhoff, S., Haug, T. T., Hellstrom, K., Holme, I., Humble, M., Madsbu, H. P., & Wold, J. E. (2001). Randomised controlled general practice trial of sertraline, exposure therapy and combined treatment in generalized social phobia. *British Journal of Psychiatry, 179*, 23–30.

Brown, E. J., Heimberg, R.G., & Juster, H.R. (1995). Social phobia subtype and avoidant personality disorder, impairment and outcome of cognitive behavioral treatment. *Behavioral Therapy, 26, 467–486.*

Chambless, D. L., Tran, G. O., & Glass, C. R. (1997). Predictors of response to cognitive-behavioral group therapy for social phobia. *Journal of Anxiety Disorders, 11, 221–240.*

Clark, D. B., & Agras, S. W. (1991). The assessment and treatment of performance anxiety in musicians. *American Journal of Psychiatry, 148, 598–605.*

Clark, D. M. (2001). A cognitive perspective on social phobia. In W. R. Crozier & L. E. Alden (Eds.), *International handbook of social anxiety: Concepts, research and interventions relating to the self and shyness* (pp. 405–430). New York: Wiley.

Clark, D. M., Ehlers, A., McManus, F., Hackmann, A., Fennell, M., Campbell, H., et al. (2003). Cognitive therapy versus fluoxetine plus self-exposure in the treatment of social phobia: A randomized, placebo-controlled trial. *Journal of Consulting and Clinical Psychology, 71, 1058–1069.*

Clark, D. M., & Wells, A. (1995). A cognitive model of social phobia. In R. G. Heimberg, M. R. Liebowitz, D. A. Hope, & F. R. Schneier (Eds.), *Social phobia: Diagnosis, assessment, and treatment* (pp. 69–93). New York: Guilford Press.

Connor, K. M., Davidson, J. R. T., Potts, N. L. S., Tupler, L. A., Miner, C. M., Malik, M. L., Book, S. W., Colke, J. T., & Ferrell, F. (1998). Discontinuation of clonazepan in the treatment of social phobia. *Journal of Psychopharmacology, 18, 373–378.*

Davidson, J. R. T. (1998). Pharmacotherapy of social anxiety disorder. *Journal of Clinical Psychiatry, 59*(Suppl. 17), 47–53.

Davidson, J. R. T., Foa, E. B., Connor, K. M., & Churchill, L. E. (2002). Hyperhidrosis in social anxiety disorder. *Progress in Neuropsychopharmacology and Biological Psychiatry, 26, 1327–1331.*

Davidson, J. R. T., Foa, E. B., Huppert, J. D., Keefer, F. J., Franklin, M. E., Compton, J., et al. (2004). Fluoxetine, comprehensive cognitive group therapy and placebo in generalized social phobia. *Archives of General Psychiatry, 61, 1005–1013.*

Davidson, J. R. T., Miner, C. M., de Veaugh-Geiss, J., Tupler, L. A., Colket, J. T., & Potts, N. L. S. (1997). The Brief Social Phobia Scale: A psychometric evaluation. *Psychological Medicine, 27, 161–166.*

Davidson, J. R. T., Potts, N. L. S., Richichi, E. A., Krishnan, K. R. R., Ford, S. M., Smith, R. D., & Wilson, W. H. (1993). Treatment of social phobia with clonazepam and placebo. *Journal of Clinical Psychopharmacology, 13, 423–428.*

Fahlen, T., Nilsson, H. L., Borg, K., Humble, M., & Pauli, U. (1995). Social phobia: The clinical efficacy and tolerability of the monoamine oxidase-A and serotonin uptake inhibitor brofaromine: A double blind placebo-controlled study. *Acta Psychiatrica Scandinavica, 92*(5), 351–358.

Falloon, I. R. H., Lloyd, G. G., & Halpin, R. E. (1981). The treatment of social phobia: Real-life rehearsal with non-professional therapists. *Journal of Nervous and Mental Disorder, 169, 180–184.*

Fedoroff, I. C., & Taylor, S. (2001). Psychological and pharmacological treatments of social phobia: A meta-analysis. *Journal of Clinical Psychopharmacology, 21, 311–324.*

Feske, U., & Chambless, D. L. (1995). Cognitive behavioral versus exposure-only treatment for social phobia: A meta-analysis. *Behavior Therapy, 26,* 695–720.

Foa, E. B., Franklin, M. E., Perry, K. J., & Herbert, J. D. (1996). Cognitive biases in generalized social phobia. *Journal of Abnormal Psychology, 105,* 433–443.

Foa, E. B., Franklin, M. E., & Kozak, M. J. (2001). Social phobia: An information processing perspective. In S. Hofman & P. M. DiBartolo (Eds.), *From social anxiety to social phobia: Multiple perspectives* (pp. 268–280). Needham, MA: Allyn & Bacon.

Foa, E. B., & Kozak, M. J. (1986). Emotional processing of fear: Exposure to corrective information. *Psychological Bulletin, 99,* 20–35

Franklin, M. E., Feeny, N. C., Abramowitz, J. S., et al. (2001). Comprehensive cognitive-behavioral therapy: A multi-component treatment for generalized social phobia. *Psychoterapia Cognitiva e Comportamentale, 7,* 211–221

Franklin, M. E., Huppert, J. D., Langner, R., Leiberg, S., & Foa, E. B. (in press). *Interpretation bias: A comparison of treated social phobics, untreated social phobics, and controls.*

Franklin, M. E, Jaycox, L. H., & Foa, E. B. (1999). Social phobia: Social skills training. In M. Hersen & A. Bellack (Eds.), *Handbook of comparative treatments for adult disorders* (2nd ed., pp. 317–339). New York: Wiley.

Furmark, T., Tillfors, M., Marteinsdottir, I., Fischer, H., Pissiota, A., Langstrom, B., & Fredrikson, M. (2002). Common changes in cerebral blood flow in patients with social phobia treated with citalopram or cognitive-behavioral therapy. *Archives of General Psychiatry, 59,* 425–433.

Gelernter, C. S., Uhde, T. W., Cimbolic, P., Arnkoff, D. B., Vottone, B. J., Tancer, M. E., & Barthlo, J. J. (1991). Cognitive-behavioral and pharmacological treatments of social phobia: A controlled study. *Archives of General Psychiatry, 48,* 938–945.

Gelernter, J., Page, G. P., Stein, M. B., & Woods, S. W. (2004). Genome-wide linkage scan for loci predisposing to social phobia: Evidence for a chromosome 16 risk locus. *American Journal of Psychiatry, 161,* 59–66.

Gilboa-Schectman, E., Franklin, M. E., & Foa, E. B. (2000). Anticipated reactions to social events: Differences among individuals with generalized social phobia, obsessive–compulsive disorder, and non-anxious controls. *Cognitive Therapy and Research, 24,* 731–746.

Goldapple, K., Segal, Z., Garson, G., Lau, M., Bieling, P., Kennedy, S., & Mayberg, H. (2004). Modulation of cortical-limbic pathways in major depression. *Archives of General Psychiatry, 61,* 34–41.

Gould, R. A., Buckminster, S., Pollack, M. H., Otto, M. W., & Yap, L. (1997). Cognitive-behavioral and pharmacological treatment for social phobia: A meta-analysis. *Clinical Psychology, Science and Practice, 4,* 291–306.

Heimberg, R. G., Liebowitz, M. R., Hope, D. A., Schneier, F. R., Holt, C. S., Welkowitz, L., et al. (1998). Cognitive-behavioral group therapy versus phenelzine in social phobia: 12-week outcome. *Archives of General Psychiatry, 55,* 1133–1141.

Herbert, J. D., Gaudiano, B. A., Rheingold, A. A., et al. (2005). *Social skills training augments the effectiveness of cognitive behavioral group therapy for social anxiety disorder.* Manuscript in preparation.

Hidalgo, R. B., Barnett, S. D., & Davidson, J. R. T. (2001). Social anxiety disorder in review: Two decades of progress. *International Journal of Neuropsychopharmacology, 4,* 279–298.

Hope, D. A., Heimberg, R. G., & Bruch, M. A. (1995). Dismantling cognitive-behavioral group therapy for social phobia. *Behavior Research and Therapy, 3*, 637–650.

Huppert, J. D., Roth, D. A., & Foa, E. B. (2003). Cognitive behavioral therapy for social phobia: New advances. *Current Psychiatry Reports, 5*, 289–296.

International Multicenter Clinical Trial Group on Moclobemide in Social Phobia. (1997). Moclobemide in social phobia: A double-blind, placebo-controlled clinical trial. *European Archives of Psychiatry and Clinical Neuroscience, 247*, 71–80.

Katzelnick, D. J., Kobak, K. A., DeLeire, T., Henk, H., Greist, J. H., Davidson, J. R. T., et al. (2001). Impact of generalized social phobia in managed care. *American Journal of Psychiatry, 151*, 1999–2007.

Katzelnick, D. J., Kobak, K. A., Greist, J. H., Jefferson, J. W., Mantle, J. M., & Serkin, R. C. (1995). Sertraline for social phobia: A double-blind, placebo-controlled crossover study. *American Journal of Psychiatry, 152*, 1368–1371.

Kessler, R. C., McGonagle, K. A., Zhao, S., Nelson, C. B., Hughes, M., Eschleman, S., et al. (1994). Lifetime and 12-month prevalence of DSM-III-R psychiatric disorders in the United States: Results from the National Comorbidity Survey. *Archives of General Psychiatry, 51*, 8–19.

Kobak, K. A., Greist, J. H., Jefferson, J. W., & Katzelnick, D. J. (2002). Fluoxetine in social phobia: A double-blind, placebo-controlled pilot study. *Journal of Clinical Psychopharmacology, 22*, 257–262.

Liebowitz, M. R., Allgulander, C., Mangano, R., & Costa, C. (2003, November). *Comparison of venlafaxine-XR and paroxetine in the short-term treatment of SAD.* Poster presented at the U.S. Psychiatric and Mental Health Congress, Orlando, FL.

Liebowitz, M. R., Schneier, F., Campeas, R., Hollander, E., Hatterer, J., & Fyer, A. J. (1992). Phenelzine vs. atenolol in social phobia: A placebo-controlled comparison. *Archives of General Psychiatry, 49*, 290–300.

Lipsitz, J. D., Markowitz, J. C., Cherry, S., & Fyer, A. J. (1999). Open-trial of interpersonal psychotherapy for the treatment of social phobia. *American Journal of Psychiatry, 156*, 1814–1816.

Lott, M., Greist, J. H., Jefferson, J. W., Kobak, K. A., Katzelnick, D. J., Katz, R. J., & Schaettle, S. C. (1997). Brofaromine for social phobia: A multicenter placebo-controlled, double-blind study. *Journal of Clinical Psychopharmacology, 17*, 255–260.

Martell, C. R., Addis, M. E., & Jacobson, N. S. (2001). *Depression in context: Strategies for guided action.* New York: Norton.

Noyes, R., Moroz, G., Davidson, J. R. T., Liebowitz, M. R., Davidson, A., Siegel, J., et al. (1997). Moclobemide in social phobia: A controlled dose–response trial. *Journal of Clinical Psychopharmacology, 17*(4), 247–254.

Otto, M. W., Pollack, M. H., Gould, R. A., Worthington, J. J., III, McArdle, E. T., & Rosenbaum, J. F. (2002). A comparison of the efficacy of clonazepam and cognitive-behavioral group therapy for the treatment of social phobia. *Journal of Anxiety Disorders, 14*, 345–358.

Pande, A. C., Davidson, J. R. T., Jefferson, J. W., Janney, C. A., Katzelnick, D. J., Weisler, R. H., et al. (1999). Treatment of social phobia with gabapentin: A placebo-controlled study. *Journal of Clinical Psychopharmacology, 19*, 341–348.

Pande, A. C., Feltner, D. C., Jefferson, J. W., Davidson, J. R. T., Pollack, M. H., Stein, M. B., et al. (2004). Efficacy of the novel anxiolytic pregabalin in social anxiety disorder: A placebo-controlled, multicenter study. *Journal of Clinical Psychopharmacology, 24,* 141–149.

Randall, C. L., Johnson, M. R., Thevos, A. K., Sonne, S. C., Thomas, S. E., Willard, S. L., et al. (2001). Paroxetine for social anxiety and alcohol use in dual-diagnosed patients. *Depression and Anxiety, 14,* 225–262.

Rapee, R. M., & Heimberg, R. G. (1997). A cognitive-behavioral model of anxiety in social phobia. *Behavior Research and Therapy, 35,* 741–756.

Roth, D. A., Huppert, J. D., Foa, E. B., Davidson, J. R. T., Keefe, F. J., & Potts, N. L. S. (2004). *The impact of depression on the treatment of generalized social anxiety disorder.* Manuscript submitted for publication.

Schneier, F. R., Goetz, D., Campeas, R., Fallon, B., Marshall, R. D., & Liebowits, M. R. (1998). Placebo-controlled trial of moclobemide in social phobia. *British Journal of Psychiatry, 172,* 70–77.

Stangier, U., Heidenreich, T., Peitz, M., Lauterbach, W., & Clark, D. M. (2003). Cognitive therapy for social phobia: Individual vs. group treatment. *Behavior Research and Therapy, 41,* 991–1007.

Stein, D. J., Versiani, M., Hair, T., & Kumar, R. (2002). Efficacy of paroxetine for relapse prevention in social anxiety disorder: A 24-week study. *Archives of General Psychiatry, 59,* 1111–1118.

Stein, M. B., Fyer, A. J., Davidson, J. R. T., Pollack, M. H., & Witte, B. (1999). Fluvoxamine treatment of social phobia (social anxiety disorder): A double-blind, placebo-controlled study. *American Journal of Psychiatry, 156,* 756–760.

Stein, M. B., Liebowitz, M. R., Lydiard, R. B., Pitts, C. D., Bushnell, W., & Gergel, I. (1998). Paroxetine treatment of generalized social phobia (social anxiety disorder): A randomized controlled trial. *Journal of American Medical Association, 280,* 708–713.

Sutherland, S. M., & Davidson, J. R. T. (1995). Beta-blockers and benzodiazepines in the treatment of social phobia. In M. B. Stein (Ed.), *Social phobia: Clinical and research perspectives* (pp. 323–346). Washington, DC: American Psychiatric Press.

Taylor, S. (1996). Meta-analysis of cognitive-behavioral treatment for social phobia. *Journal of Behavior Therapy and Experimental Psychiatry, 27,* 1–9.

Turner, S. M., Beidel, D. C., & Jacob, R. G. (1994). Social phobia: A comparison of behavior therapy and atenolol. *Journal of Consulting and Clincial Psychology, 62,* 350–358.

Uren, T. H., Szabo, M., & Lovibond, P. F. (2004). Probability and cost estimates for social and physical outcomes in social phobia and panic disorder. *Journal of Anxiety Disorders, 18,* 481–490

Van Ameringen, M. A., Lane, R. M., Walker, J. R., Bowen, R. C., Chokka, P. R., Goldner, E. M., et al. (2001). Sertraline treatment of generalized social phobia: A 20-week, double-blind, placebo-controlled study. *American Journal of Psychiatry, 158,* 275–281.

van Vliet, I. M., den Boer, J. A., & Westenberg, H.G. M. (1994). Psychopharmacological treatment of social phobia: A double-blind placebo-controlled study with fluvoxamine. *Psychopharmacology, 115,* 128–134.

Van Vliet, I. M., Westenberg, H. G., & den Boer, J. A. (1992). Psychopharmacological treatment of social phobia: Clinical and biochemical effects of brofaromine, a selective MAO-A inhibitor. *European Neuropsychopharmacology*, *2*, 21–29.

Van Vliet, I. M., den Boer, J. A., Westenberg, H. G., & Pian, K. L. (1997). Clinical effects of buspirone in social phobia: A double-blind, placebo-controlled study. *Journal of Clinical Psychiatry*, *58*, 164–168.

Versiani, M., Nardi, A. E., Figueira, I., & Marques, C. (1997). Double-blind placebo-controlled trial with bromazepam in social phobia. *Journal Brasileiro de Psiquiatria*, *46*, 167–171.

Versiani, M., Nardi, A. E., Mundim, F. D., Alves, A. A., Liebowitz, M. R., & Amrein, R. (1992). Pharmacotherapy of social phobia: A controlled study of moclobemide and phenelzine. *British Journal of Psychiatry*, *161*, 353–360.

Walker, J. R., Van Ameringen, M. A., Swinson, R., Bowen, R. C., Chokka, P. R., Goldner, E., et al. (2000). Prevention of relapse in generalized social phobia: Results of a 24-week study in responders to 20 weeks of sertraline treatment. *Journal of Clinical Psychopharmacology*, *20*, 636–644.

Zaider, T. I., & Heimberg, R. G. (2003). Non-pharmacological treatments for social anxiety disorder. *Acta Psychiatrica Scandinavica*, *108*(Suppl. 417), 72–84.

8

Best Practice in Treating Obsessive–Compulsive Disorder

What the Evidence Says

HELEN BLAIR SIMPSON
MICHAEL R. LIEBOWITZ

For more than 10 years, the Center for the Treatment and Study of Anxiety, directed by Edna Foa, and the Anxiety Disorders Clinic, directed by Michael Liebowitz, have collaboratively studied how to treat adults with obsessive–compulsive disorder (OCD). The Center for the Treatment and Study of Anxiety is known for its expertise in psychosocial treatments; the Anxiety Disorders Clinic is known for its expertise in pharmacological treatments. Therefore, these two sites originally joined forces to compare the efficacy of the then (and arguably still today) two best treatments for OCD: cognitive-behavioral therapy consisting of exposure and response (or ritual) prevention (EX/RP) and pharmacotherapy with clomipramine. This first collaborative study led to two subsequent studies: one to evaluate residual impairment in treated OCD patients and another to examine whether EX/RP can augment a partial response to serotonin reuptake inhibitors (SRIs; i.e., clomipramine and the selective SRIs). Together, these studies have helped determine the best treatments for adults with OCD.

These three studies are described in detail in this chapter. Key findings include the following:

1. EX/RP and SRI treatment are both efficacious treatments for adults with OCD.

2. EX/RP can be superior to SRI treatment when delivered intensively by skilled therapists.
3. EX/RP can be more durable than SRI treatment.
4. Many SRI responders continue to have clinically significant OCD symptoms and require additional treatment.
5. EX/RP may be one of the safest and most effective ways to augment a partial SRI response.
6. Despite state-of-the-art treatments such as EX/RP and SRIs, many OCD patients continue to have impaired functioning and poor quality of life.

We conclude by discussing the advantages and disadvantages of EX/RP and SRIs for the treatment of adults with OCD.

CLOMIPRAMINE VERSUS EX/RP IN THE TREATMENT OF OCD

By 1990, controlled trials had proven that two treatments were efficacious for OCD: psychotherapy consisting of EX/RP and pharmacotherapy with SRIs such as clomipramine. However, the relative and combined efficacy of these treatments had not been directly compared. Thus, with funding from the National Institutes of Mental Health (NIMH), the Center for the Treatment and Study of Anxiety and the Anxiety Disorders Clinic conducted a multisite randomized controlled trial to compare the efficacy and durability of EX/RP, clomipramine, their combination, and pill placebo for adults with OCD (Foa et al., 2005; Simpson et al., 2004). To increase the credibility of the results and to guard against investigator bias, the study was conducted at three centers: the Center for the Treatment and Study of Anxiety, the Anxiety Disorders Clinic, and a third site knowledgeable in both treatment modalities (St. Boniface General Hospital, Winnipeg, Manitoba, Canada). Each site conducted all treatments after training and with ongoing supervision. It was hypothesized that after 12 weeks of treatment (1) EX/RP, clomipramine, and their combination would each be superior to pill placebo; (2) the combination of EX/RP and clomipramine would be superior to either treatment alone; and (3) EX/RP alone would be superior to clomipramine alone. It was also hypothesized that patients who responded to EX/RP with or without clomipramine would be less likely to relapse 12 weeks after treatment discontinuation than responders to clomipramine alone.

Patients in this study were adult outpatients with primary OCD and clinically significant OCD symptoms. OCD severity was measured using the Yale–Brown Obsessive Compulsive Scale (Y-BOCS; Goodman, Price, Rasmussen, Mazure, Fleischmann, et al., 1989; Goodman, Price, Rasmussen, Mazure, Delgado, et al., 1989); this scale has a range from 0 to 40, and a score of 16 or more indicates clinically significant OCD. Patients were without significant depression or substance abuse or dependence and had never been treated previously with EX/RP or clomipramine.

During the acute phase (Weeks 0–12), patients were randomly assigned to EX/RP, clomipramine, their combination, or pill placebo. Patients receiving medication were seen weekly by a psychopharmacologist. Dosing was fixed for the first 5 weeks, starting at 25 mg (or half a pill) per day and increasing to 200 mg (or four pills) per day, with an optional increase thereafter to 250 mg (or five pills) per day if necessary. EX/RP followed the standard procedures outlined by Kozak and Foa (1997). Specifically, patients were taught to confront what they feared (i.e., exposure) and to refrain from performing compulsions (i.e., ritual prevention). Exposures included live confrontations with feared situations and imaginal confrontations with feared consequences. The aim was for patients to face their fears for a prolonged period without ritualizing, allowing the initial anxiety to dissipate on its own (i.e., habituation). The goal was to weaken the connections between feared stimuli and distress and between ritualizing and relief from distress and, in the process, to correct mistaken OCD beliefs (e.g., that rituals prevent harm, that anxiety or discomfort will persist forever, that feared consequences will occur). EX/RP was delivered intensively during the first 4 weeks (i.e., two information-gathering sessions, fifteen 2-hour exposure sessions over 3 weeks, and two home visits); for the remaining 8 weeks, patients met weekly with their therapists for 45 minutes to review EX/RP procedures. Patients receiving the combination of EX/RP and clomipramine met individually with a therapist and a psychopharmacologist.

After 12 weeks of treatment, those judged by an independent evaluator to be much or very much improved relative to Week 0 as measured by the Clinical Global Impression–Improvement Scale (Guy, 1976) were eligible to enter the discontinuation phase. During the discontinuation phase (Weeks 12–24), EX/RP was stopped, medication was tapered and stopped, but patients still met with their psychopharmacologist and/or therapist for general support and monitoring of clinical status. Patients on medication were seen weekly for the first 4 weeks while tapering off their medication (decreasing by 50 mg, or one pill, per week) and every 2 weeks thereafter. EX/RP patients met with their therapist every 2 weeks. In all cases, sessions lasted 20 minutes or less. Relapse was defined a priori as (1) a return to pretreatment (i.e., Week 0) severity or worse in the preceding week on the Clinical Global Impression–Severity Scale (Guy, 1976); and/or (2) a clinical state that made further study participation unsafe.

Results from the Acute Phase (Weeks 0–12)

Of the 122 OCD patients who entered the acute phase, 87 patients completed it, and 48 patients responded to 12 weeks of treatment (Table 8.1).

The treatment groups did not differ significantly in baseline demographic or clinical characteristics; on average, patients had chronic OCD (e.g., mean duration = 16 years) of moderate severity. The mean daily medication doses during the last week in the acute phase for all who entered and all who completed treatment, respectively, were 196 (standard deviation [SD] = 82) and 235 (SD = 34) mg for the clomipramine group, 163 (SD = 65) and 194 (SD = 48) mg for the combination group, and 209 (SD = 76) and 245 (SD = 23) for the placebo group. Most clomipramine completers (77%)—but only some completers in the combination group (38%)—received the maximum dose of 250 mg per day. The dropout rates did not differ significantly between the treatment groups.

The change in OCD severity as measured by the Y-BOCS is shown in Figure 8.1 for each of the treatment groups. In analyses using mixed effects models, all active treatments reduced OCD symptoms significantly more than placebo treatment. At Week 12, the effects of EX/RP did not differ from those of EX/RP combined with clomipramine, but both were superior to clomipramine alone at reducing OCD symptoms. On average, patients receiving EX/RP with or without clomipramine had only mild OCD symptoms (observed mean Y-BOCS = 11) after 12 weeks of treatment, whereas patients receiving clomipramine alone still had clinically significant symptoms (observed mean Y-BOCS = 18).

The treatment groups also differed in the proportion of patients who responded to 12 weeks of treatment, when response was defined as a rating of much or very much improved on the Clinical Global Impression–Improvement Scale (Guy, 1976). For the treated and completer samples, respectively, the proportions of responders were 62% and 86% for EX/RP, 42% and 48% for clomipramine, 70% and 79% for combination treatment, and 8% and 10% for placebo (overall $p < .001$). In pairwise comparisons, there were significantly more responders to EX/RP than to clomipramine in the completer ($p < .01$) but not the treated sample ($p =$

TABLE 8.1. Study Sample and Descriptive Outcome

Treatment group	Acute Phase entrants	Completers to Week 12	Responders at Week 12	Entrants to the Discontinuation Phase	Completers to Week 24 without relapse	Entrants who relapsed	Entrants who dropped
EX/RP	29	21	18	18	16	2	0
CMI	36	27	13	11	6	5	0
EX/RP + CMI	31	19	15	15	12	2	1
PBO	26	20	2	2	1	0	1
Total	122	87	48	46	35	9	2

Note. EX/RP, exposure and ritual prevention; CMI, clomipramine; PBO, pill placebo.

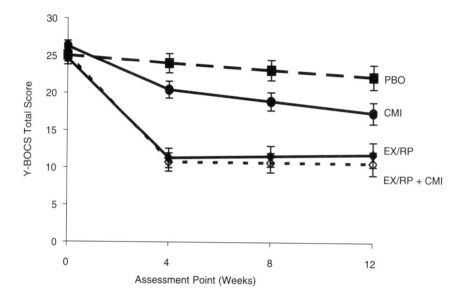

FIGURE 8.1. OCD severity. Mean Yale–Brown Obsessive Compulsive Scale (Y-BOCS) scores (and standard errors) based on mixed-effect models during 12 weeks of treatment by pill placebo (PBO), clomipramine (CMI), exposure and ritual prevention (EX/RP), or their combination (EX/RP + CMI).

.10); there were significantly more responders to combination treatment than to clomipramine alone in both samples ($p < .05$).

Conclusions from the Acute Phase

These data support the following conclusions. First, all active treatments (intensive EX/RP, clomipramine, their combination) are superior to placebo. Second, EX/RP alone can produce as good an outcome as combination treatment. Third, EX/RP with or without clomipramine is superior to clomipramine alone, both in the magnitude of response and in the proportion of responders.

Several factors may have limited the ability to detect significant benefits of combined treatment over EX/RP alone. First, most patients in the combination group (unlike the clomipramine group) did not achieve the maximum dose of clomipramine. Second, the potency of intensive EX/RP alone left little room for further improvement. Third, the simultaneous instigation of intensive EX/RP and slow upward titration of clomipramine meant that the intensive phase of EX/RP was completed (within the first 4 weeks) before the full impact of clomipramine could be realized. Finally, OCD patients with comorbid depression were excluded.

As is true of any clinical trial, this study had several limitations, including the fact that only the medication groups were double-blinded and the lack of systematic data on prior treatment history. Nonetheless, this study provides empirical support for the superiority of intensive EX/RP with or without clomipramine over clomipramine monotherapy in patients with OCD and without comorbid depression when EX/RP is delivered by skilled therapists. The results also highlight the substantial OCD symptoms that remain even if patients respond to clomipramine treatment, a problem the selective SRIs have as well (Pigott & Seay, 1999).

Results from the Discontinuation Phase (Weeks 12–24)

Of the 46 patients who completed and responded to 12 weeks of active treatment, 44 entered the discontinuation phase (Table 8.1). There were two significant differences between the active treatment groups: first, the Week 12 mean clomipramine dose was significantly lower for the combination group than for the clomipramine group (186 [$SD = 44$] vs. 236 [$SD = 23$] mg per day, $p = .001$); second, all patients who received EX/RP (with or without clomipramine) had significantly lower mean Week 12 Y-BOCS scores than patients who received clomipramine alone (8 [$SD = 5$] vs. 12 [$SD = 5$], $p = .02$).

During the 12-week discontinuation phase, nine patients relapsed (Table 8.1). As hypothesized, significantly fewer responders to EX/RP with or without clomipramine relapsed after treatment discontinuation than responders to clomipramine alone (4/33 = 12% vs. 5/11 = 45%; $p = .031$). Responders to EX/RP with or without clomipramine also showed a significantly longer time-to-relapse than responders to clomipramine alone ($p = .017$). OCD severity at entry to the discontinuation phase had a significant effect on the time-to-relapse ($p = 0.031$). Specifically, among responders to EX/RP with or without clomipramine, those with higher Week 12 Y-BOCS scores were more likely to relapse. In contrast, among responders to clomipramine alone, those with lower Week 12 Y-BOCS scores were more likely to relapse.

Conclusions from the Discontinuation Phase

This study was the first to compare the posttreatment effects of EX/RP and clomipramine in OCD by following treatment responders after sustained treatment discontinuation and by assessing relapse blind to the original treatment. Responders to intensive EX/RP (with or without clomipramine) fared better than responders to clomipramine alone. They had less severe OCD at the start of the discontinuation phase, were less likely to relapse during the discontinuation phase, and showed a significantly longer time-to-relapse if they did relapse.

Among responders to EX/RP with or without clomipramine, those with greater OCD severity after treatment were at a higher risk of relapsing, confirming prior findings (Foa et al., 1983). These data suggest that maximizing EX/RP outcome in the short term may prevent relapse in the long term. In contrast, responders to clomipramine alone with less severe OCD after treatment were at greater risk of relapsing, perhaps because these patients had a true (vs. a placebo) response, which was lost once clomipramine was discontinued.

The discontinuation phase was limited by a small sample size (such that there was sufficient power to compare relapse rates only when the two groups receiving EX/RP were combined), a short treatment period (12 weeks) prior to treatment discontinuation, and a short follow-up period (12 weeks) after treatment discontinuation. Moreover, the results were based on an a priori and conservative definition of relapse (a return to pretreatment severity) and on one OCD measure (the Clinical Global Impression-Severity scale). On the other hand, a post hoc analysis of relapse using various relapse definitions found similar results (Simpson, Franklin, Cheng, Foa, & Liebowitz, 2005), supporting these findings. Despite these limitations, the data suggest that EX/RP treatment with or without clomipramine is more durable 12 weeks after treatment discontinuation than clomipramine alone.

Overall Conclusions

In this sample of outpatients with OCD seeking care at specialty research centers, patients receiving intensive EX/RP alone or EX/RP with clomipramine each showed superior outcome after 12 weeks of treatment to patients receiving clomipramine alone; responders to EX/RP with or without clomipramine also had a lower relapse rate and longer time-to-relapse 12 weeks after treatment discontinuation than responders to clomipramine alone. We conclude that EX/RP should be adapted for wider use in the treatment of OCD, given the magnitude and durability of improvement it can produce. Moreover, effective ways to augment SRI response are needed.

RESIDUAL IMPAIRMENT IN TREATED
PATIENTS WITH OCD

The preceding study demonstrated the efficacy of intensive EX/RP and clomipramine in the treatment of adults with OCD. However, the results also highlighted that some patients with OCD, even with state-of-the-art treatment, continued to have residual symptoms and functional impairment. With NIMH funding, the Center for the Treatment and Study of Anxiety and the Anxiety Disorders Clinic evaluated in more detail the nature of this residual impairment by conducting a follow-up assessment of patients in the preceding study. The assessment focused on neuropsychological functioning because several studies at the time reported that patients with OCD (including those on medications) had specific deficits in executive functioning and visual memory and/or motor slowing (Purcell, Maruff, Kyrios, & Pantelis, 1998; Savage et al., 1999; Savage et al., 2000); we hypothesized that these deficits might be contributing to these residual symptoms and/or to functional impairment. Therefore, the aim was first to explore the presence of these neuropsychological deficits in our large clinical sample (Simpson, Rosen, et al., 2005); our ultimate goal was to design rehabilitative strategies for these putative deficits.

Patients with OCD who had finished their participation in the clinical trial described previously were recruited at least 6 months and up to 10 years after study completion for a 1-day follow-up assessment. Healthy controls were also recruited who had no psychiatric history and were matched to the patients as closely as possible on age, sex, ethnicity, and years of education. Participants received the following: (1) a psychiatric interview by experienced clinicians; (2) an assessment by independent raters that included the Structured Clinical Interview for DSM-IV (First, Spitzer, Gibbon, & Williams, 2002) and the Y-BOCS; and (3) a neuropsychological assessment by trained examiners. Participants filled out self-rating forms to assess functional impairment (using the Social Adjustment Scale; Weissman & Bothwell, 1976) and quality of life (using the Quality of Life Enjoyment and Satisfaction Scale; Endicott, Nee, Harrison, & Blumenthal, 1993).

The neuropsychological battery included: (1) the Rey–Osterrieth Complex Figure Test (Osterrieth, 1944); (2) several tasks from the Cambridge Neuropsychological Test Automated Battery (CANTAB, 1999), including tasks of Spatial Working Memory, Stockings of Cambridge, and Attentional Set-Shifting; (3) the Benton Visual Retention Test (Benton, 1974); (4) the Wechsler Abbreviated Scale of Intelligence (WASI; Wechsler, 1999); and (5) a computerized version of the Wisconsin Card Sorting Test (Heaton, 1993). Because we wanted our findings to be applicable to real-world clinical settings, neuropsychological tasks were chosen that had shown strong effects in prior studies and that would be relatively easy to use in clinical practice; several tasks that had shown discrepant results in prior OCD studies were also included.

Of 65 patients with OCD who participated in person, 30 met DSM-IV criteria for current OCD only (Current-OCD), 15 met DSM-IV criteria for current OCD and another Axis I disorder (Comorbid-OCD), and 15 had a history of OCD and no other Axis I disorder (History-of-OCD). The Comorbid-OCD group had the most severe OCD and the most depressive symptoms. Some of the patients were on medication at the time of testing (8 Comorbid-OCD, 11 Current-OCD, 4 History-of-OCD). All of the 11 patients with Current-OCD on medication were on a selective SRI.

To our surprise, when we compared the three OCD groups and healthy controls ($n = 35$), we found no significant ($p < .05$) overall group differences on any neuropsychological tests, when the four groups were compared in analyses that covaried for education. On some tasks (e.g., the Attention Set-Shifting task, the Wisconsin Card Sorting Test), this lack of difference was consistent with the literature (Basso, Bornstein, Carona, & Morton, 2001; Moritz et al., 2001; Purcell et al., 1998), supporting the conclusion that set-shifting deficits attributed to OCD in prior studies may not be specific to OCD. On other tasks (e.g., Spatial Working Memory, Stockings of Cambridge, Rey–Osterrieth Complex Figure Test), the lack of difference between patients with OCD and healthy controls contradicted the literature. The reasons for this discrepancy were not obvious, but they were not due to insufficient power to detect a statistical difference or to the fact that some of our patients were on medication, because prior studies had found deficits on these tasks in OCD samples with a higher proportion of patients on medication.

Although few neuropsychological differences appeared between patients with OCD and healthy controls in our sample, patients with OCD had significantly more functional impairment and lower quality of life than healthy controls. Of the patients, patients with Comorbid-OCD had the greatest functional impairment and lowest quality of life.

This study relied on a sample of convenience: willing patients who had participated in a prior clinical trial. As a result, the patients had different treatment histories and different types of OCD symptoms, and some were on medication at the time of testing. However, the findings were clear: In this clinical sample, there were few differences between patients with OCD and healthy controls in their performance on these neuropsychological tasks. The results do not support the idea that deficits on these tasks of executive functioning, nonverbal memory, and motor speed are characteristic of all patients with OCD. However, given the clinical heterogeneity of our sample, we cannot exclude the possibility that homogeneous OCD subtypes (e.g., one symptom dimension) might have specific neuropsychological deficits. Although we did not identify neuropsychological deficits in our OCD sample, we did confirm that many patients with OCD, despite the availability of state-of-the-art treatments, have residual OCD symptoms, functional impairment, and inferior quality of life (Huppert et al., in preparation). Continued efforts to improve the long-term outcome of patients with OCD are needed.

CBT AUGMENTATION OF SRI PHARMACOTHERAPY

SRIs are used widely in clinical practice to treat adults with OCD (Blanco et al., submitted). However, as described earlier, only some patients respond to these medications, and even those who benefit are typically left with substantial residual symptoms (Foa et al., 2005; Pigott & Seay, 1999). The only medications demonstrated in randomized controlled trials to augment a partial SRI response are antipsychotic medications such as risperidone (McDougle, Epperson, Pelton, Wasylink, & Price, 2000). An open trial of twice-weekly EX/RP found that EX/RP could also augment SRI response (Simpson, Gorfinkle, & Liebowitz, 1999). Thus, with NIMH funding, the Center for the Treatment and Study of Anxiety and the Anxiety Disorders Clinic are currently conducting a randomized controlled trial to examine whether adjunctive EX/RP benefits patients with residual symptoms despite an adequate SRI trial. In this study, EX/RP is compared with stress management training (SMT), a credible comparison treatment that controls for the nonspecific effects of therapy. The primary hypothesis is that adjunctive EX/RP will produce clinically significant improvements in OCD when compared with SMT. We are also examining whether patients who benefit acutely from adjunctive treatment can maintain their gains up to 1 year later.

Patients in this study are adult outpatients with primary OCD and clinically significant symptoms (Y-BOCS total score ≥ 16) despite having benefited from an adequate trial of an SRI. An adequate trial is defined as an adequate SRI dose (e.g., fluoxetine 60 mg, paroxetine 60 mg, fluvoxamine 250 mg, sertraline 200 mg, clomipramine 225 mg per day) for at least 12 weeks. Comorbid psychiatric and medical conditions are allowed unless they dominate the clinical picture and/or render participation unsafe.

During the 2-month acute phase, participants continue their medication at the same dose and are randomly assigned to receive adjunctive EX/RP or SMT. Both adjunctive therapies are delivered twice per week for a total of seventeen 2-hour sessions. EX/RP follows the standard protocol of Kozak and Foa (1997) and consists of two information-gathering sessions and fifteen exposure sessions. SMT also consists of two information-gathering sessions and fifteen sessions, during which patients are taught stress reduction techniques, including controlled breathing, progressive muscle relaxation, positive imagery, assertiveness skills, and structured problem solving. Patients with at least a 6-point Y-BOCS decrease enter a 6-month maintenance and then a 6-month follow-up phase.

This study is ongoing. The total sample has not yet been entered, a definitive analysis of the data has not been performed, and all findings are thus preliminary. With these caveats in mind, several observations can be made. First, preliminary data suggest that many patients who receive adjunctive EX/RP achieve a clinically significant improvement in their OCD symptoms (i.e., at least a 6-point decrease in their pretreatment Y-BOCS scores). Second, despite the fact that SRIs are more widely available than EX/RP, many patients with OCD screened for this study have not received an adequate SRI trial despite published OCD treatment guidelines (March, Frances, Carpenter, & Kahn, 1997). In some cases, the reason is that the patients did not want medication or could not tolerate SRI side effects. However, in other cases, providers apparently never offered SRI medication at an optimal dose for a sufficient duration. Third, patients in this study are not terminated for poor EX/RP adherence, enabling us to collect preliminary data on the association between adherence and outcome. These data suggest the following: (1) patient adherence to the EX/RP procedures is variable; (2) only good adherence is associated with excellent response; and (3) patients who complete and adhere to EX/RP procedures can achieve superior EX/RP outcome regardless of their baseline severity.

Several tentative conclusions can be made. First, even though SRI treatment is widely available, many patients with OCD are not receiving an adequate SRI trial. The reasons are complex but include both patient and provider barriers. Second, twice-weekly EX/RP appears to be an effective and safe way to augment SRI pharmacotherapy; we are currently examining whether patients who benefit acutely from adjunctive EX/RP can maintain these gains long term. Third, if patients do not adhere to treatment, an excellent response to EX/RP treatment is unlikely. Determinants of EX/RP adherence and methods for increasing EX/RP adherence are needed.

SUMMARY AND FUTURE DIRECTIONS

Directed by Dr. Foa, the Center for the Treatment and Study of Anxiety has collaborated with the Anxiety Disorders Clinic for over a decade to help determine how best to treat adults with OCD. Based on these data and the findings of others, we conclude that both SRI pharmacotherapy and EX/RP are efficacious treatments for OCD, but each treatment has advantages and disadvantages. One of the main advantages of SRIs is that they are readily available; moreover, unlike clomipramine, the selective SRIs have minimal side effects and few that are dangerous. SRI limitations include the following. First, up to 50% of patients with OCD do not respond to an SRI trial. Second, the degree of response is modest: The mean reduction in OCD symptoms from SRI treatment across randomized controlled trials is only 20–40% (Pigott & Seay, 1999). Third, relapse can occur after SRI discontinuation (Simpson et al., 2004).

Compared with SRIs, EX/RP treatment has several advantages. It can be more efficacious when delivered by skilled therapists and when patients adhere to the procedures (Foa et al., 2005), and it results in lower short-term relapse rates after treatment discontinuation (Simpson, Franklin, et al., 2005; Simpson et al., 2004). EX/RP limitations include: (1) a substantial proportion of patients refuse, drop out of, or only partially adhere to EX/RP treatment; (2) not all patients maintain their gains long term; and (3) EX/RP is not widely available.

Foa et al. (2005) found that the combination of SRI and EX/RP was superior to SRI alone but not to EX/RP alone. However, as described earlier the design may have limited the ability to detect the benefits of combination treatment. Other research data and clinical experience suggest that combination treatment is more effective than EX/RP alone in certain clinical situations, such as when there is severe comorbid depression, when patients are too fearful to try EX/RP alone, or when intensive EX/RP is not available (Franklin & Simpson, in press). In addition, preliminary data from our ongoing trial indicate that EX/RP may be one of the most helpful (and safest) augmentation strategies for patients with a partial SRI response.

We know more about how to treat adults with OCD than ever before: We have two established treatments for adults with OCD (EX/RP and SRIs) and proven methods for augmenting SRI response (adjunctive EX/RP or antipsychotic medications). However, much work remains. First, only some patients with OCD are receiving SRIs at appropriate doses (Fireman, Koran, Leventhal, & Jacobson, 2001), and few patients are receiving EX/RP. Methods for disseminating these evidence-based treatments to real-world settings are needed. Second, to maximize outcome from our current treatments, interventions to increase treatment entry, retention, and adherence are needed; this is especially true for EX/RP, a treatment that can result in superior outcome if patients adhere to the procedures. Third, even with SRI and/or EX/RP treatment, patients with OCD can have substantial residual symptoms, ongoing functional impairment, and inferior quality of life. Thus future treatment efforts need to focus on helping patients with OCD achieve not only sustained remission but also improved functioning and quality of life. Finally, although several brain models of OCD have been proposed (Saxena, Bota, & Brody, 2001) and are actively being examined with modern brain imaging techniques (Simpson et al., 2003), we know very little about what causes OCD, how SRIs or EX/RP work, or why these treatments fail in some patients. Armed with improved knowledge about the pathophysiology of OCD, we potentially could develop even better treatments than we currently have for people with this disabling disorder.

ACKNOWLEDGMENTS

Dr. Edna Foa, Director of the Center for the Treatment and Study of Anxiety has been a principal investigator and our collaborator on the three studies described herein. This chapter was written to honor her many contributions to the field of anxiety disorders, including this work on OCD. We thank the staff at both the Anxiety Disorder Clinic and the Center for the Treatment and Study of Anxiety who helped conduct these studies; the patients who participated; and the National Institutes of Mental Health for funding (Grant Nos. RO1 MH45436 [Principal Investigator: Dr. Michael Liebowitz], R01 MH45404 [Principal Investigator: Dr. Edna Foa], and K23 MH01907 [Principal Investigator: Dr. Helen Blair Simpson]).

REFERENCES

Basso, M. R., Bornstein, R. A., Carona, F., & Morton, R. (2001). Depression accounts for executive function deficits in obsessive–compulsive disorder. *Neuropsychiatry, Neuropsychology, and Behavioral Neurology, 14*(4), 241–245.

Benton, A. L. (1974). *Revised Visual Retention Test* (4th ed.). San Antonio, TX: The Psychological Corporation.

Blanco, E., Olfson, M., Stein, D. J., Simpson, H. B., Gameroff, M. I., & Narrow, W. (submitted). Treatment of OCD by U.S. psychiatrists. *Journal of Clinical Psychiatry.*

CANTAB. (1999). *CANTAB for Windows.* Cambridge, UK: CeNeS.

Endicott, J., Nee, J., Harrison, W., & Blumenthal, R. (1993). Quality of Life Enjoyment and Satisfaction Questionnaire: A new measure. *Psychopharmacology Bulletin, 29*(2), 321–326.

Fireman, B., Koran, L. M., Leventhal, J. L., & Jacobson, A. (2001). The prevalence of clinically recognized obsessive–compulsive disorder in a large health maintenance organization. *American Journal of Psychiatry, 158*(11), 1904–1910.

First, M. B., Spitzer, R. L., Gibbon, M., & Williams, J. B. (2002). *Structured Clinical Interview for DSM-IV-TR Axis I Disorders—Patient Edition (SCID-I/P).* New York: New York State Psychiatric Institute, Biometrics Research Department.

Foa, E. B., Grayson, J. B., Steketee, G. S., Doppelt, H. G., Turner, R. M., & Latimer, P. R. (1983). Success and failure in the behavioral treatment of obsessive–compulsives. *Journal of Consulting Clinical Psychology, 51*(2), 287–297.

Foa, E. B., Liebowitz, M. R., Kozak, M. J., Davies, S., Campeas, R., Franklin, M. E., et al. (2005). Randomized, placebo-controlled trial of exposure and ritual prevention, clomipramine, and their combination in the treatment of obsessive–compulsive disorder. *American Journal of Psychiatry, 162*(1), 151–161.

Franklin, M. E., & Simpson, H. B. (in press). Combined treatment of obsessive–compulsive disorder: Research findings and clinical application. *Journal of Cognitive Psychotherapy.*

Goodman, W. K., Price, L. H., Rasmussen, S. A., Mazure, C., Delgado, P., Heninger, G. R., et al. (1989). The Yale–Brown Obsessive Compulsive Scale: II. Validity. *Archives of General Psychiatry, 46*(11), 1012–1016.

Goodman, W. K., Price, L. H., Rasmussen, S. A., Mazure, C., Fleischmann, R. L., Hill, C. L., et al. (1989). The Yale–Brown Obsessive Compulsive Scale: I. Development, use, and reliability. *Archives of General Psychiatry, 46*(11), 1006–1011.

Guy, W. (1976). *ECDEU Assessment Manual for Psychopharmacology.* Rockville, MD: U.S. Department of Health, Education, and Welfare.

Heaton, R. K. (1993). *Wisconsin Card Sorting Test: Computer Version—2.* Odessa, FL: Psychological Assessment Resources.

Kozak, M. J., & Foa, E. B. (1997). *Mastery of obsessive–compulsive disorder: A cognitive-behavioral approach*. San Antonio, TX: The Psychological Corporation.

March, J. S., Frances, A., Carpenter, L. L., & Kahn, D. (1997). Expert Consensus Treatment Guidelines for Obsessive–Compulsive Disorder: A guide for patients and families. *Journal of Clinical Psychiatry, 58*(Suppl. 4), 65–72.

McDougle, C. J., Epperson, C. N., Pelton, G. H., Wasylink, S., & Price, L. H. (2000). A double-blind, placebo-controlled study of risperidone addiction in serotonin reuptake inhibitor-refractory obsessive–compulsive disorder. *Archives of General Psychiatry, 57*(8), 794–801.

Moritz, S., Birkner, C., Kloss, M., Jacobsen, D., Fricke, S., Boethern, A., et al. (2001). Impact of comorbid depressive symptoms on neuropsychological performance in obsessive–compulsive disorder. *Journal of Abnormal Psychology, 110*(4), 653–657.

Osterrieth, P. (1944). Test of copying a complex figure: Contribution to the study of perception and memory. *Archives de Psychologie, 30,* 206–356.

Pigott, T. A., & Seay, S. M. (1999). A review of the efficacy of selective serotonin reuptake inhibitors in obsessive–compulsive disorder. *Journal of Clinical Psychiatry, 60*(2), 101–106.

Purcell, R., Maruff, P., Kyrios, M., & Pantelis, C. (1998). Neuropsychological deficits in obsessive–compulsive disorder: a comparison with unipolar depression, panic disorder, and normal controls. *Archives of General Psychiatry, 55*(5), 415–423.

Savage, C. R., Baer, L., Keuthen, N. J., Brown, H. D., Rauch, S. L., & Jenike, M. A. (1999). Organizational strategies mediate nonverbal memory impairment in obsessive–compulsive disorder. *Biological Psychiatry, 45*(7), 905–916.

Savage, C. R., Deckersbach, T., Wilhelm, S., Rauch, S. L., Baer, L., Reid, T., et al. (2000). Strategic processing and episodic memory impairment in obsessive–compulsive disorder. *Neuropsychology, 14*(1), 141–151.

Saxena, S., Bota, R. G., & Brody, A. L. (2001). Brain–behavior relationships in obsessive–compulsive disorder. *Seminars in Clinical Neuropsychiatry, 6*(2), 82–101.

Simpson, H. B., Franklin, M. E., Cheng, J., Foa, E. B., & Liebowitz, M. R. (2005). Standard criteria for relapse are needed in obsessive–compulsive disorder. *Depression and Anxiety, 21*(1), 1–8.

Simpson, H., Gorfinkle, K., & Liebowitz, M. R. (1999). Cognitive–behavioral therapy as an adjunct to serotonin reuptake inhibitors in obsessive–compulsive disorder: An open trial. *Journal of Clinical Psychiatry, 60*(9), 584–590.

Simpson, H., Rosen, W., Huppert, J. D., Lin, S. H., Foa, E., & Liebowitz, M. R. (submitted). *Are there reliable neuropsychological deficits in OCD?* Manuscript submitted for publication.

Simpson, H. B., Liebowitz, M. R., Foa, E. B., Kozak, M. J., Schmidt, A. B., Rowan, V., et al. (2004). Post-treatment effects of exposure therapy versus clomipramine in OCD. *Depression and Anxiety, 19,* 225–233.

Simpson, H. B., Lombardo, I., Slifstein, M., Huang, H. Y., Hwang, D. R., Abi-Dargham, A., et al. (2003). Serotonin transporters in obsessive-compulsive disorder: A positron emission tomography study with [(11)C]McN 5652. *Biological Psychiatry, 54*(12), 1414–1421.

Simpson, H. B., Rosen, W., Huppert, J. H., Lin, S., Foa, E. B., & Liebowitz, M. R. (in press). Are there reliable neuropsychological deficits in OCD? *Journal of Psychiatric Research*.

Wechsler, D. (1999). *Wechsler Abbreviated Scale of Intelligence: Manual*. San Antonio, TX: The Psychological Corporation.

Weissman, M. M., & Bothwell, S. (1976). Assessment of social adjustment by patient self-report. *Archives of General Psychiatry, 33*(9), 1111–1115.

9

Cognitive-Behavioral Therapy for Pediatric Obsessive–Compulsive Disorder

JOHN S. MARCH
MARTIN E. FRANKLIN

At any given time, between ½ and 1% of children and adolescents suffers from clinically significant obsessive–compulsive disorder (OCD; Flament et al., 1988), and up to one-half of adults with OCD develop the disorder during childhood or adolescence (Rasmussen & Eisen, 1990). Thus, besides reducing morbidity associated with pediatric OCD, improvements in treating the disorder early in life have the potential to reduce adult morbidity. Despite this readily apparent advantage of earlier intervention, the treatment literature in pediatric OCD has generally lagged behind the adult literature; hence, the development and empirical evaluation of treatments for pediatric OCD is an issue of paramount public health importance. Fortunately, significant advances in this direction have been made over the past 15 years and, as is the case with adult OCD, cognitive-behavioral therapy (CBT) has emerged as the initial treatment of choice for OCD across the lifespan (March, Frances, Kahn, & Carpenter, 1997). Moreover, the evidence base on which these expert opinions are built has strengthened considerably in the past few years, lending further credence to the experts' recommendation that families should be vigorously encouraged to seek CBT for children and adolescents suffering from this often disabling condition.

Following a brief discussion of the assessment of pediatric OCD, this chapter moves on to review the current status of CBT for OCD in children and adolescents. We begin by reviewing the principles that underlie the treatment and provide a brief review of our CBT protocol as used in both clinical and research settings (March & Mulle, 1998) that was derived from the work of Foa and colleagues with adult OCD. Next we discuss empirical studies supporting the use of CBT with children and adolescents, summarize findings from our recently completed randomized controlled trial in pediatric OCD (Pediatric OCD Treatment Study Team, 2004), and recommend directions for future research.

ASSESSMENT

An adequate assessment of pediatric OCD should include a comprehensive evaluation of current and past OCD symptoms, current OCD symptom severity and associated functional impairment, and a survey of comorbid psychopathology. In addition, the strengths of the child and family should be evaluated, as well as their knowledge of OCD and its treatment. There are many self-report and clinician-administered instruments that can be used to guide this type of assessment. We typically mail several relevant self-report questionnaires for the family to complete prior to the intake visit and then review these materials prior to meeting with the child. If it is apparent from these materials that comorbid depression or other anxiety problems besides OCD are prominent, we focus on these symptoms as well in the intake. The Anxiety Disorders Interview Schedule for Children (ADIS-C) is a semistructured interview that can be used to examine comorbid problems in greater detail; we used the ADIS in our collaborative study examining the relative efficacy of CBT, sertraline, combined treatment, and pill placebo (Franklin, Foa, & March, 2003; Pediatric OCD Treatment Study Team, 2004). For documenting past and current OCD symptoms and current symptom severity, we use the Children's Yale–Brown Obsessive–Compulsive Scale (CY-BOCS) checklist and severity scale (Scahill et al., 1997). Before administering this scale, it is important to determine whether the child should be interviewed with or without the parent present. The decision can be informed by discussing the alternatives with the parent in advance or by observing the child and family's behavior in the waiting area and even during the interview itself if necessary. For example, if it becomes clear that a patient is reluctant to discuss certain symptoms with a parent present (e.g., sexual obsessions), the therapist can skip that item on the CY-BOCS checklist and save some time at the end of the interview to revisit these potentially sensitive issues alone with the patient. Our mantra in the clinic is "get the information," meaning that if parental presence increases the validity of the assessment, then do that; if not, then interview the child alone.

Prior to administering the CY-BOCS, the therapist should explain the concepts of obsessions and compulsions, using examples if the child or parent has difficulty grasping the concepts. We also take this opportunity to tell children and adolescents about the prevalence, nature, and treatment of OCD, which may increase their willingness to disclose their specific symptoms. Children may be particularly vulnerable to feeling as if they are the only ones on earth with obsessive fears of hurting a loved one, so they may preface the examples with, "I once met a kid who . . ." in order to dispel this myth and minimize the accompanying sense of isolation. During the intake, it is also important to observe the child's behavior and inquire whether certain behaviors (e.g., unusual movements, vocalizations) are compulsions designed to neutralize obsessions or to reduce distress. Tic disorders are commonly comorbid with OCD, and it is important clinically to make a differential diagnosis of such behaviors as compulsions or tics, as different treatment procedures might be used depending on how the behavior is categorized. Further, as mentioned earlier, some children who are aware of their obsessional content may be fearful of speaking about the fears aloud. Surveying common obsessions with a checklist instead of asking the child to disclose the fears tends to help with this problem, as does encouragement on the part of the therapist (e.g., "Lots of the kids I see have a hard time talking about these kinds of fears"). We have found that flexibility in the manner of disclosing the obsession is warranted. Thus, for example, we allow the child to write down the fears or to nod his or her head as the therapist describes examples of similar fears in order to help the child share his or her OCD problems. In this way we can convey to the child and family that we recognize the difficulty associated with disclosure. We also use examples from children we have evaluated in the past (e.g., "I remember a few months ago when a kid about your age told me she would be scared to touch her dog for fear she might lose control and hurt him"), although we let the children and families know we are careful not to violate confidentiality when citing such examples. Following are brief descriptions of our core assessments.

Children's Yale–Brown Obsessive–Compulsive Scale (CY-BOCS)

The primary instrument for assessing OCD is the Y-BOCS, which assess obsessions and compulsions separately on time consumed, distress, interference, degree of resistance, and control. We use the pediatric version (Scahill et al., 1997) to record past and present OCD symptoms, initial severity, total OCD severity, relative preponderance of obsessions and compulsions, and degree of insight. The CY-BOCS is a clinician-rated instrument merging data from clinical observation and parent and child report.

Anxiety Disorders Interview for Children (ADIS-C)

The child and adolescent ADIS is a semistructured interview for assessing DSM-IV anxiety disorders in youth (Silverman & Albano, 1996). Relative to other available instruments, such as the Diagnostic Interview Schedule for Children (DISC), it has excellent psychometric properties for internalizing conditions. The ADIS-C uses an interviewer–observer format, thereby allowing the clinician to draw information from the interview and from clinical observations. Scores are derived regarding (1) specific diagnoses and (2) level of diagnosis-related interference. Adequate psychometric properties have been demonstrated.

Children's OCD Impact Scale (COIS)

We also obtain child and parent versions of the OCD Impact Scale, which shows preliminary evidence favoring psychometric adequacy and sensitivity to change, for use in analyses of functional impairment from OCD (Piacentini, Jaffer, Bergman, McCracken, & Keller, 2001). This instrument enables us to estimate whether the CY-BOCS improvements result in normalization as assessed by functional impairment. A new and shorter version of this scale has been developed recently, and the psychometric properties of this scale appear to be favorable (Piacentini et al., 2001).

Multidimensional Anxiety Scale for Children (MASC)

The MASC has four factors and six subfactors—Physical Anxiety (tense/restless, somatic/autonomic), Harm Avoidance (perfectionism, anxious coping), Social Anxiety (humiliation/rejection, performance anxiety), and Separation Anxiety—and is in use in a variety of treatment outcome studies funded by the National Institute of Mental Health (NIMH). The MASC shows high test–retest reliability using the intraclass correlation coefficient (ICC) in clinical (ICC > .92) and school samples (ICC > .85); convergent/divergent validity is similarly superior (March, 1998).

Children's Depression Inventory (CDI)

The CDI is a 27-item self-report scale that measures cognitive, affective, behavioral, and interpersonal symptoms of depression (Kovacs, 1996). Each item consists of three statements, of which the child is asked to select the one statement that best describes his or her current functioning. Items are scored from 0 to 2 so scores on the CDI can range from 0 to 54. The CDI shows adequate reliability and validity. This scale is useful to assess symptoms of depression, which assists in tailoring the treatment plan.

Medical History

Pediatric OCD patients' medical histories should also be examined, with particular attention to the presence of recurrent streptococcal infection. Although children with streptococcal-precipitated OCD (pediatric autoimmune neuropsychiatric disorders associated with streptococcal infection; PANDAS) may require somewhat different treatment(s), experts agree that the base rate of PANDAS given OCD is currently unknown and that the diagnosis cannot be assigned retrospectively at this juncture (Swedo et al., 1998), although it is likely to be fairly common (Giulino et al., 2002). Current research diagnostic criteria for PANDAS require at least two prospectively documented episodes of exacerbations in OCD and tic symptoms associated with streptococcal infection. Unfortunately, an unambiguous retrospective diagnosis of PANDAS is next to impossible in a clinically referred population of youths with OCD (Giulino et al., 2002). Clinically, children who have unambiguous evidence of PANDAS should be referred for appropriate treatment of their group A β-hemolytic streptococcal (GABHS) infection. Once treated for the infection, the clinician should then also consider the CBT and/or selective serotonin reuptake inhibitor (SSRI) pharmacotherapy strategies described subsequently.

In brief, the aforementioned scales, interviews, and questionnaires may be useful to help generate relevant clinical information at pretreatment and in helping us to evaluate treatment outcome. In our research-oriented settings, this is part of routine clinic practice. We hope the development of an efficient package for evaluating outcome may stimulate effectiveness research in real-world clinical settings; we view this as an important next step in the pediatric OCD research agenda now that several randomized clinical trials have been completed and have underscored the fact that we have developed several treatment options that are likely to be efficacious. Until our measurements have been streamlined and boiled down to their essential components, however, financial, time, and personnel constraints may limit the more general usefulness of the current assessment battery.

THE APPLICATION OF CBT FOR PEDIATRIC OCD

Overview

In adults, the cognitive-behavioral treatment of OCD generally involves a three-stage approach: (1) information gathering; (2) therapist-assisted exposure and response (or ritual) prevention (EX/RP), including homework assignments; and (3) generalization training and relapse prevention. Component analyses suggest that both exposure and response prevention are active ingredients of treatment, with exposure reducing phobic anxiety and response prevention reducing rituals (Foa, Steketee, Grayson, Turner, & Latimer, 1984). Relaxation has been shown to be an inert component of behavioral treatment for OCD and has been used as an active placebo in brief (4–6 weeks) studies in adults (e.g., Fals-Stewart, Marks, & Schafer, 1993). Cognitive interventions, though found efficacious in some studies (e.g., van Balkom et al., 1998), may be generally less potent than EX/RP in reducing OCD symptoms. A recent study comparing EX/RP plus cognitive therapy to EX/RP plus relaxation found that the addition of cognitive therapy with EX/RP reduced dropout but did not enhance outcome as examined using an intent-to-treat analysis (Vogel, Stiles, & Gotestam, 2004).

Tools

Exposure and Ritual Prevention

As applied to OCD, the exposure principle relies on the fact that anxiety usually attenuates after sufficient duration of contact with a feared stimulus. Thus a child with fear of germs must confront relevant feared but low-risk situations until his or her anxiety decreases. Repeated exposure is associated with decreased anxiety across exposure trials, with anxiety reduction largely specific to the domain of exposure, until the child no longer fears contact with specifically targeted phobic stimuli. Adequate exposure depends on blocking the negative reinforcement effect of rituals or avoidance behavior, a process termed response or ritual prevention. For example, a child with germ worries must not only touch "germy things" but must also refrain from ritualized washing until his or her anxiety diminishes substantially. EX/RP is typically implemented in a gradual fashion (sometimes termed graded exposure), with exposure targets under the control of the patient or, less desirably, the therapist. Intensive approaches may be especially useful for treatment-resistant OCD or for patients who desire a very rapid response (Franklin et al., 1998).

Cognitive Techniques

A wide variety of cognitive interventions have been used to provide the child with a "tool kit" to facilitate compliance with EX/RP (Soechting & March, 2002). The goals of cognitive techniques, which may be more or less useful or necessary depending on the child and nature of OCD, typically include increasing a sense of personal efficacy, predictability, controllability, and self-attributed likelihood of a positive outcome within EX/RP tasks. Specific interventions include: (1) constructive self-talk, (2) cognitive restructuring, and (3) cultivating nonattachment or, stated differently, recognizing obsessions and allowing them to come and go of their own accord instead of engaging in inherently futile thought suppression attempts. Each must be individualized to match the specific OCD symptoms that afflict the child and must mesh with the child's cognitive abilities, developmental stage, and individual differences in preference among the three techniques. Such methods are often incorporated into EX/RP programs, in which the cognitive procedures are used to support and complement EX/RP rather than to replace it (Franklin & Foa, 2002).

Ritual Prevention

Because preventing rituals or avoidance behaviors removes the negative reinforcement effect of the rituals or avoidance, ritual prevention technically is an extinction procedure. By convention, however, extinction is usually defined as the elimination of OCD-related behaviors through removal of parental positive reinforcement for rituals. For example, with a child with reassurance-seeking rituals, the therapist may ask parents to refrain from gratifying the child's reassurance seeking. Extinction frequently produces rapid effects, but it can be hard to implement when the child's behavior is bizarre (e.g., screaming out "God forgive me" in response to obsessional thoughts about the devil, regardless of the social context) or very frequent (e.g., counting every breath). In addition, nonconsensual extinction procedures often produce unmanageable distress on the part of the child, disrupt the therapeutic alliance, miss important EX/RP targets that are not amenable to extinction procedures, and, most important, fail to help the child internalize a strategy for resisting OCD. Hence, as with EX/RP, placing the extinction program under the child's control leads to increased compliance and improved outcomes.

Modeling and Shaping

Modeling—whether overt (the child understands that the therapist is demonstrating more appropriate or adaptive coping behaviors) or covert (the therapist informally models a behavior)—may help improve compliance with in-session EX/RP and generalization to between-session EX/RP homework. Intended to increase motivation to comply with EX/RP, shaping involves positively reinforcing successive approximations to a desired target behavior. Modeling and shaping reduce anticipatory anxiety and provide an opportunity for practicing constructive self-talk before and during EX/RP.

Operant Procedures

Clinically, positive reinforcement seems not to directly alter OCD symptoms but rather helps to encourage compliance with EX/RP and so produces a noticeable if indirect clinical benefit. In contrast, punishment (defined as imposition of an aversive event) and response-cost (defined as removal of a positive event) procedures have shown themselves to be unhelpful in the treatment of OCD. Most CBT programs use liberal positive reinforcement for EX/RP and proscribe aversive contingency management procedures unless they are targeting disruptive behavior outside the domain of OCD. Because OCD itself is a powerful tonic aversive stimulus, successful EX/RP promotes willingness to engage in further EX/RP via negative reinforcement (e.g., elimination of OCD symptoms boosts compliance with EX/RP) as manifested by unscheduled generalization to new EX/RP targets as treatment proceeds.

Involvement of the Family in Treatment

Family psychopathology is neither necessary nor sufficient for the onset of OCD; nonetheless, families affect and are affected by the disorder (Amir, Freshman, & Foa, 2000). Hence, although empirical data is lacking, clinical observations suggest that a combination of individual and family sessions is best for most patients. In our protocol we included several sessions that involved the whole family and typically included the family at the end of each session in order to ensure that the parent and child both understood the EX/RP homework assignment and their respective roles in implementing it. Some investigators have emphasized family work even more in the development of their CBT protocols (e.g., Piacentini et al., 2002), and a recent study found that group cognitive-behavioral family CBT was as good as individual CBT at reducing OCD symptoms (Barrett, Healy-Farrell, 8 March, 2004).

A Typical CBT Protocol

The protocol that we used in our NIMH study (Franklin et al., 2003; Pediatric OCD Treatment Study Team, 2004), which is fairly typical of a gradual-exposure regimen (March & Mulle, 1998), consists of 14 visits over 12 weeks spread across five phases: (1) psychoeducation, (2) cognitive training, (3) mapping OCD, (4) exposure and ritual prevention, and (5) relapse prevention and generalization training. Except for weeks 1 and 2, when patients come twice weekly, all visits are administered on a once-per-week basis, last 1 hour, and include one between-visit 10-minute telephone contact scheduled during Weeks 3–12. Psychoeducation, defining OCD as the identified problem, cognitive training, and development of a stimulus hierarchy (mapping OCD) take place during sessions 1–4; EX/RP take up sessions 5–12, with the last two sessions incorporating generalization training and relapse prevention. Each session includes a statement of goals, a review of the previous week, provision of new information, therapist-assisted practice, homework for the coming week, and monitoring procedures.

Parents are centrally involved at Sessions 1, 7, and 11, with the latter two sessions devoted to guiding the parents about their central role in assisting their child to accomplish the homework assignments. Sessions 13 and 14 also require significant parental input. Parents check in with the therapist at each session, and the therapist provides feedback describing the goals of each session and the child's progress in treatment. The therapist works with parents to assist them in refraining from insisting on inappropriate EX/RP tasks, which is a common problem in pediatric OCD treatment. The therapist also encourages parents to praise the child for resisting OCD, while at the same time refocusing their attention on positive elements in the child's life, an intervention technically termed differential reinforcement of other behavior (DRO). In some cases, extensive family involvement in rituals and/or the developmental level of the child require that family members play a more central role in treatment. It is important to note that the CBT protocol provides sufficient flexibility to accommodate variations in family involvement dictated by the OCD symptom picture.

Crucial to the success of any CBT protocol is the ability to deliver protocol-driven treatments in a developmentally appropriate fashion (Clarke, 1995). In our hands, CBT has been shown effective in children as young as 5. We promote developmental appropriateness by allowing flexibility in CBT within the constraints of fixed session goals. More specifically, the therapist adjusts the level of discourse to the cognitive functioning, social maturity, and capacity for sustained attention of each patient. Younger patients require more redirection and activities in order to sustain attention and motivation. Adolescents are generally more sensitive to the effects of OCD on peer interactions, which in turn require more discussion. Cognitive interventions in particular require adjustment to the developmental level of the patient, so, for example, adolescents are less likely to appreciate giving OCD a "nasty nickname" than are younger children. Developmentally appropriate metaphors relevant to the child's areas of interest and knowledge are also used to promote active involvement in the treatment process. For instance, an adolescent male football player treated with CBT was better able to grasp treatment concepts by casting them in terms of offensive and defensive strategies employed during football games (e.g., picking up blitzes). Patients whose OCD symptoms entangle family members will require more attention to family involvement in treatment planning and implementation than those without as much family involvement. On the other hand, although the CBT manual (March & Mulle, 1998) includes a section on developmental sensitivity that is specific for each treatment session, the general format and goals of the treatment sessions will be the same for all children.

EMPIRICAL STUDIES OF CBT TREATMENT OUTCOME

As has typically been the case with pediatric anxiety and mood disorders, the building of the CBT outcome literature in pediatric OCD began with age-downward extension of protocols found efficacious with adults, then continued with publication of single-case studies, case series, and open clinical trials involving these protocols. Collectively, the published uncontrolled evaluations (e.g., Franklin et al., 1998; March, Mulle, & Herbel, 1994; Piacentini, Bergman, Jacobs, McCracken, & Kretchman, 2002; Wever & Rey, 1997) yielded remarkably similar and encouraging findings: At posttreatment, the vast majority of patients were responders, with mean CY-BOCS reductions ranging from 50 to 67%. This pilot work set the stage for controlled studies evaluating the efficacy of CBT, one of which was published in the late 1990s (deHaan, Hoogduin, Buitelaar, & Keijsers, 1998), two that have been published more recently (Barrett et al., 2004; Pediatric OCD Treatment Study Team, 2004), and one that has recently been completed (J. Piacentini, personal communication). Following we review some of the key findings from the empirical literature that fueled design decisions on our recently completed NIMH collaborative study.

Dose and Time Response

Most of the studies of CBT outcome in pediatric OCD have employed a weekly therapy regimen. In contrast, Wever and Rey (1997) used an intensive CBT protocol that included two information gathering sessions followed by 10 daily sessions of CBT over 2 weeks. Franklin et al. (1998) found no differences between 14 weekly sessions over 12 weeks or 18 sessions over 4 weeks, but interpretation of this finding is hampered by the lack of random assignment. As yet, no study has evaluated the relative efficacy of weekly versus intensive treatment using randomization to condition. Taken together, the available studies suggested that patients respond well to CBT delivered either weekly or intensively. Given the greater acceptability of weekly treatment for patients and providers alike, we chose to examine a weekly CBT protocol in our recently completed and current NIMH studies, described later in the chapter.

Durability

Epidemiological studies suggest that OCD is a chronic condition. On the other hand, clinical research in adults shows that long-term outcomes for patients successfully treated with CBT alone or with CBT plus medication are generally favorable. Foa and Kozak (1996) concluded that gains achieved with EX/RP persist without continuing treatment, whereas those achieved with medication alone require continuing medication for maintenance. As in adults, OCD in children and adolescents is a chronic mental illness in many patients. For example, in the first NIMH follow-up study, 68% of patients had clinical OCD at follow-up (Flament et al., 1990). In a subsequent, more systematic 2- to 7-year follow-up study (Leonard et al., 1993), 43% still met diagnostic criteria for OCD; only 11% were totally asymptomatic. Seventy percent continued to take medication at the time of follow-up, clearly illustrating the limitations of the treatments received by these patients. The three pediatric OCD pilot studies that have included a follow-up evaluation (Franklin et al., 1998; March et al., 1994; Wever & Rey, 1997) support the durability of CBT, with therapeutic gains maintained up to 9 months posttreatment. Moreover, because relapse commonly follows medication discontinuation, the finding of March et al. (1994) that improvement persisted in six of nine responders following the withdrawal of medication provides limited support for the hypothesis that CBT inhibits relapse when medications are discontinued. A direct comparison of maintenance of gains following treatment discontinuation was needed, and this design element was included in our collaborative study.

Availability, Acceptability, and Tolerability

Experts have recommended CBT with a strong emphasis on EX/RP as a first-line treatment for OCD in children and adolescents (March et al., 1997), yet several barriers may limit its widespread use. First, few therapists have extensive experience with CBT for pediatric OCD; thus, CBT, if available at all, typically is obtainable only in areas associated with major medical centers. Second, even when the treatment is available, some patients and families reject the treatment as "too difficult." Once involved in CBT, some patients find the initial distress when confronting feared thoughts and situations while simultaneously refraining from rituals so aversive that they drop out of treatment. In our protocol we use hierarchy-driven EX/RP, actively involve the patient in choosing exposure exercises, and include anxiety management techniques for the few who need them. As a result, the dropout rates in our pilot studies and in our now completed comparative treatment trial are quite low, which in turn suggests that the vast majority of children and adolescents can tolerate and will benefit from CBT when delivered in a clinically informed and developmentally sensitive fashion.

Modifiers of Treatment Outcome

The question of paramount interest to clinicians and to researchers attempting to refine and improve treatment outcome is "Which treatment for which child with what characteristics?" Conventional wisdom holds that patients with OCD who benefit from CBT and medication differ in important if ill-understood ways. However, other than comorbid schizotypy (Baer et al., 1992) and tic disorders (McDougle et al., 1993), which may represent treatment impediments and possible indications for neuroleptic augmentation, the meager empirical literature on moderators of treatment outcome in adults provides no clear support for any of the putative predictors proposed by Goodman and colleagues in their review of pharmacotherapy trial methodology in OCD (Goodman, Rasmussen, Foa, & Price, 1994). Conversely, predictors of a successful response to behavior therapy include the presence of rituals, the desire to eliminate symptoms, ability to monitor and report symptoms, absence of complicating comorbidities, willingness to cooperate with treatment, and psychophysiological indicators (Foa & Emmelkamp, 1983).

Although many have suggested that the presence of comorbidity, especially with the tic disorders, lack of motivation or insight, and the presence of family psychopathology might predict a poor outcome in children undergoing CBT, there is as yet little or no empirical basis on which to predict treatment outcome in children undergoing psychosocial treatment. In contrast, a rather extensive literature on prediction of outcome for drug treatment has failed to identify any predictor variables. For example, in a recently published multicenter trial of sertraline and pill placebo in children and adolescents with OCD (March, Biederman, et al., 1998), neither age, race, gender, body weight, baseline OCD score, baseline depression score, comorbidity, socioeconomic status, nor plasma sertraline or desmethylsertraline level predicted the outcome of treatment. We will examine moderators and mediators of response in the context of the NIMH Collaborative Study, although we recognize that limited statistical power will likely render their exploration an exercise in hypothesis generation rather than a definitive evaluation of the influence of these variables on treatment outcome.

NIMH-FUNDED COMPARATIVE TREATMENT TRIAL

Funded in 1997 under the R01 mechanism by NIMH, the Pediatric OCD Treatment Study (POTS) evolved out of a collaborative relationship between John March (Duke University Medical Center) and Edna Foa (University of Pennsylvania), the study's principal investigators, and their respective clinical research teams. Brown University School of Medicine later joined the collaboration as a third clinical site, under the direction of Henrietta Leonard. The POTS was the first randomized trial in pediatric obsessive–compulsive disorder (OCD) to directly compare the efficacy of an established medication (sertraline; SER), OCD-specific cognitive-behavior therapy (CBT), and their combination (COMB) to a control condition, pill placebo (PBO), in the acute treatment of pediatric OCD. It is also the first study to allow for a direct comparison of relapse rates in children who respond to serotonin reuptake inhibitor (SRI) medication treated with and without concomitant CBT; these discontinuation data have yet to be fully analyzed. Experimental design decisions made in the early stages of the collaboration were guided by the principles of maximizing generalizability without sacrificing internal validity. This balance between efficacy and effectiveness design elements was considered essential in order to encourage ready dissemination of scientifically credible study findings to the real-world clinical settings in which most pediatric patients with OCD receive care.

The background and rationale for the POTS has been described elsewhere (March, Franklin, Nelson, & Foa, 2001) and thus will be discussed only briefly here. The efficacy of SRI pharmacotherapy for pediatric OCD has been well established; Food and Drug Administration (FDA) indication for pediatric OCD has been obtained for clomipramine, sertraline, fluoxetine, and fluvoxamine following multicenter registration trials (DeVeaugh-Geiss et al., 1992; Geller et al., 2001; March et al., 1998; Riddle et al., 2001). Inspection of posttreatment outcomes from these controlled pharmacotherapy trials, however, indicates that SRI pharmacotherapy is neither completely nor universally effective, and the need to develop other treatments and augmentation strategies remains apparent (March et al., 1997). Concerns about relapse on discontinuation of SRIs in OCD (Leonard et al., 1991) and the unknown risks associated with long-term SRI pharmacotherapy (Leonard, March, Rickler, & Allen, 1997) generated interest in whether combining SRI pharmacotherapy with CBT, which appears to be a more durable treatment (March et al., 1994), may protect against loss of treatment gains when the medication is discontinued. One direct comparison of CBT versus the SRI clomipramine for pediatric OCD found that both produced significant symptom reductions on the CY-BOCS at posttreatment and also found an advantage for CBT (de Haan et al., 1998), but there were no controlled studies comparing monotherapy with CBT, pharmacotherapy with an SSRI, and their combination in the same patient population.

Study Design

The POTS was a multicenter, randomized, clinical trial designed to evaluate the relative benefit and durability of four treatments for children and adolescents with OCD: (1) SER, (2) CBT; (3) COMB; and (4) PBO. To this end, POTS employed a balanced 2 (site)× 1 (time) × 4 (treatment) experimental design in Stage I, followed by open discontinuation design in Stage II. Stage I (12 weeks) was a balanced randomized comparison of these four treatments. Notably, patients and treatment providers were blind in the "pills only" conditions of SER or PBO, whereas patients and treatment providers were aware that COMB participants were receiving active medicine. In Phase II, responders to any Stage I treatment advanced to 16 weeks of open follow-up in their assigned condition, during which time all active treatment was discontinued. Nonresponders to treatment at the end of Stage I, any patient relapsing in Stage II, and all Stage I PBO patients at the end of Stage II (if not before) received open treatment tailored to the patient needs.

A volunteer sample of 112 participants between the ages of 7 and 17 inclusive with a primary DSM-IV diagnosis of OCD entered the study; the sample was evenly split between males and females and approximately equal with respect to adolescents ages 12–17 and younger children ages 7–11. Consistent with an intent-to-treat (ITT) analytic model, all patients, regardless of responder status, returned for all scheduled assessments, with the main dependent variables assessed by an independent evaluator. Specifically, in Stage I (12 weeks), patients were assessed at baseline and at Weeks 4, 8, and 12; in Stage II, patients were evaluated in Phase II at weeks 16, 20, 24, and 28. POTS received Institutional Review Board approval at each of the three participating sites.

Results

Results of our ITT analyses indicated a significant advantage for all three active treatments—combined treatment, CBT, and sertraline—compared with placebo (Pediatric OCD Treatment Study Team, 2004). With respect to comparisons of the active treatments, overall combined treatment was particularly effective; it proved superior to CBT and to sertraline, which did not differ from one another. Reflecting the ordering of effect sizes on the scalar CY-BOCS, approximately 54% of the patients who received combined treatment and 39% of those who received CBT alone achieved excellent response (posttreatment CY-BOCS $\leq$ 10), in comparison with approximately 21% of those who received sertraline and 3% who received placebo. We also detected site-by-treatment effects on the CY-BOCS such that CBT alone at the University of Pennsylvania was superior to CBT at Duke University, whereas the reverse was true for sertraline alone; notably, no site-by-treatment effects were found for combined treatment or for placebo, suggesting that the effects of combined treatment are relatively less vulnerable to site effects.

Based on these results, we recommend that children and adolescents with obsessive–compulsive disorder begin treatment with either the combination of CBT and an SSRI or with CBT alone. The addition of medication to CBT alone may be particularly important when CBT is attenuated for some reason; subsequent studies from this same data set will be aimed at determining whether patient factors, therapist effects, or differences in implementing the protocols underlie the observed site effects.

FOUNDATIONS FOR FUTURE STUDIES

Over the course of conducting the POTS, we observed that a substantial proportion of initial inquiries did not progress because the children were already receiving pharmacotherapy with an SRI, which the parents were unwilling to discontinue for the purpose of entering a study. Indeed, for most pediatric patients with OCD treated in the community, the first-line treatment is monotherapy with an SRI. Unfortunately, recommended doses of these medications leave the great majority of patients with clinically significant residual symptoms (March, 1999), and the chances for excellent response (as defined earlier) are lower with medication alone—for example, the results of our study indicate that rates of excellent response in children treated with sertraline only was just 21%. Accordingly, our next phase of research, which has also been funded by NIMH (J. S. March, Duke University; M. E. Franklin, University of Pennsylvania; H. L. Leonard, Brown University, principal investigators), addresses the issue of treatment augmentation (adding an additional treatment to a current treatment), as well as treatment transportability (bringing a treatment developed in a research setting to the community). This study will evaluate the effectiveness of two 12-week treatments that will be added to ongoing medication management for childhood OCD—either full CBT by a psychologist or instructions in CBT by a psychiatrist in the context of medication management. The primary questions of interest to be addressed are: (1) Can CBT augment medication management? and (2) Is a more transportable treatment, in the form of psychiatrist-delivered instructions in CBT, as effective as full CBT by a psychologist? We are currently recruiting children ages 7–17 who are taking an SSRI for OCD and who still experience clinical impairment from OCD.

Using the POTS as a stepping stone, current research efforts in the field of pediatric OCD are now (or shortly will be) focusing on the following eight key areas:

1. More controlled trials comparing medications, CBT, and combination treatment to determine whether medications and CBT are synergistic or additive in their effects on symptom reduction.
2. Follow-up studies to evaluate relapse rates, including examining the utility of booster CBT in reducing risk for relapse.
3. Component analyses, such as a comparison of EX/RP, cognitive therapy, and their combination, to evaluate the relative contributions of specific treatment components to symptom reduction and treatment acceptability.
4. Comparisons of individual- and family-based treatments to determine which is more effective in which children.

5. Development of innovative treatment for OCD subtypes, such as obsessional slowness, primary obsessional OCD, and tic-like OCD, that do not respond well to EX/RP.
6. Targeting treatment innovations to factors, such as family dysfunction, that constrain the application of CBT to patients with OCD.
7. Exporting research treatments to divergent clinical settings and patient populations in order to judge the acceptability and effectiveness of CBT as a treatment for child and adolescent OCD in real-world settings.
8. Once past initial treatment, the management of partial response, treatment resistance, and treatment maintenance and discontinuation.

Edna Foa has set the standard in the field with respect to the development of a programmatic line of research that moves from the study of psychopathology to empirically informed treatment development to evaluation of treatment efficacy and effectiveness. We hope that this same systematic and scientifically informed approach will be widely adopted as we collectively endeavor to better understand, treat, and reach children and adolescents who suffer from OCD.

REFERENCES

Amir, N., Freshman, M., & Foa, E. B. (2000). Family distress and involvement in relatives of obsessive–compulsive disorder patients. *Journal of Anxiety Disorders, 14*(3), 209–217.

Baer, L., Jenike, M. A., Black, D. W., Treece, C., Rosenfeld, R., & Greist, J. (1992). Effect of Axis II diagnoses on treatment outcome with clomipramine in 55 patients with obsessive–compulsive disorder. *Archives of General Psychiatry, 49*(11), 862–866.

Barrett, P., Healy-Farrell, L., & March, J. S. (2004). Cognitive-behavioral family treatment of childhood obsessive–compulsive disorder: A controlled trial. *Journal of the American Academy of Child and Adolescent Psychiatry, 43*, 46–62.

Clarke, G. N. (1995). Improving the transition from basic efficacy research to effectiveness studies: Methodological issues and procedures. *Journal of Consulting and Clinical Psychology, 63*(5), 718–725.

de Haan, E., Hoogduin, K. A., Buitelaar, J. K., & Keijsers, G. P. (1998). Behavior therapy versus clomipramine for the treatment of obsessive–compulsive disorder in children and adolescents. *Journal of the American Academy of Child and Adolescent Psychiatry, 37*(10), 1022–1029.

DeVeaugh-Geiss, J., Moroz, G., Biederman, J., Cantwell, D., Fontaine, R., Greist, J. H., et al. (1992). Clomipramine hydrochloride in childhood and adolescent obsessive–compulsive disorder: A multicenter trial. *Journal of the American Academy of Child and Adolescent Psychiatry, 31*(1), 45–49.

Fals-Stewart, W., Marks, A. P., & Schafer, J. (1993). A comparison of behavioral group therapy and individual behavior therapy in treating obsessive–compulsive disorder. *Journal of Nervous and Mental Disease, 181*(3), 189–193.

Flament, M. F., Koby, E., Rapoport, J. L., Berg, C. J., Zahn, T., Cox, C., et al. (1990). Childhood obsessive–compulsive disorder: A prospective follow-up study. *Journal of Child Psychology and Psychiatry and Allied Disciplines, 31*(3), 363–380.

Flament, M. F., Whitaker, A., Rapoport, J. L., Davies, M., Berg, C. Z., Kalikow, K., et al. (1988). Obsessive–compulsive disorder in adolescence: An epidemiological study. *Journal of the American Academy of Child and Adolescent Psychiatry, 27*(6), 764–771.

Foa, E., & Emmelkamp, P. (1983). *Failures in behavior therapy.* New York: Wiley.

Foa, E. B., & Kozak, M. J. (1996). Psychological treatment for obsessive–compulsive disorder. In M. R. Mavissakalian & R. F. Prien (Eds.), *Long-term treatments of anxiety disorders* (pp. 285–309). Washington, DC: American Psychiatric Press.

Foa, E. B., Steketee, G., Grayson, B., Turner, M., & Latimer, P. (1984). Deliberate exposure and blocking of obsessive–compulsive rituals: Immediate and long-term effects. *Behavior Therapy, 15*(5), 450–472.

Franklin, M. E., & Foa, E. B. (2002). Cognitive-behavioral treatment of obsessive–compulsive disorder. In P. Nathan & J. Gorman (Eds.), *A guide to treatments that work* (2nd ed., pp. 367–386). Oxford, UK: Oxford University Press.

Franklin, M. E., Foa, E. B., & March, J. S. (2003). The Pediatric OCD Treatment Study (POTS): Rationale, design and methods. *Journal of Child and Adolescent Psychopharmacology, 13*(Suppl. 1), 39–52.

Franklin, M. E., Kozak, M. J., Cashman, L. A., Coles, M. E., Rheingold, A. A., & Foa, E. B. (1998). Cognitive-behavioral treatment of pediatric obsessive-compulsive disorder: An open clinical trial. *Journal of the American Academy of Child and Adolescent Psychiatry, 37*(4), 412–419.

Geller, D. A., Hoog, S. L., Heiligenstein, J. H., Ricardi, R. K., Tamura, R., Kluszynski, S., & Jacobson, J. G. (2001). Fluoxetine treatment for obsessive–compulsive disorder in children and adolescents: A placebo-controlled clinical trial. *Journal of the American Academy of Child and Adolescent Psychiatry, 40*, 773–779.

Giulino, L., Gammon, P., Sullivan, K., Franklin, M., Foa, E., Maid, R., & March, J. S. (2002). Is parental report of upper respiratory infection at the onset of obsessive–compulsive disorder suggestive of pediatric autoimmune neuropsychiatric disorder associated with streptococcal infection? *Journal of Child and Adolescent Psychopharmacology, 12*(2), 157–164.

Goodman, W., Rasmussen, S., Foa, E., & Price, L. (1994). Obsessive–compulsive disorder. In R. Prien & D. Robinson (Eds.), *Clinical evaluation of psychotropic drugs: Principles and guidelines* (pp. 431–466). New York: Raven Press.

Kovacs, M. (1996). *The Children's Depression Inventory.* Toronto, Ontario, Canada: Multi-Health Systems.

Leonard, H. L., March, J., Rickler, K. C., & Allen, A. J. (1997). Pharmacology of the selective serotonin reuptake inhibitors in children and adolescents. *Journal of the American Academy of Child and Adolescent Psychiatry, 36*(6), 725–736.

Leonard, H. L., Swedo, S. E., Lenane, M. C., Rettew, D. C., Cheslow, D. L., Hamburger, S. D., & Rapoport, J. L. (1991). A double-blind desipramine substitution during long-term clomipramine treatment in children and adolescents with obsessive–compulsive disorder. *Archives of General Psychiatry, 48*(10), 922–927.

Leonard, H. L., Swedo, S. E., Lenane, M. C., Rettew, D. C., Hamburger, S. D., Bartko, J. J., & Rapoport, J. L. (1993). A 2- to 7-year follow-up study of 54 obsessive–compulsive children and adolescents. *Archives of General Psychiatry, 50*(6), 429–439.

March, J. (1998). *Manual for the Multidimensional Anxiety Scale for Children (MASC).* Toronto, Ontario, Canada: Multi-Health Systems.

March, J. (1999). Current status of pharmacotherapy for pediatric anxiety disorders. In D. Beidel (Ed.), *Treating anxiety disorders in youth: Current problems and future solutions* (pp. 42–62). Washington, DC: Anxiety Disorders Association of America.

March, J., Frances, A., Kahn, D., & Carpenter, D. (1997). Expert consensus guidelines: Treatment of obsessive–compulsive disorder. *Journal of Clinical Psychiatry, 58*(Suppl. 4), 1–72.

March, J., & Mulle, K. (1998). *OCD in children and adolescents: A cognitive-behavioral treatment manual.* New York: Guilford Press.

March, J. S., Biederman, J., Wolkow, R., Safferman, A., Mardekian, J., Cook, E. H., et al. (1998). Sertraline in children and adolescents with obsessive–compulsive disorder: A multicenter randomized controlled trial [see comments]. *Journal of the American Medical Association, 280*(20), 1752–1756.

March, J. S., Franklin, M., Nelson, A., & Foa, E. (2001). Cognitive-behavioral psychotherapy for pediatric obsessive–compulsive disorder. *Journal of Clinical Child Psychology, 30*(1), 8–18.

March, J. S., Mulle, K., & Herbel, B. (1994). Behavioral psychotherapy for children and adolescents with obsessive–compulsive disorder: An open trial of a new protocol-driven treatment package. *Journal of the American Academy of Child and Adolescent Psychiatry, 33*(3), 333–341.

McDougle, C. J., Goodman, W. K., Leckman, J. F., Barr, L. C., Heninger, G. R., & Price, L. H. (1993). The efficacy of fluvoxamine in obsessive–compulsive disorder: Effects of comorbid chronic tic disorder. *Journal of Clinical Psychopharmacology, 13*(5), 354–358.

Pediatric OCD Treatment Study Team. (2004). Cognitive-behavioral therapy, sertraline, and their combination for children and adolescents with obsessive–compulsive disorder: The Pediatric OCD Treatment Study (POTS) randomized controlled trial. *Journal of the American Medical Association, 292,* 1969–1976.

Piacentini, J., Bergman, R. L., Jacobs, C., McCracken, J. T., & Kretchman, J. (2002). Open trial of cognitive behavior therapy for childhood obsessive–compulsive disorder. *Journal of Anxiety Disorders, 16,* 207–219.

Piacentini, J., Jaffer, M., Bergman, R. L., McCracken, J., & Keller, M. (2001). *Measuring impairment in childhood OCD: Psychometric properties of the COIS.* Paper presented at the annual meeting of the American Academy of Child and Adolescent Psychiatry, Honolulu, HI.

Rasmussen, S. A., & Eisen, J. L. (1990). Epidemiology of obsessive–compulsive disorder. *Journal of Clinical Psychiatry, 53,* 10–13.

Riddle, M. A., Reeve, E. A., Yaryura-Tobias, J. A., Yang, H. M., Claghorn, J. L., Gaffney, G., et al. (2001). Fluvoxamine for children and adolescents with obsessive–compulsive disorder: A randomized, controlled, multicenter trial. *Journal of the American Academy of Child and Adolescent Psychiatry, 40*(2), 222–229.

Scahill, L., Riddle, M. A., McSwiggin-Hardin, M., Ort, S. I., King, R. A., Goodman, W. K., et al. (1997). Children's Yale–Brown Obsessive–Compulsive Scale: Reliability and validity. *Journal of the American Academy of Child and Adolescent Psychiatry, 36*(6), 844–852.

Silverman, W., & Albano, A. (1996). *The Anxiety Disorders Interview Schedule for DSM-IV, Child and Parent Versions.* San Antonio, TX: The Psychological Corporation.

Soechting, I., & March, J. (2002). Cognitive aspects of obsessive–compulsive disorder in children. In R. Frost & G. Steketee (Eds.), *Cognitive approaches to obsessions and compulsions: Theory, assessment, and treatment* (pp. 299–314). Amsterdam, The Netherlands: Pergamon/Elsevier Science.

Swedo, S. E., Leonard, H. L., Garvey, M., Mittleman, B., Allen, A. J., Perlmutter, S., et al. (1998). Pediatric autoimmune neuropsychiatric disorders associated with streptococcal infections: Clinical description of the first 50 cases. *American Journal of Psychiatry, 155*(2), 264–271.

van Balkom, A. J. L. M., de Haan, E., van Oppen, P., Spinhoven, P., Hoogduin, K. A. L., Vermeulen, A. W. A., & van Dyck, R. (1998). Cognitive and behavioral therapies alone and in combination with fluvoxamine in the treatment of obsessive–compulsive disorder. *Journal of Nervous and Mental Disease, 186,* 492–499.

Vogel, P. A., Stiles, T. C., & Gotestam, K. G. (2004). Adding cognitive therapy elements to exposure therapy for obsessive–compulsive disorder: A controlled study. *Behavioral and Cognitive Psychotherapy, 32,* 275–290.

Wever, C., & Rey, J. M. (1997). Juvenile obsessive–compulsive disorder. *Australian and New Zealand Journal of Psychiatry, 31,* 105–113.

10

Treatment of Panic Disorder

Outcomes and Basic Processes

LAURA B. ALLEN
DAVID H. BARLOW

Panic disorder is one of the most widely studied anxiety disorders. Research on the phenomenon of panic dates back to the 1960s, and these early investigations have laid the groundwork for how we conceptualize and treat anxiety and its disorders. The essential feature of panic disorder is the experience of repeated, unexpected "panic attacks," which are defined as discrete episodes of intense fear or discomfort, accompanied by a number of physical and cognitive changes. At least four of the physical changes listed in the fourth edition of the *Diagnostic and Statistical Manual of Mental Disorders* (DSM-IV; American Psychiatric Association, 1994) must be present during a typical, full-blown panic attack; three or fewer symptoms accompanying the same rush of fear or discomfort is considered a limited-symptom panic attack. Although heightened levels of anxiety may exist prior to or following a panic attack, the attack itself is unique in that the intense rush of fear and physical symptoms usually peaks in less than 15 minutes. However, many individuals may experience repeated panic attacks over the course of several hours, which can often feel like a single episode.

Although panic attacks are common in other anxiety disorders (e.g., worry-triggered panic attacks in generalized anxiety disorder, or panic attacks in social situations in social phobia), panic disorder can be distinguished from other anxiety disorders by the apparent lack of a trigger that causes the attack. "Out of the blue" attacks happen for no apparent reason, or in unexpected situations, such that an individual may find it difficult to identify a clear trigger. Often, the lack of a definable trigger results in fear and/or avoidance of situations that the individual assumes may induce a panic attack or that would not allow for escape if a panic attack should occur—a condition known as agoraphobia. However, not all individuals who experience panic attacks develop agoraphobia (Craske & Barlow, 1988). Although the diagnosis requires that the individual has experienced at least several unexpected panic attacks, as the disorder progresses, someone with panic disorder will typically panic in situations or contexts that have previously been associated with panic.

INITIAL STUDIES ON PANIC DISORDER AND AGORAPHOBIA

Beginning in the 1960s, psychological approaches to treating agoraphobia (panic disorder) began to develop out of an emerging understanding of the interaction between cognitive, physiological, and behavioral factors contributing to the development and maintenance of anxiety disorders. Yet the dominating psychological theories of the time still supported relaxation strategies as a way of overcoming fearful responses. Joseph Wolpe first identified the concept of systematic desensitization (SD), and his work focused on implementing progressive relaxation strategies in the context of feared stimuli as a way of conditionally associating relaxation with the stimulus (Wolpe, 1958, 1973). In addition, some patients with anxiety and phobias were also asked to inhale mixtures of 40–65% CO_2 and air, so the relaxation after blowing off the CO_2 would be enhanced. Although his aim was to provide the participants with greater relaxation, he was more likely providing a context for experiencing intense physiological arousal that had been previously associated with anxiety (what we now refer to as interoceptive exposure). These techniques proved moderately helpful for treating specific phobias but were less effective in modifying more broad-ranging, complex phobias such as agoraphobia.

More specific exposure strategies for treating phobias began to develop in the next decade. Agras, Leitenberg, and Barlow (1968) examined the impact of selective social reinforcement on agoraphobic behavior. The treatment was based on an understanding of learning theory and the assumption that the avoidance of fearful stimuli (i.e., agoraphobia) could be changed through incorporating positive reinforcement. Therapists would alternate patterns of reinforcement and no reinforcement to examine the impact of positive social reinforcement on two different behavioral measures: time spent away and distance walked from the clinic. As expected, patients improved significantly on either behavioral measure during reinforcement periods (as compared with nonreinforced trials), and one patient even modified her behavior according to a differential pattern of reinforcement (i.e., alternating reinforcement for time spent away and then for distance walked). However, perhaps the most interesting finding was that individuals began to improve even during the baseline phase of the study, prior to the implementation of any reinforcement strategies. It appeared as though mere exposure to feared stimuli was resulting in some improvement and that positive social reinforcement may have facilitated this process.

Although these and other studies (e.g., Watson & Marks, 1971) paved the way for a new understanding of the principles of exposure to anxiety and panic, efficacious treatments for these and other disorders were virtually nonexistent. Even though research demonstrated fear reduction in the laboratory, most of the patients undergoing these procedures still continued to suffer from significant levels of anxiety, panic, and residual avoidance. In a 1982 review of 24 exposure-based treatment studies for panic disorder with agoraphobia (PDA), it was clear that 35% of those in treatment received little or no benefit (Jansson & Öst, 1982). It was not until several years later that cognitive-behavioral therapy (CBT) for PDA was introduced.

COGNITIVE-BEHAVIORAL CONCEPTUALIZATION OF PANIC DISORDER

In the 1980s, several areas of research allowed us to refine our conceptualization of panic disorder, providing answers about how biological and psychological vulnerabilities and conditioning experiences contribute to the development and maintenance of panic disorder and agoraphobia. This era proved to be a revolution in treatment development for anxiety disorders, as standardized, efficacious treatments were finally implemented in laboratories and clinics (e.g., Barlow, 1986; Barlow et al., 1984). Although these much-needed treatments improved significantly on the strategies used in earlier decades, questions still remained about how complex conditioning processes factored into the development of panic disorder and why some individuals did not improve after treatment.

Vulnerabilities to Developing PDA

Biological, or physiological, vulnerabilities are generally referred to as elevated autonomic response and reactivity (Barlow, 2002; Bouton, Mineka, & Barlow, 2001). Enhanced autonomic arousal may be caused by a number of factors, including changes in a variety of neurotransmitter systems and nonspecific genetic transmission (see Barlow, 2002, for a comprehensive review of biological vulnerabilities). One psychological vulnerability implicated in the development of panic disorder (PD) or PDA that has received considerable attention and empirical support in the laboratory is known as "anxiety sensitivity" (Reiss, Peterson, Gursky, & McNally, 1986). Anxiety sensitivity refers to an individual's attentiveness to and perception of physical changes associated with anxiety. Generally, individuals with high anxiety sensitivity are highly attuned to physiological changes in the body and have the tendency to focus anxiety on these physical sensations. Scores on a measure of anxiety sensitivity, the Anxiety Sensitivity Index (ASI; Peterson & Reiss, 1987), have been shown to predict panic attack history beyond trait anxiety and negative affect (Lilienfeld, 1997). In two separate studies using military participants, scores on the ASI predicted the development of spontaneous panic attacks 5 weeks after a highly stressful period (basic training), and anxiety sensitivity was symptom-specific for anxiety and not depression (Schmidt, Lerew, & Jackson, 1997, 1999). These data implicate the role of anxiety sensitivity in the pathogenesis of panic disorder. This vulnerability, in turn, may be part of what we have termed a "generalized psychological vulnerability" to experience salient external and internal events as uncontrollable as a function of early learning experiences (Barlow, 2002). Biological and psychological vulnerabilities may then synergize in the genesis of panic disorder.

Conditioning Experiences

The term "fear of fear" refers to the fear of bodily sensations associated with panic attacks (e.g., heart palpitations, dizziness, sweating; Goldstein & Chambless, 1978). Even a single, unexpected panic attack can be frightening enough to produce fear of bodily sensations, depending on the contextual and experiential factors present at the time of the attack. "Interoceptive conditioning" happens when physiological arousal and bodily sensations become paired with intense fear, pain, or distress, such that the physiological sensations themselves can elicit a fear response. This is consistent with the traumatic nature of panic attacks, as an "unexpected" panic attack has no definable external trigger, so the focus of the fear is directed internally—toward the individual's own body. Interoceptive conditioning often occurs at an unconscious level, where even subtle, undetectable somatic changes may precipitate panic. As a result, panic attacks may appear to be "out of the blue." Fear of bodily sensations is also related to a cognitive misappraisal of the meaning or consequences of the sensations. For example, physiological arousal may be perceived as a sign of imminent danger or loss of control, and this evaluation may happen at both an unconscious and a conscious level.

In an attempt to bring emerging research on the pathophysiology of panic together with current understandings of learning theory in the etiology of panic disorder, Bouton and colleagues (2001) suggest that initial panic attacks become associated with a variety of contextual factors—both internal and external—present at the time of the attack. When these contextual cues are present in a nonpanic situation, cognitive, behavioral, and physiological changes occur. This preparatory response in anticipation of future danger is what we call "anxiety." Panic, however, is a surge of physiological responding that occurs only in the presence of an immediate threat. Although these two emotional states can be distinguished by the quality and intensity of physiological changes, panic and anxiety are not necessarily mutually exclusive. Modern learning theory suggests that anxiety may in fact precipitate panic, as the physiological changes experienced during anxiety become conditioned stimuli for the pending attack (Bouton et al., 2001). This process happens at both conscious and unconscious levels, whereby an individual may experience mild innocuous physiological changes (e.g., increase in heart rate) and begin to worry about panicking. In addition, virtually undetectable levels of increased physiological arousal can initiate a panic attack through the conditioned associations, even though the individual is unaware of it. Subtle conditioning events then begin to influence behavior, such that the association between physiological activity and fear (panic) become strengthened (LeDoux, 1996). These hypotheses are supported by brain imaging techniques that have demonstrated both conscious and unconscious conditioning processes (Öhman, 1999). As the associations between the physical sensations of anxiety and the experience of panic become strengthened, there is greater risk for panic, as normal fluctuations in the body begin to initiate attacks. Subsequently, the occurrence of frightening, unexpected panic attacks becomes associated with a number of external stimuli, particularly situations in which the individual has experienced a panic attack before or situations that may not allow for easy escape if panic were to occur (e.g., public transportation, crowds, long-distance driving), resulting in substantial avoidance of these cues (i.e., agoraphobia). As such, modern learning theory suggests that the experience of fear becomes paired with a variety of contextual factors, including both internal body sensations and external situations (Bouton et al., 2001). Theoretically, eliciting any one of the contextual cues associated with panic should produce some fear, depending on the strength of the association and other factors (e.g., physiological arousal) present at the time of the exposure.

Emotion Provocation

In the late 1970s and 1980s, emotional processing theories of anxiety reduction were being developed and drawing from emerging data in the fields of learning, cognitive science, and neuroscience (Lang, 1977a, 1977b, 1979, 1985). Although these accounts agreed that exposure was a necessary component to anxiety reduction, proponents of emotional processing theories viewed emotional processing *during* exposure as the key ingredient to successful treatment. According to this model, anxiety and fear are responses stored in the memory and are composed of a number of different components, including stimulus, response, and emotional meaning. To ensure successful fear reduction, each of the components that make up the fear structure must be accessed. Thus, even if the association between a stimulus and fear response (panic) is activated and physiological arousal decreases (habituation), it is still possible that subjective fear will remain high. Emotional processing theory would explain these findings by stating that the emotional meaning component (subjective fear) was not fully accessed during the exposure, thus preventing the subjective fear from decreasing and inhibiting a full decrease in anxiety.

Foa and Kozak (1986) presented a theory of emotional processing that added an additional twist to traditional accounts. They suggested that successful fear reduction can occur only when the fear network (association) is accessed and the individual receives information incompatible with the existing association (emotional meaning component) in memory. Emotional change results from the integration of this new information in the fear structure, and any circumstances that inhibit the intake of the new nonfearful information will prevent full habituation and extinction of the fearful association.

In a practical context, Foa and Kozak's (1986) theory suggests that exposures must be conducted so that the individual is not being distracted in any way and is fully attentive to all the emotional, cognitive, and physiological changes during the exposure. Craske, Street, and Barlow (1989) examined whether patients who were instructed to focus on physiological and cognitive changes during exposure did better over the course of treatment than patients who were instructed to actively distract themselves during exposure. Although the groups did not differ at posttreatment or follow-up, the focused exposure group improved significantly from posttreatment to follow-up, whereas the distraction group deteriorated somewhat. Similar results were found in a study of patients with obsessive–compulsive disorder (Grayson, Foa, & Steketee, 1982), suggesting the importance of attending to all contextual experiences during an exposure task.

CURRENT APPROACHES TO TREATMENT

With an increasingly greater understanding of the causes of and maintaining factors for panic disorder, the development of cognitive-behavioral treatments proved to be a revolutionary breakthrough for individuals suffering from anxiety and panic. Cognitive therapy, which was originally developed to treat depression (Beck, 1972; Beck, Rush, Shaw, & Emery, 1979), was modified for anxious cognitions and became a staple of anxiety reduction procedures. In addition to situational exposures, induction of feared somatic sensations in the laboratory or office to allow for extinction of conditioned somatic cues (interoceptive exposure) proved to be beneficial for panic sufferers (Barlow, 1986; Barlow & Cerny, 1988). Finally, controlled studies using manualized treatment protocols were able to provide empirical support for the efficacy of cognitive-behavioral treatments for PDA (Barlow & Craske, 1988).

Cognitive-Behavioral Treatment

CBT is considered the "gold standard" treatment for panic disorder (Craske & Barlow, 2001). The strategies used are derived directly from learning theory and emotional processing theory, whereby the goal of treatment is for the individual to experience anxiety and panic in a variety of feared contexts and learn that the physical sensations of panic are not harmful. The process is not one of "unlearning" the panic response but rather learning to change responses (action tendencies) to the feared stimuli, such that a new, nonfearful association with the stimuli is learned.

Modern learning theory refers to this process as extinction, in which repeated exposure to previous conditioned stimuli (somatic sensations, agoraphobic situations) without escape or avoidance allows the patient to learn that those stimuli are not dangerous or harmful. According to this theory, exposing an individual to as many contextual cues as possible will provide the most significant anxiety reduction, as the panic response following exposure to conditioned stimuli is eventually extinguished (Bouton et al., 2001). In this case, contextual factors include both external triggers and internal cues. As such, successful treatment may also include interoceptive exposure (exposure to physical sensations in the body), providing another opportunity for new learning of a nonfearful association to take place.

Current approaches to treating panic disorder with CBT have also been based on Foa and Kozak's (1986) emotional processing theory. During *in vivo* exposure, patients enter agoraphobic situations and are asked to stay in the situation until their anxiety decreases. However, it is essential that the patient experience significant levels of anxiety and/or panic to allow for habituation, which is consistent with Foa and Kozak's model. Most important, the patient must never escape from the situation; this would prevent the subjective experience of fear (emotional meaning component of the fear structure) from decreasing. Furthermore, patients are encouraged to experience anxiety to its fullest, without attempting to avoid or control it in any way, such that the fear structure can be accessed completely. As such, all "safety signals" (i.e., any item the patient carries that makes him or her feel "safe" in case of panic—typically medication, water bottles, reading materials) and "safety behaviors" (i.e., any behavior that reduces anxiety in a situation, such as distraction, deep breathing, and seeking reassurance from others) are eliminated during an exposure. These precautions allow for full access to the fear structure in the memory of the patient, as well as an opportunity for the patient to take in new information (panic attacks are not dangerous) that is incompatible with the existing association in the fear network.

Medication

The use of psychopharmacological treatments, such as benzodiazepines and antidepressants, is another approach to treating individuals with PDA. Benzodiazepines such as lorazepam and clonazepam act quickly on the central nervous system by reducing the body's physiological arousal, and antidepressants are taken on a regular basis and exert their effects by altering a variety of neurotransmitter, particularly serotonin, systems in an undetermined manner. Many individuals receiving CBT for panic disorder are also receiving some form of concurrent psychopharmacological treatment, although the use of benzodiazepines on an "as needed" basis is discouraged when receiving CBT. Using a short-acting medication to reduce anxiety may be conceptualized as a safety signal, which may interfere with fully accessing fear during an exposure. Use of the medication during panic episodes may also subtly reinforce the idea that panic and anxiety are dangerous emotions, which would prevent learning of nonfearful associations from taking place.

A large-scale, multisite clinical trial examined the efficacy of CBT, imipramine (a tricyclic antidepressant), and their combination on treatment for panic disorder (Barlow, Gorman, Shear, & Woods, 2000). Patients were randomly assigned to one of five groups: CBT alone, CBT plus imipramine, imipramine alone, pill placebo, or CBT plus pill placebo. All patients received 3 months of weekly treatment. After treatment, "responders" (rated "much improved" and having no more than "mild" severity of panic symptoms by an independent evaluator) participated in a "maintenance phase," in which treatments were continued and they were seen monthly for the next 6 months. After maintenance, treatments were discontinued, and these individuals were then followed for another 6 months (see Figure 10.1).

After acute treatment, all active treatments were significantly more effective than placebo, with no differences among treatments. Thus combination treatments (CBT plus imipramine) did not confer an advantage over monotherapy. After the maintenance phase, the combined (CBT plus imipramine) group appeared to have improved more than the other groups, including CBT plus placebo, on at least one measure, supporting the hypothesis that the combined treatment would prove effective; but the differential clinical effect was not dramatic. When follow-up data were analyzed (6-month treatment-free period after the maintenance phase), only two groups—CBT alone and CBT plus placebo—were significantly better than placebo. The effects of the two medication conditions had diminished once

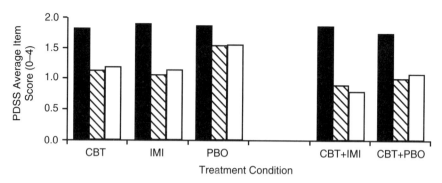

FIGURE 10.1. Comparison of baseline, acute, and maintenance treatment for in-tent-to-treat (ITT) sample based on PDSS average item score ($n = 312$). CBT, cogni-tive-behavioral treatment; IMI, imipramine; PBO, placebo. From Barlow, Gorman, Shear, & Woods (2000). Copyright 2000 by the American Medical Association. Reprinted by permission.

treatment was withdrawn. In addition, the combined-treatment group had the highest relapse rate at follow-up (48.28%), followed by imipramine alone (40%). Relapse rates for CBT plus placebo were comparable to those of CBT alone (16.67% vs. 17.86%, respectively). Therefore, none of the data suggested that either medication alone or combined treatment was su-perior to CBT once treatment was removed. In fact, the findings suggest just the opposite, in that CBT seemed to provide a more durable effect.

DESCRIPTION OF CBT FOR PDA

Before beginning any psychological treatment, a careful assessment of the patient's presenting concerns is an essential first step. Because the occur-rence of panic attacks is common in other anxiety disorders, it is important that the clinician be able to appropriately diagnose the patient based on the description of current symptoms. Once differential diagnoses have been made and a principal diagnosis of panic disorder with or without agora-phobia has been assigned, treatment can commence. The description of treatment provided here is a modification of the treatment manual *Mastery of Your Anxiety and Panic, 3rd Edition* (MAP-3; Craske, Barlow, & Meadows, 2000).

The first treatment session helps therapist and patient develop a working conceptualization of the patient's current difficulties, including frequency of panic, interoceptive sensitivity, and degree of agoraphobic avoidance. An overview of the treatment structure, including treatment components, is pro-vided, and the importance of session attendance, self-monitoring, and home-work completion between sessions are emphasized. Therapist and patient build rapport through discussion of the patient's anxious patterns of responding and how attempts to avoid situations and other triggers for panic have interfered in the patient's life. Using the patient's own examples, the therapist weaves specific descriptions of panic situations into the "three-component model" of anxiety and panic, which presents the interrelation of physiological sensations, cognitions, and behaviors as contributing to the cycle of anxious responding. Treatment focuses on targeting each of these components to help break the cycle, beginning with physiological arousal, then cognitions, and then behaviors. Finally, the therapist provides some general psychoeducation about the physiological differences between anxiety and panic and how the physical changes that occur in the body during the "fight-or-flight" response are necessary for protection in case of an actual threat. Although the clinician may want to briefly address a patient's inquiry about the causes of anxiety and panic, it is important to keep the discussion focused on the present moment. For homework, the patient is asked to complete several monitoring forms, including a Daily Panic Attack and Anxiety Record (DPAAR; Craske et al., 2000), as well as an illustration of the three-component model with examples from a recent panic episode.

The next several sessions are devoted to exploring the patient's sensitivity to interoceptive (somatic) cues. The therapist conducts a "symptom induction test" during a session, consisting of the patient engaging in a number of activities designed to induce physiological responses similar to those experienced during a panic attack. Some of these activities include: breathing through a thin straw for 120 seconds, spinning while standing for 60 seconds, hyperventilating for 60 seconds, and maintaining complete body muscle tension for 120 seconds. Following each task, the patient is asked to rate his or her anxiety level on a 0–8 scale (0 = *no anxiety*, 8 = *extreme anxiety*), to describe the physical sensations experienced during the task, and to rate the similarity of the physical sensations to those during a naturally occurring panic attack. The therapist selects the three activities that produced the most anxiety and assigns the symptom induction test for homework. The patient is encouraged to practice the three assigned symptom induction activities in a variety of setting and contexts, noting how the perceived dangerousness of the situation can alter the response to the same activity.

The next session focuses on conducting interoceptive exposure using the three most difficult symptom induction tests. The therapist and patient practice several trials of interoceptive exposure during session, although the patient benefits most from practicing interoceptive exposure for homework. During interoceptive exposure, the patient is asked to repeatedly engage in the symptom induction test until his or her *anxiety* about the physical sensations has decreased to a 2 or less. It is important to remind the patient that, although the physiological arousal may remain high, his or her subjective experience of the physical changes will decrease in between trials and between sessions. For homework, the patient is assigned daily interoceptive exposure practices, as well as a monitoring form for tracking anxious cognitions prior to or during panic attacks.

Sessions 4 and 5 are typically devoted to identifying cognitive misappraisals of the dangerousness and feared consequences of panic attacks and to implementing cognitive restructuring strategies. In these sessions, it is important that the clinician push the patient to identify the frightening cognitions associated with a panic attack (e.g., that he or she will die, have a heart attack, crash the car, etc.). Once several "core" fears have been identified, the therapist assists the patient in challenging these fears. The therapist explains two cognitive errors common to individuals experiencing anxiety and panic: probability overestimation and catastrophizing. "Probability overestimation" refers to the tendency of anxious individuals to overestimate the likelihood of feared events actually occurring. For example, a patient with panic disorder may estimate the likelihood of having a car accident while panicking in the car at 50%, despite having always been able to safely pull off to the side of the road. "Catastrophizing," on the other hand, refers to the tendency of anxious individuals to think that the worst possible outcome will come true. A patient may automatically assume that he or she will die in a car accident caused by panic, even though less catastrophic outcomes are much more likely. The therapist helps the patient challenge these cognitive errors by examining the actual likelihood of the feared event occurring, based on evidence from the patient's past experience. In addition, the patient is instructed on how to assess his or her ability to cope with the worst possible outcome, should it actually occur. For homework, the patient is asked to monitor anxious cognitions, identify appropriate cognitive errors, and challenge cognitions through cognitive restructuring strategies. Interoceptive exposures are also practiced for homework.

Midtreatment (Session 6) focuses on reviewing the patient's progress and preparing for situational exposures. Successes with interoceptive exposure and cognitive strategies are emphasized, and areas in which the patient needs to continue to apply the skills are highlighted. The rationale for situational, or *in vivo*, exposures is presented, and the importance of preventing avoidance of emotional or physiological arousal is also stressed. In an effort to plan appropriate exposures, the patient is asked to construct a fear and avoidance hierarchy (FAH; Craske et al., 2000). The FAH is a list of 10 feared situations, allowing for a range from mild to severe fear and avoidance. The patient is also asked to write a list of safety signals and safety behaviors, so the therapist can prevent the patient's use of these avoidance strategies.

The final six sessions are spent designing and implementing *in vivo* exposures, based on the patient's success with previous exposures and progression on the FAH. Ideally, all safety signals and safety behaviors are eliminated prior to any exposure, and an exposure to a situation lower on the hierarchy done without safety signals or behaviors is more effective than one higher on the hierarchy done with safety signals or behaviors. Effective exposures elicit significant anxiety and/or panic, while the patient is able to remain in the situation until anxiety decreases. Escape from an exposure should always be prevented, as leaving a situation during the height of panic can serve to reinforce the situation as dangerous. Several exposure tasks are assigned for homework after each session, and the patient is instructed to increase the difficulty of the tasks, if necessary, by adding interoceptive cues (e.g., drinking caffeine, hyperventilating, etc.) during the situational exposure.

At the final session (Session 12), the therapist reviews the patient's progress and reminds the patient that continued practice and application of skills learned is essential to maintaining gains made and improving functioning. Residual agoraphobia is a predictor of relapse (Fava, Zielezny, Savron, & Grandi, 1995), so the patient is urged to tackle all fears listed on the FAH. Finally, the patient is reminded that some symptoms of panic may return during times of stress and that implementation of the treatment strategies is essential to preventing relapse.

Intensive Treatment Program

Although most CBT protocols for PDA suggest 12 to 15 sessions as an appropriate treatment schedule, our clinic has also developed an intensive treatment program for PDA that condenses the 12-session treatment into 8 days. The same components of psychoeducation, interoceptive exposure, and cognitive restructuring are used, although the primary focus of the treatment is on *in vivo* exposure. On the fourth and fifth days of treatment, the therapist spends all day with the patient in a variety of situations outside the clinic. From elevators to subways to airplanes, the therapist pushes the patient to tackle the most feared situation on the hierarchy as early as possible. Although this is a relatively new treatment, data from our clinic suggest that individuals who participated in the intensive treatment program have comparable response rates to those who participated in the standard 12 session treatment and have maintained their gains at follow-up (Morrissette, Spiegel, & Heinrichs, 2005).

FUTURE DIRECTIONS

Decades of research on the nature and treatment of anxiety have begun to illuminate the complex interplay between emotional, behavioral, and neurobiological factors that contribute to the development and maintenance of panic disorder. We now have efficacious treatments for PDA that provide significant improvement for 70–80% of patients. Of course, this means that 20–30% of people still suffer from anxiety and panic, and others may not be entirely free of symptoms.

We will continue to advance in deepening our understanding of the nature of emotional disorders, and this will spark additional innovations in treatment. As schools of therapy disappear with the emergence of evidence-based, empirically supported treatment principles (Barlow, 2004), we will focus our efforts on principles of emotion regulation and dysregulation, and most likely arrive at a set of therapeutic procedures widely applicable to emotional disorders (Barlow, Allen, & Choate, 2004). These advances will be due, in no small part, to some of the pioneering work of Edna Foa.

REFERENCES

Agras, W. S., Leitenberg, H., & Barlow, D. H. (1968). Social reinforcement in the modification of agoraphobia. *Archives of General Psychiatry, 19,* 423–427.

American Psychiatric Association. (1994). *Diagnostic and statistical manual of mental disorders* (4th ed.). Washington, DC: Author.

Barlow, D. H. (1986). Behavioral conception and treatment of panic. *Psychopharmacology Bulletin, 22,* 802–806.

Barlow, D. H. (2002). *Anxiety and its disorders: The nature and treatment of anxiety and panic* (2nd ed.). New York: Guilford Press.

Barlow, D. H. (2004). Psychological treatments. *American Psychologist, 59,* 869–878.

Barlow, D. H., Allen, L. B., & Choate, M. L. (2004). Towards a unified treatment for emotional disorders. *Behavior Therapy, 35,* 205–230.

Barlow, D. H., & Cerny, J. A. (1988). *Psychological treatment of panic.* New York: Guilford Press.

Barlow, D. H., Cohen, A. S., Waddell, M., Vermilyea, J. A., Klosko, J. S., Blanchard, E. B., & Di Nardo, P. A. (1984). Panic and generalized anixety disorders: Nature and treatment. *Behavior Therapy, 15,* 431–449.

Barlow, D. H., & Craske, M. G. (1988). *Master of your anxiety and panic.* Albany, NY: Graywind.

Barlow, D. H., Gorman, J. M., Shear, M. K., & Woods, S. W. (2000). Cognitive-behavioral therapy, imipramine, or their combination for panic disorder: A randomized controlled trial. *Journal of the American Medical Association, 283,* 2529–2536.

Beck, A. T. (1972). *Depression: Causes and treatment.* Philadelphia: University of Pennsylvania Press. (Original work published 1967)

Beck, A. T., Rush, A. J., Shaw, B. F., & Emery, G. (1979). *Cognitive therapy of depression.* New York: Guilford Press.

Bouton, M. E., Mineka, S., & Barlow, D. H. (2001). A modern learning theory perspective on the etiology of panic disorder. *Psychological Review, 108,* 4–32.

Craske, M. G., & Barlow, D. H. (1988). A review of the relationship between panic and avoidance. *Clinical Psychology Review, 8,* 667–685.

Craske, M. G., & Barlow, D. H. (2001). Panic disorder and agoraphobia. In D. H. Barlow (Ed.), *Clinical handbook of psychological disorders* (3rd ed., pp. 1–59). New York: Guilford Press.

Craske, M. G., Barlow, D. H., & Meadows, E. A. (2000). *Mastery of your anxiety and panic: Therapist guide for anxiety, panic, and agoraphobia* (3rd ed.). Boulder, CO: Graywind.

Craske, M. G., Street, L., & Barlow, D. H. (1989). Instructions to focus upon or distract from internal cues during exposure treatment for agoraphobic avoidance. *Behaviour Research and Therapy, 27,* 663–672.

Fava, G. A., Zielezny, M., Savron, G., & Grandi, S. (1995). Long-term effects of behavioural treatment for panic disorder and agoraphobia. *British Journal of Psychiatry, 166,* 87–92.

Foa, E., & Kozak, M. (1986). Emotional processing of fear: Exposure to corrective information. *Psychological Bulletin, 99,* 20–35.

Goldstein, A., & Chambless, D. (1978). A reanalysis of agoraphobia. *Behavior Therapy, 9,* 47–59.

Grayson, J. B., Foa, E. B., & Steketee, G. (1982). Habituation during exposure treatment: Distraction versus attention-focusing. *Behaviour Research and Therapy, 20,* 323–328.

Jansson, L., & Öst, L.-G. (1982). Behavioral treatments for agoraphobia: An evaluative review. *Clinical Psychology Review, 2,* 311–336.

Lang, P. J. (1977a). Imagery in therapy: An information processing analysis of fear. *Behavior Therapy, 8,* 862–886.

Lang, P. J. (1977b). Physiological assessment of anxiety and fear. In J. D. Cone & R. A. Hawkins (Eds.), *Behavioral assessment: New directions in clinical psychology* (pp. 178–195). New York: Brunner/Mazel.

Lang, P. J. (1979). A bio-informational theory of emotional imagery. *Psychophysiology, 16,* 495–512.

Lang, P. J. (1985). The cognitive psychophysiology of emotion: Fear and anxiety. In A. H. Tuma & J. D. Maser (Eds.), *Anxiety and the anxiety disorders* (pp. 131–170). Hillsdale, NJ: Erlbaum.

LeDoux, J. E. (1996). *The emotional brain: The mysterious underpinnings of emotional life.* New York: Simon & Schuster.

Lilienfeld, S. O. (1997). The relation of anxiety sensitivity to higher and lower order personality dimensions: Implications for the etiology of panic attacks. *Journal of Abnormal Psychology, 106,* 539–544.

Morrissette, S. B., Spiegel, D. A., & Heinrichs, N. (2005). Sensation-focused intensive treatment for panic disorder with moderate to severe agoraphobia. *Cognitive and Behavioral Practice, 12,* 17–29.

Öhman, A. (1999). Distinguishing unconscious from conscious emotional processes: Methodological considerations and theoretical implications. In T. Dalgleish & M. Power (Eds.), *Handbook of cognition and emotion* (pp. 321–352). Chichester, UK: Wiley.

Peterson, R. A., & Reiss, S. (1987). *Anxiety Sensitivity Index manual.* Worthington, OH: IDS.

Reiss, S., Peterson, R. A., Gursky, D. M., & McNally, R. J. (1986). Anxiety sensitivity, anxiety frequency, and the prediction of fearfulness. *Behaviour Research and Therapy, 24,* 1–8.

Schmidt, N. B., Lerew, D. R., & Jackson, R. J. (1997). The role of anxiety sensitivity in the pathogenesis of panic: Prospective evaluation of spontaneous panic attacks during acute stress. *Journal of Abnormal Psychology, 106,* 355–364.

Schmidt, N. B., Lerew, D. R., & Jackson, R. J. (1999). Prospective evaluation of anxiety sensitivity in the pathogenesis of panic: Replication and extension. *Journal of Abnormal Psychology, 108,* 532–537.

Watson, J. P., & Marks, I. M. (1971). Relevant and irrelevant fear in flooding: A crossover study of phobic patients. *Behavior Therapy, 2,* 275–293.

Wolpe, J. (1958). *Psychotherapy by reciprocal inhibition.* Stanford, CA: Stanford University Press.

Wolpe, J. (1973). *The practice of behavior therapy* (2nd ed.). Elmsford, NY: Pergamon Press.

11

The Nature and Treatment of Generalized Anxiety Disorder

EVELYN BEHAR

T. D. BORKOVEC

Three decades of scientific research on worry has equipped us with considerable information not only about this process in particular but also about the nature of human anxiety in general. Such knowledge has informed our understanding of other anxiety syndromes and has been valuable in developing clinical practice guidelines for the treatment of all DSM-IV anxiety disorders. In this chapter, we present specific techniques utilized by our laboratory group in the treatment of generalized anxiety disorder (GAD). These techniques are based on empirical information regarding the nonadaptive patterns in living displayed by individuals with GAD. These habitual patterns reduce their quality of life, and the learning of more adaptive ways of living can increase the quality of life of many clients who suffer from anxiety disorders.

The definition of GAD has changed substantially across editions of the DSM. GAD first appeared as a diagnosis in DSM-III (American Psychiatric Association, 1980) and required that individuals experience symptoms in at least three of four symptom categories (tension, startle, and restlessness; autonomic hyperactivity; apprehensive expectation; and hypervigilance). A hierarchical approach to diagnosis was also instituted, such that a diagnosis of GAD was considered appropriate only when an individual failed to meet criteria for any of the other anxiety disorders. The definition of GAD changed considerably with the publication of DSM-III-R (American Psychiatric Association, 1987). Excessive anxiety and worrying about more than one topical domain became the central feature of GAD, and associated symptoms were drawn from three categories (motor tension, autonomic hyperactivity, and hypervigilance). Furthermore, the hierarchical approach was discarded in that one could be diagnosed with GAD and another anxiety disorder simultaneously. The DSM-IV (American Psychiatric Association, 1994) changed the definition yet again based on the scientific literature that had emerged since the previous edition's publication. Excessive worry remained the central feature, but due to research showing that autonomic hyperactivity evidenced the lowest diagnostic reliability (Marten et al., 1993), only the associated symptoms of muscle tension and vigilance were retained. Moreover, difficulty controlling worry became a diagnostic criterion for GAD, given evidence that individuals with GAD experience their worry as uncontrollable relative to individuals without GAD (Craske, Rapee, Jackel, & Barlow, 1989). The worrying must occur more days than not for at least 6 months and be associated with at least three of six associated symptoms (restlessness, fatigue, difficulty concentrating, irritability, muscle tension, and sleep disturbance). Moreover, the anxiety and worry must not occur exclusively during the course of a mood disorder or during posttraumatic stress disorder, and it must not be the result of another Axis I disorder, a general medical condition, or a substance abuse disorder. Finally, the anxiety and worry must lead to significant distress or impairment in functioning.

Much of our group's theoretical foundation underlying treatment of GAD rests on Mowrer's (1947) two-stage theory of fear, a theoretical conceptualization of the neurotic paradox based on animal conditioning research. Mowrer's theory asserts that fear emerges via classical conditioning and is maintained via the operant negative reinforcement of avoidance responses that result in fear maintenance. Modern exposure-based therapies arose from this theory and seek to reduce anxiety via repeated exposures to feared stimuli while avoidance reactions (e.g., avoidance of fear cues) are prevented.

Most anxiety disorders are characterized by motoric avoidance of fear cues. For example, individuals with panic disorder frequently avoid and/or escape situations that cause them to experience somatic arousal and to feel anxious, and individuals with social phobia often go to great lengths to avoid situations in which they are likely to be evaluated. However, individuals with GAD rarely avoid behaviorally discrete disorder-specific situations that cause them to feel anxious. Instead, current theoretical models conceptualize worry as a *cognitive* avoidance response to threatening material. When the threat has to do with some future event and no behavioral avoidance response is possible, the person is left with only cognitive operations to try to solve this problem. Moreover, worry is primarily a verbal–linguistic, as opposed to imagery-based, activity (Borkovec & Inz, 1990; Behar, Zuellig, & Borkovec, 2005), and this verbal nature makes it remote from physiological and affective experience (Borkovec, Alcaine, & Behar, 2004). Indeed, experimental data show that relative to a period of relaxation, a period of worrying decreases the physiological activity elicited by a subsequent anxiety-eliciting task (i.e., images of giving a speech; Borkovec & Hu, 1990). When viewed in light of theoretical assertions by Edna Foa (Foa & Kozak, 1986) that physiological activation is an important index of emotional processing, a conceptualization of worry as a cognitive avoidance response that precludes emotional processing emerges.

Indeed, it is apparent from other lines of research that cognitive avoidance can serve to maintain fear responses. For instance, Grayson and Borkovec (1978) found that participants who imagined avoiding a phobic stimulus reported greater increases in fear over hierarchy scenes than did participants who imagined effectively coping with the feared situations. Grayson, Foa, and Steketee (1982) found a similar phenomenon in treatment of obsessive–compulsive disorder with respect to attention. Habituation of heart rate and subjectively reported fear across two sessions was more successful for participants who were given exposure with attention-focusing followed by exposure with distraction, relative to participants who were treated with the opposite order of exposure techniques. Therefore, *cognitive* avoidance may contribute to maintenance of anxiety and may also mitigate the habituation that otherwise ensues from repeated exposure to the anxiety-provoking material. Worriers experience repeated exposure to their worries due to the ruminative nature of worrisome thinking, but such repeated exposure does not lead to habituation of the anxiety response. Individuals with GAD likely employ cognitive avoidance in an attempt to mitigate the anxiety resulting from the perception of future threat.

Closely related to this avoidance conceptualization, GAD is characterized by a host of nonadaptive patterns involving physiological, behavioral, cognitive, and emotional systems. Current treatment approaches draw on knowledge regarding these patterns in order to treat individuals living with this condition. In this chapter, we present each of these classes of habitual nonadaptive patterns and the techniques employed to establish new habits that can enhance quality of life.

NONADAPTIVE PATTERNS OF AWARENESS AND SELF-MONITORING

Clients with GAD live in a busy internal world. They are highly focused on future negative events and are engaged in high levels of internal verbal activity that makes them feel anxious and depressed (Borkovec & Inz, 1990; Behar et al., 2005). This constant focus on ruminative mental activity strips such individuals of the attentional resources needed to attend to external aspects of the environment and the reality around them. The result is that they fail to escape the illusory world created in their thoughts and images and rarely experience the present moment that possesses the potential to bring them joy.

One of the first skills taught to clients with GAD, one that lays the foundation for the other skills taught in therapy, is self-monitoring. A core component of behavior therapy, this basic skill teaches clients to closely observe the external situations related to their concerns; the thoughts, feelings, physiological activity, and behaviors they experience in reaction to those situations and concerns; and the consequences that emerge from their reactions. Self-monitoring achieves three basic goals. First, it provides rich information about the causal relationships between clients' cognitions, emotions, and behaviors and the internal and external problems in their lives. Such functional analytic information makes it clear to clients that their anxiety is more likely a result of their personal choices than it is a necessary product of the external situations in which they find themselves. This offers what is perhaps the first indication that they have the power to reduce their own discomfort. Second, self-monitoring teaches clients to detect the first signs of escalating anxiety. The therapist can then have clients repeatedly recall in imagery the sequence of events surrounding the anxiety and worry in order to help them to detect the earliest possible onset of anxious responding. The earlier clients can detect this onset, the more capable they will be of choosing and implementing coping responses that shift them away from that spiraling and their self-perpetuating worrisome and anxious state. Finally, self-monitoring lays the groundwork for teaching clients to focus on the present moment. Focusing on the present allows clients to attend to the reality of the world around them as opposed to the illusory world they have otherwise created in their thoughts and images and contains the potential for genuineness, connectedness to the environment and people around them, and joy.

As clients become capable of monitoring themselves, they become ready to learn and use the other components of treatment. As therapy progresses, clients are further taught to process positive information in their present moments, in addition to negative information, as well as to identify positive experiences each day. Because individuals with emotional disorders often filter information and attend only to the negative aspects of situations, and because many individuals are susceptible to confirmatory biases (Faust, 1984), encouraging clients to process positive information gives them the gift of flexibility and frees them from automatically attending only to the negative. As is discussed throughout this chapter, self-monitoring also allows clients to observe more objectively their physiological states, interpersonal behaviors, and emotional responses, and all of these areas of functioning contribute to the ultimate goal of living in the present moment.

NONADAPTIVE PHYSIOLOGICAL FUNCTIONING

Whereas self-monitoring lays the foundation for attending to the present moment, training in relaxation methods lays the foundation for attending specifically to the *pleasant* present moment. Individuals with GAD differ from other anxious clients in their physiological reactions to fear-relevant stimuli in that GAD and worry are characterized by a *lack* of sympathetic activation and reduced cardiovascular variability (Hoehn-Saric, McLeod, & Zimmerli, 1989), increased muscle tension (Hazlett, McLeod, & Hoehn-Saric, 1994), and reduced EMG variability (Hazlett et al., 1994).

Because muscle tension is the only symptom shown to be elevated in the physiological experiences of clients with GAD, relaxation training is used as a means of reducing this tension. Specifically, progressive muscle relaxation (PMR; Bernstein, Borkovec, & Hazlett-Stevens, 2000) entails teaching clients to tense and subsequently let go of the tension in muscle groups. PMR is used to (1) achieve greater cognizance of the pleasantness associated with letting go as it is juxtaposed with prior increased tension; (2) achieve greater control over levels of muscular tension so that clients can decrease those levels quickly and deeply as needed in their everyday lives; and (3) extend the metaphor of "letting go" to include letting go of reactions that involve negative thoughts, images, and feelings and a focus on the future. In addition to PMR training, slowed, paced, diaphragmatic breathing, pleasant relaxing imagery, and meditation are all used to enhance relaxation. Upon detection of early cues indicating incipient anxiety or worry, clients are encouraged to flexibly apply their different relaxation skills depending on the situation, their preferences, and how successful each skill is.

In addition to its effects on muscle tension and cardiovascular invariability, one of the largest benefits of relaxation may lie in its facilitation of other mechanisms of treatment. For example, past research (Borkovec & Sides, 1979) has shown that relaxation facilitates the vividness of fearful imagery, thereby potentially increasing the effectiveness of imagery interventions (e.g., self-control desensitization, described later) and facilitates physiological reactivity to fear cues and its decline with repeated exposure, which is argued to be an important component of emotional processing (Foa & Kozak, 1986). Relaxation may also facilitate cognitive flexibility. We are currently examining whether a period of deep relaxation is associated with the generation of a greater number of potential outcomes of worries relative to neutral mentation and worrisome rumination (Behar, Zalewski, & Borkovec, 2004). Taken together, extant findings indicate that relaxation may increase the potency of other components of treatment for anxiety. They also illustrate that areas of functioning in human beings (cognition, affect, physiology, and behavior) are not independent and that we can begin to influence habitual areas of functioning by loosening other areas.

NONADAPTIVE BEHAVIOR

Although behavioral avoidance of a specific stimulus is not typically a central characteristic of GAD, some individuals with GAD do show subtle signs of behavioral avoidance to various situations (Butler, Cullington, Hibbert, Klimes, & Gelder, 1987). Therefore, therapists do encourage such clients to approach whatever situations they fear and to practice their coping skills (e.g., relaxation) before, during, and after these situations. However, the most salient fears in GAD have to do with apprehensions about numerous potential (but nonexistent) future events. Given the general lack of circumscribed fear triggers and behavioral avoidance of such stimuli, *in vivo* exposure frequently used in the treatment of other anxiety conditions is not as central in GAD treatment. Instead, therapists have a number of tools at their disposal to help clients overcome nonadaptive behavioral patterns that limit their quality of life.

In self-control desensitization (SCD; Goldfried, 1971), clients are taught to vividly imagine stressful or worrisome situations until that imagery has elicited anxious feelings. Upon detection of this anxiety, clients are instructed to continue imagining the anxiety-inducing situations while they imagine deploying their relaxation skills in that situation. Once the anxiety has dissipated, clients are instructed to continue imagining themselves relaxing in the situation before terminating the image and focusing solely on their relaxed state. The procedure is repeated until an anxious response is either quickly eliminated or fails to arise altogether in response to imagery of the stressful situation or to an incipient worrisome process.

Clients' nonadaptive behavioral patterns extend to their interpersonal relationships, in which they exhibit rigid ways of relating to those around them (Pincus & Borkovec, 1994). Because the presence of interpersonal problems subsequent to cognitive-behavioral treatment of GAD predicts poor short-term and long-term outcome (Borkovec, Newman, Pincus, & Lytle, 2002), helping clients to learn more flexible and adaptive interpersonal behavior would be valuable for clients' overall improvement. To address rigid interpersonal behavior, Newman (Newman, Castonguay, Borkovec, & Molnar, 2004) developed an interpersonal and emotional processing (IEP) component of therapy based on the work of Safran and Segal (1990) that employs functional analysis of clients' interpersonal behaviors. Specifically, clients are asked to observe the impact of their behaviors on others, and therapists directly observe and provide feedback about such behaviors in session in order to provide information to clients about how their behavior affects the therapist. Identification of clients' interpersonal needs based on their emotions when with others and how they are behaving in order to fulfill those needs allows the therapist to assess how and when those behaviors are nonadaptive for achieving the clients' goals and the learning of new interpersonal behaviors that better accomplish those goals.

Finally, because worry can take place anytime and anywhere, chronic worriers often come to associate many environmental cues with worry and therefore experience an onset of worrisome activity when they come into contact with those external cues. To address the problem of worry becoming a diffuse experience with a potentially high number of environmental triggers, we use a stimulus control procedure (derived from Bootzin's stimulus control treatment for insomnia; Bootzin & Epstein, 2000). Clients are instructed to set aside a daily half-hour worry period at a specific time and in a specific location. Using their self-monitoring skills to detect the start of worry early in its cycle, they are encouraged to postpone worrying until the prescribed time and place and to focus their attention back to the present moment. Although clients can certainly use the half-hour period for worrying, they are encouraged to engage in adaptive problem solving and to apply the various coping skills they have learned in therapy (e.g., SCD, cognitive therapy, relaxation) in order to deal more effectively with their worrying. Scientific investigations have documented empirical support for the use of stimulus control techniques with worry (Borkovec, Wilkinson, Folensbee, & Lerman, 1983; Behar, Tishk, & Zalewski, 2002).

An alternative but related method is the use of worry-free zones, in which clients create a time and/or place (e.g., while having dinner, while in their cars) during which they temporarily let go of and postpone all incipient worry until they are out of the zone. Over time, additional worry-free zones are added. The goal is to decrease the number of places and situations associated with worrisome activity so that progressively fewer situations come to elicit anxiety.

NONADAPTIVE COGNITION

Clients with GAD display nonadaptive ways of perceiving, interpreting, and predicting events. Evidence from the Dysfunctional Attitudes Scale suggests that clients with GAD endorse nonadaptive core beliefs (Behar & Borkovec, 2002), providing empirical evidence for the clinical observation that they hold inflexible and inaccurate views of themselves, their pasts, their futures, and the world. Traditional cognitive therapy (Beck, 1976) is used in our treatment of GAD in order to help clients identify their nonadaptive automatic thoughts and beliefs, assess the accuracy of those cognitions, create perspectives that are more accurate, and test their new views in their everyday lives.

The rigidity seen in clients with GAD is perhaps most insidious in their cognitive activity. In addition to spending so much of their time engaged in worrisome thinking, individuals with GAD display rigid cognitive biases. Specifically, they show biases in (1) their attention to threat cues (Bradley, Mogg, White, Groom, & de Bono, 1999), (2) their interpretations of ambiguous information as threatening (Mogg, Bradley, Miller, & Potts, 1994), and (3) their perceptions of a higher than average subjective risk of bad things occurring in the future (Butler & Mathews, 1987). Worry is also characterized by a lack of flexibility in thinking during streams of consciousness, as evidenced by significant decreases in topical shifts during this process (Molina, Borkovec, Peasely, & Person, 1998). Moreover, given that worrying involves the repetition of anxiety-relevant words and that the repetition of a word temporarily leads to a relative inaccessibility to associative networks of meaning (Smith, 1984), worrying likely results in decreased flexible access to other (e.g., affective) elements of meaning. Finally, individuals with GAD experience more thinking than imagery while worrying (indicating rigidity in the pathway by which they experience cognition), and the images that do occur are often catastrophic and negatively valenced (Borkovec & Inz, 1990). Based on these known areas of nonadaptiveness, our treatment includes various components aimed at loosening these rigid structures and providing more adaptive ways of seeing things.

Multiple, Flexible Perspectives

In our treatment of GAD, we encourage clients to generate multiple perspectives and to remain open to adopting different perspectives based on the idea that the adaptiveness of a given perspective depends on the specific situation and specific environment. The first step in therapy is to teach clients to consider many possible perspectives for a neutral situation in order to get them accustomed to the concept of multiple perspective generation, without regard to any one perspective's accuracy and using situations that are unlikely to bring forth their rigid patterns of responding. Once clients have been introduced to the concept of multiple perspective generation, the therapist shifts to employing this skill with clinically relevant material. Traditional cognitive therapy methods for assessing each perspective's accuracy, adaptiveness, and impact on affect can then be applied.

Rehearsal of Multiple Perspectives

Most clients with GAD have held their nonadaptive perceptions and interpretations for many years. Simply asking them to generate multiple perspectives in sessions is unlikely to help them break their habitual accessing of negative perspectives during challenging, anxiety-provoking situations.

Therefore, the frequent rehearsal of new perspectives in everyday life is vital to their learning to generate multiple (and more adaptive) ways of viewing things. Accordingly, clients are asked to shift their perspectives to those new views upon detection of incipient anxiety. Practice in doing this is provided during self-control desensitization, wherein clients vividly imagine changing perspectives during anxiety-inducing or worrisome scenes, in addition to deploying their relaxation responses. The more clients rehearse the generation of multiple perspectives, the more habitual the accession of those perspectives can become.

Worry Outcome Diary

Human beings do not always process all of the information available to them. Even therapists are guilty of failing to test alternative hypotheses and of falling prey to illusory correlations, confirmatory biases, and other errors of judgment (e.g., Alloy & Tabachnik, 1984). Therapists usefully show clients how to consider evidence that contradicts their often tightly held assumptions, beliefs, and expectations. One method that facilitates this goal is the use of worry outcome diaries, on which clients record the specific worries they experience during the day and the feared outcome(s) of each worry. Each evening, clients review the previous diary entries to assess whether those feared outcomes have indeed occurred and, if so, rate whether the outcome turned out better than they expected, as badly as they expected, or worse than they expected. For outcomes with a bad result, they further rate how well they coped with the actual outcome. Each week, the therapist reviews the outcomes with the client and reinforces the client's creation of a new, alternative reality based on the accurate evidence provided by them.

The use of daily worry outcome diaries has several advantages. First, research we conducted shows that the worrisome outcomes recorded by clients rarely end up actually happening and that, in those cases in which they do, clients report handling the situation much better than they expected they would (Borkovec, Hazlett-Stevens, & Diaz, 1999). Second, the use of the diaries reinforces clients' newly learned skills of attending to the present moment and processing events objectively and accurately as they occur. Third, clients are also asked to relive actual outcomes in imagery and can, therefore, over time more easily access new ways of generating predictions or expectations about the future that are more accurate and adaptive. Fourth, the process of generating predictions and expectations, collecting data, and comparing predictions to objective reality helps clients to create new general narratives for themselves regarding their worries and ways of reacting to potential future events. The generation of new narratives goes beyond the alteration of individual, specific worries and equips clients with the schemas needed to interpret future events and situations in more adaptive ways.

Imagery

Imagery is a powerful cognitive process in several ways. First, imagery is incipient action (efferent command into physiology, behavior, and affect; Lang, 1985). Imagining something is paramount to engaging internally in that behavior, and this influences later actual performance. For example, imaginal rehearsal enhances the quality of subsequent behavioral performance (e.g., in sports; Murphy, 1994). Also, laboratory research has shown that when individuals are asked to imagine a stressful event that in fact never actually happened (e.g., getting stuck in a tree as a child), they are more likely to later believe that the event actually occurred (Garry, Manning, Loftus, & Sherman, 1996). Additionally, imagining scenes from a fearful film elicits a stronger physiological response than does engaging in other types of cognitive activity (i.e., verbal thought) about the same stimulus (Vrana, Cuthbert, & Lang, 1986), suggesting that imagery is highly realistic and elicits internal reactions similar to those occurring in response to actual events (Lang, Levin, Miller, & Kozak, 1983).

The power of imagery has important implications for the lives of clients with GAD. Although most of the cognitive activity experienced during worry is of a verbal–linguistic, thought-based nature, negatively valenced images do find their way into the worry process. One aspect of the avoidance theory of GAD (Borkovec et al., 2004) posits that worriers react to perceptions of threat (including catastrophic images) by shifting to verbal thought (which is less closely tied to physiological activation; Vrana et al., 1986) and that their worrying is negatively reinforced by the resulting decrease in somatic anxious experience. Given the realistic quality of imagery, however, catastrophic images that do occur are stored in the client's memory as evidence that such bad things have actually occurred. Evidence from the social psychology literature shows that imagining a future event increases the subjective probability that the event will actually occur (Carroll, 1978). Futhermore, the term "imagination inflation" (coined by Elizabeth Loftus and her colleagues) describes the phenomenon that imagining a past event promotes increased confidence that the event actually has occurred, even when in reality it did not transpire. Given that the information from catastrophic images has a high likelihood of being stored in memory, it is unlikely that clients will process new information in ways that are inconsistent with the cognitive schemas that result from those imagined events.

Given the importance of imagery discussed herein, we include an imagery rehearsal component in our protocol treatment for GAD. This takes place within the SCD procedures as described earlier, but the SCD procedure is supplemented with repeated rehearsals of images of the most likely outcomes of a worrisome situation (based on logical analysis contained in in-session cognitive therapy), and clients are encouraged to substitute most likely outcome images as soon as they detect a worry in their daily lives. When practiced upon detection of incipient anxiety or worry cues in conjunction with other coping skills, it is likely to reduce the frequency and intensity of catastrophic images that would otherwise enter the worry cycle. Recent evidence from our laboratory suggests that rehearsal of imagined worst-case scenarios (akin to imaginal exposure) may also be useful in the treatment of worry. Evidence using analogue GAD participants has shown that relative to three comparison conditions (verbal rehearsal of worst-case scenarios, verbal rehearsal of best-case scenarios, and imaginal rehearsal of best-case scenarios), imaginal rehearsal of worst-case scenarios produced the greatest subjective decrease in anxiety (Behar & Yamasaki, 2002). There was also evidence for emotional processing of fear in that participants in this condition evidenced increases in both subjective fear (Behar & Yamasaki, 2002) and autonomic arousal (Behar, Yamasaki, Borkovec, & Ray, 2003) while viewing pictures intended to elicit arousal. Therefore, imaginal exposure to feared outcomes in worry does indeed facilitate accessing of the fear structure that is otherwise precluded in GAD. Although this investigation was conducted on an analogue GAD sample, the use of imaginal exposure to catastrophic outcomes may be similarly useful in the treatment of clients with GAD. Future research using formally diagnosed samples will clarify whether this technique contains active mechanisms of change in that population.

Expectancy-Free Living

Another method used to address faulty information processing (e.g., confirmatory biases) is to encourage clients to let go of the expectations and predictions that cause them distress in the first place. Having preexisting assumptions, beliefs, and expectations is in many ways adaptive. It allows us to organize the vast amounts of incoming information from the environment. However, those schemas can also color how we process new information such that objective present-moment reality becomes difficult to access. From a therapeutic standpoint, it therefore is clear that the greatest amount of new learning and loosening of rigid belief structures would take place if we could let go of those preexisting assumptions, beliefs, and expectations. If instead of habitually accessing their negative expectations, clients with GAD could live moment to moment perceiving and processing the objective reality before them, they could effectively let go of the very biases in perception that predispose them to interpret events in negative ways. In therapy, this translates to helping clients move from their habitual negative expectations to more accurate expectations and eventually to no expectations at all. Therefore, as is the case for self-monitoring, relaxation, and behavioral interventions, the ultimate goal of our cognitive therapy procedures listed herein is freedom: freedom from expectations and predictions, freedom from the past and the future, and the freedom to experience and process each moment as it occurs.

Intrinsic Motivation in the Present Moment

Once our clients are having successful experiences in living more in the present, our therapists encourage them to begin bringing intrinsically motivated behaviors into those present moments. Given the amount of avoidance and defensive responding in their lives, we wish to help them cultivate instead ways of approaching each moment, not just behaviorally but with cognitive perspectives and emotions that are synchronous with a true, "whole organism" approach. Engaging present environments (tasks, other people) from value-directed perspectives allows clients to create joy in those moments, because the resulting intrinsically motivated behaviors are reinforcing in and of themselves, irrespective of the ultimate outcome. Moreover, the likelihood of favorable outcomes increases when so motivated because value-directed perspectives increase the likely quality and adaptiveness of the ensuing behaviors (see Borkovec & Sharpless, 2004).

NONADAPTIVE EMOTIONAL EXPERIENCING

Individuals with GAD experience frequent negative emotionality. As a result of their high levels of worrisome thinking, they experience high levels of anxious affect and also commonly report high levels of depression, both diagnostically (Brown & Barlow, 1992) and as a mood state (Andrews & Borkovec, 1988). Moreover, there is evidence that individuals with GAD experience difficulties with emotions in general. They report difficulty in identifying and describing their emotions on the Toronto Alexithymia Scale (Yamas, Hazlett-Stevens, & Borkovec, 1997), and they find emotions in general to be aversive (Turk, Heimberg, Luterek, Mennin, & Fresco, 2005). Clients with GAD may be avoiding fully processing emotion and/or they may not notice changes in affect throughout the day because their attentional resources are occupied by their worrisome thought activity.

Three elements of our therapy address clients' nonadaptive experiencing of emotion. First, the self-monitoring skills described earlier enable clients to attend to and fully experience all emotions as they occur in reaction to present-moment events. Second, our cognitive techniques place a strong emphasis on generating perspectives that facilitate experiencing genuine joyfulness in daily life (e.g., cultivation of a value-directed approach to present-moment tasks and the processing of positive information available in each present moment). Third, Newman's (Newman et al., 2004) interpersonal and emotional processing therapy (described earlier) comprises techniques designed to intensify genuine, primary affect. Through repeated exposure to emotional experiences, therapists help clients lessen their fear and avoidance of affect. The ultimate goal of this component of therapy, then, is to aid clients in the identification and processing of all types of emotional experiences (positive and negative) such that, over time, the accessing of such experiences is habitual and allows for a more genuine life experience. Emotional deepening methods also contribute to adaptiveness in clients' interpersonal functioning. Experiencing authentic emotions leads to authentic behaviors (e.g., responses that show assertiveness or vulnerability), which are more likely than nongenuine behaviors to lead to close interpersonal connections.

ACKNOWLEDGMENT

Preparation of this chapter was supported in part by National Institute of Mental Health Research Grant No. RO1 MH58593 to T. D. Borkovec.

REFERENCES

Alloy, L. B., & Tabachnik, N. (1984). Assessment of covariation by humans and animals: The joint influence of prior expectations and current situational information. *Psychological Review, 91*, 112–149.

American Psychiatric Association. (1980). *Diagnostic and statistical manual of mental disorders* (3rd ed.). Washington, DC: Author.

American Psychiatric Association. (1987). *Diagnostic and statistical manual of mental disorders* (3rd ed., rev.). Washington, DC: Author.

American Psychiatric Association. (1994). *Diagnostic and statistical manual of mental disorders* (4th ed.). Washington, DC: Author.

Andrews, V. H., & Borkovec, T. D. (1988). The differential effects of induction of worry, somatic anxiety, and depression on emotional experience. *Journal of Behavior Therapy and Experimental Psychiatry, 19*, 21–26.

Beck, A. T. (1976). *Cognitive therapy and the emotional disorders.* New York: New American Library.

Behar, E., & Borkovec, T. D. (2002, November). *Cognitive-behavioral therapy for generalized anxiety disorder: Changes in dysfunctional attitudes.* Poster presented at the annual meeting of the Association for Advancement of Behavior Therapy, Reno, NV.

Behar, E., Tishk, L., & Zalewski, M. (2002, November). *Stimulus control of worry among high and low worriers.* Poster presented at the annual meeting of the Association for Advancement of Behavior Therapy, Reno, NV.

Behar, E., & Yamasaki, A. S. (2002, November). *Imagery vs. thought training: Which treatment component best targets emotional processing for GAD?* Paper presented at the annual meeting of the Association for Advancement of Behavior Therapy, Reno, NV.

Behar, E., Yamasaki, A. S., Borkovec, T. D., & Ray, W. J. (2003, November). *Physiological processing of emotional material following imaginal exposure for GAD.* Paper presented at the annual meeting of the Association for Advancement of Behavior Therapy, Boston, MA.

Behar, E., Zalewski, M., & Borkovec, T. D. (2004, November). *The effects of relaxation on cognitive flexibility in worrisome and depressive thoughts.* Poster presented at the annual meeting of the Association for Advancement of Behavior Therapy, New Orleans, LA.

Behar, E., Zuellig, A. R., & Borkovec, T. D. (2005). Thought and imaginal activity during worry and trauma recall. *Behavior Therapy, 36,* 157–168.

Bernstein, D. A., Borkovec, T. D., & Hazlett-Stevens, H. (2000). *New directions in progressive relaxation training: A guidebook for helping professionals.* Wesport, CT: Praeger.

Bootzin, R. R., & Epstein, D. R. (2000). Stimulus control instructions. In K. L. Lichstein & C. M. Morin (Eds.), *Treatment of late-life insomnia* (pp. 167–184). Thousand Oaks, CA: Sage.

Borkovec, T. D., Alcaine, O., & Behar, E. (2004). Avoidance theory of worry and generalized anxiety disorder. In R. G. Heimberg, C. L. Turk, & D. S. Mennin (Eds.), *Generalized anxiety disorder: Advances in research and practice* (pp. 77–108). New York: Guilford Press.

Borkovec, T. D., Hazlett-Stevens, H., & Diaz, M. L. (1999). The role of positive beliefs about worry in generalized anxiety disorder and its treatment. *Clinical Psychology and Psychotherapy, 6,* 126–138.

Borkovec, T. D., & Hu, S. (1990). The effect of worry on cardiovascular response to phobic imagery. *Behaviour Research and Therapy, 28,* 69–73.

Borkovec, T. D., & Inz, J. (1990). The nature of worry in generalized anxiety disorder: A predominance of thought activity. *Behaviour Research and Therapy, 28,* 153–158.

Borkovec, T. D., Newman, M. G., Pincus, A. L., & Lytle, R. (2002). A component analysis of cognitive behavioral therapy for generalized anxiety disorder and the role of interpersonal problems. *Journal of Consulting and Clinical Psychology, 70,* 288–298.

Borkovec, T. D., & Sharpless, B. (2004). Generalized anxiety disorder: Bringing cognitive behavioral therapy into the valued present. In S. Hayes, V. Follette, & M. Linehan (Eds.), *New directions in behavior therapy* (pp. 209–242). New York: Guilford Press.

Borkovec, T. D., & Sides, J. K. (1979). The contribution of relaxation and expectancy to fear reduction via graded, imaginal exposure to feared stimuli. *Behaviour Research and Therapy, 17,* 529–540.

Borkovec, T. D., Wilkinson, L., Folensbee, R., & Lerman, C. (1983). Stimulus control applications to the treatment of worry. *Behaviour Research and Therapy, 21,* 247–251.

Bradley, B. P., Mogg, K., White, J., Groom, C., & de Bono, J. (1999). Attentional bias for emotional faces in generalized anxiety disorder. *British Journal of Clinical Psychology, 38,* 267–278.

Brown, T. A., & Barlow, D. H. (1992). Comorbidity among anxiety disorders: Implications for treatment and DSM-IV. *Journal of Consulting and Clinical Psychology, 60,* 835–844.

Butler, B., Cullington, A., Hibbert, G., Klimes, I., & Gelder, M. (1987). Anxiety management for persistent generalized anxiety. *British Journal of Psychiatry, 151,* 535–542.

Butler, G., & Mathews, A. (1987). Anticipatory anxiety and risk perception. *Cognitive Therapy and Research, 11,* 551–565.

Carroll, J. S. (1978). The effect of imagining an event on expectations for the event: An interpretation in terms of the availability heuristic. *Journal of Personality and Social Psychology, 36,* 1501–1511.

Craske, M. G., Rapee, R. M., Jackel, L., & Barlow, D. H. (1989). Qualitative dimensions of worry in DSM-III-R generalized anxiety disorder subjects and nonanxious controls. *Behaviour Research and Therapy, 27,* 397–402.

Faust, D. (1984). *The limits of scientific reasoning.* Minneapolis: University of Minnesota Press.

Foa, E. B., & Kozak, M. J. (1986). Emotional processing of fear: Exposure to corrective information. *Psychological Bulletin, 99,* 20–35.

Garry, M., Manning, C. G., Loftus, E. F., & Sherman, S. J. (1996). Imagination inflation: Imagining a childhood event inflates confidence that it occurred. *Psychonomic Bulletin and Review, 3,* 208–214.

Goldfried, M. R. (1971). Systematic desensitization as training in self-control. *Journal of Consulting and Clinical Psychology, 37,* 228–234.

Grayson, J. B., & Borkovec, T. D. (1978). The effects of expectancy and imagined response to phobic stimuli on fear reduction. *Cognitive Therapy and Research, 22,* 11–24.

Grayson, J. B., Foa, E. B., & Steketee, G. (1982). Habituation during exposure treatment: Distraction vs. attention-focusing. *Behaviour Research and Therapy, 20,* 323–328.

Hazlett, R. L., McLeod, D. R., & Hoehn-Saric, R. (1994). Muscle tension in generalized anxiety disorder: Elevated muscle tonus or agitated movement? *Psychophysiology, 31,* 189–195.

Hoehn-Saric, R., McLeod, D. R., & Zimmerli, W. D. (1989). Somatic manifestations in women with generalized anxiety disorder: Physiological responses to psychological stress. *Archives of General Psychiatry, 46,* 1113–1119.

Lang, P. J. (1985). The cognitive psychophysiology of emotion: Fear and anxiety. In A. H. Tuma & J. D. Maser (Eds.), *Anxiety and the anxiety disorders* (pp. 131–170). Hillsdale, NJ: Erlbaum.

Lang, P. J., Levin, D. N., Miller, G. A., & Kozak, M. J. (1983). Fear behavior, fear imagery, and the psychophysiology of emotion: The problem of affective response integration. *Journal of Abnormal Psychology, 92,* 276–306.

Marten, P. A., Brown, T. A., Barlow, D. H., Borkovec, T. D., Shear, M. K., & Lydiard, R. B. (1993). Evaluation of the ratings comprising the associated symptom criterion of DSM-III-R generalized anxiety disorder. *Journal of Nervous and Mental Disease, 181,* 676–682.

Mogg, K., Bradley, B. P., Miller, T., & Potts, H. (1994). Interpretation of homophones related to threat: Anxiety or response bias effects? *Cognitive Therapy and Research, 18,* 461–477.

Molina, S., Borkovec, T. D., Peasley, C., & Person, D. (1998). Content analysis of worrisome streams of consciousness in anxious and dysphoric participants. *Cognitive Therapy and Research, 22,* 109–123.

Mowrer, O. H. (1947). On the dual nature of learning: A re-interpretation of "conditioning" and "problem-solving." *Harvard Educational Review, 17,* 102–148.

Murphy, S. (1994). Imagery interventions in sport. *Medicine and Science in Sports and Exercise, 26,* 334–345.

Newman, M. G., Castonguay, L. G., Borkovec, T. D., & Molnar, C. (2004). Integrative therapy for generalized anxiety disorder. In R. G. Heimberg, C. L. Turk, & D. S. Mennin (Eds.), *Generalized anxiety disorder: Advances in research and practice* (pp. 320–350). New York: Guilford Press.

Pincus, A. L., & Borkovec, T. D. (1994, June). *Interpersonal problems in generalized anxiety disorder: Preliminary clustering of patients' interpersonal dysfunction.* Paper presented at the annual meeting of the American Psychological Society, New York, NY.

Safran, J., & Segal, Z. V. (1990). *Interpersonal process in cognitive therapy.* New York: Basic Books.

Smith, L. C. (1984). Semantic satiation affects category membership decision time but not lexical priming. *Memory and Cognition, 12,* 483–488.

Turk, C. L., Heimberg, R. G., Luterek, J. A., Mennin, D. S., & Fresco, D. M. (2005). Emotion dysregulation in generalized anxiety disorder: A comparison with social anxiety. *Cognitive Therapy and Research, 29,* 89–106.

Vrana, S. R., Cuthbert, B. M., & Lang, P. J. (1986). Fear imagery and text processing. *Psychophysiology, 23,* 247–253.

Yamas, K., Hazlett-Stevens, H., & Borkovec, M. (1997, November). *Alexithymia in generalized anxiety disorder.* Paper presented at the annual meeting of the Association for Advancement of Behavior Therapy, Miami Beach, FL.

12

Cognitive-Behavioral Perspectives on Theory and Treatment of Posttraumatic Stress Disorder

ELIZABETH A. HEMBREE
NORAH C. FEENY

In this chapter, we review the diagnostic criteria for and prevalence of posttraumatic stress disorder (PTSD). Next, we discuss conceptualizations of the development and maintenance of PTSD, with emphasis on emotional processing theory as presented by Foa and colleagues (Foa & Kozak, 1986; Foa & Riggs, 1993; Foa, Steketee, & Rothbaum, 1989). We then describe several cognitive-behavioral approaches to the treatment of PTSD and provide a brief summary of current empirical support for these. Finally, we describe a specific treatment for PTSD that has received extensive empirical support—prolonged exposure therapy (PE; Foa & Rothbaum, 1998)—and present a case example that illustrates this effective and efficient treatment.

PTSD DIAGNOSTIC CRITERIA AND PREVALENCE

PTSD entered the formal diagnostic system as an anxiety disorder in the third revision of the *Diagnostic and Statistical Manual* (DSM-III; American Psychiatric Association, 1980). In comparison to other anxiety disorders, PTSD is unique in that it originates from a specific triggering event or events: exposure to trauma. In the current DSM-IV (American Psychiatric Association, 1994), this is an event that involves real or perceived threat to life or physical integrity that is experienced or witnessed with "horror, terror, or helplessness." Three clusters of symptoms characterize PTSD: reexperiencing (e.g., intrusive, upsetting trauma-related thoughts or images, nightmares), avoidance (of trauma-related memories or stimuli; decreased interest, restricted range of emotion or numbing, social detachment), and hyperarousal (e.g., sleep disturbance, irritability, concentration problems, hypervigilance).

These symptoms are quite common immediately after traumatic events and typically decrease in intensity and frequency over the course of natural recovery. For those who develop PTSD, the posttrauma pathology becomes persistent and disruptive. According to DSM-IV, diagnosis of PTSD can be made when symptoms have been present for more than 1 month following the trauma and cause clinically significant distress or impairment.

Exposure to traumatic events is unfortunately quite frequent (e.g., Breslau et al., 1998). However, although many individuals do experience symptoms of PTSD in the immediate aftermath of traumatic events, most do not develop long term psychopathology (e.g., Riggs, Rothbaum, & Foa, 1995; Rothbaum, Foa, Riggs, Murdock, & Walsh, 1992). In the general U.S. population, rates of PTSD range from approximately 8 to 14% (Breslau, Davis, Andreski, & Peterson, 1991; Breslau et al., 1998; Kessler, Sonnega, Bromet, Hughes, & Nelson, 1995), whereas rates are higher in samples of trauma survivors (e.g., 24%; Breslau et al., 1991). Among those who have experienced traumatic events, rates of current PTSD vary, ranging from 25% of Rwandans following the 1994 genocide (Pham, Weinstein, & Longman, 2004), up to 40% of those in serious motor vehicle accidents (Taylor & Koch, 1995), 15% among Vietnam combat veterans (Kulka et al., 1990), and between 12 and 47% of female assault survivors (Norris et al., 2003; Resnick, Kilpatrick, Dansky, Saunders, & Best, 1993; Rothbaum et al., 1992). It is of note that women appear to be twice as likely to develop PTSD than men (10.4% of women vs. 5% of men in the general population; Kessler et al., 1995). Once established, its course is commonly chronic and unremitting (e.g., Norris et al., 2003; Kessler et al., 1995).

As is evident from these data, PTSD is a fairly common disorder with considerable negative impact on the individual and on society. As such, it has merited a good deal of treatment research over the past two decades. In addition, research has focused on why PTSD develops in some but not all trauma survivors. The consistent finding across various types of trauma that only a minority of survivors develop PTSD leads to one of the interesting questions addressed by trauma theorists and researchers: Why do some recover and others do not?

CONCEPTUALIZATIONS OF PTSD: A FOCUS
ON EMOTIONAL PROCESSING THEORY

Conceptualizations of the development and maintenance of PTSD have changed over time. Early conceptualizations were primarily behavioral, building on Mowrer's (1960) two-factor conditioning theory, whereas later conceptualizations incorporated the role of cognition in the development of PTSD (e.g., Ehlers & Clarke, 2000; Foa & Rothbaum, 1998; Janoff-Bulman, 1992; Resick & Schnicke, 1992).

In Foa and Kozak's (1986) seminal paper, "Emotional processing of fear: Exposure to corrective information," emotional processing theory was advanced to integrate both learning and cognitive theories of anxiety disorders within an information-processing framework. The idea that fear/anxiety signals the activation of a cognitive structure that serves as a program for escaping danger is central to this theory. Further, building on Peter Lang's work (1977, 1979), Foa and Kozak proposed that this cognitive structure includes specific pieces of information: information about the feared stimulus (e.g., dog growling with bared teeth); information about verbal, physiological, and behavioral responses (e.g., "I screamed and tried to run," "My heart was racing"); and information about the meaning of the stimulus and response elements of the structure ("growling dogs are dangerous").

Foa and Kozak (1986) posited that fear becomes pathological when the structure includes (1) excessive response elements, so that the fear is very intense (e.g., extensive avoidance and hyperarousal); (2) associations among stimuli and responses that do not accurately represent reality (e.g., "all dogs bite people," "all dogs should be avoided"); and (3) incorrect interpretations such as "going outside is never safe." They suggested that treatment of such pathological fear requires modification of the fear structure, the core of what has been termed "emotional processing" (Lang, 1977; Rachman, 1980). Thus treatment must (1) access the fear structure and, (2) provide corrective information that serves to modify its erroneous or unrealistic elements. In our example of the dog phobic, such treatment would likely entail (1) repeated and prolonged exposure to many dogs until anxiety decreases around the dogs, and (2) not being harmed by these dogs, thus modifying the belief that all dogs bite and are dangerous.

Foa and her colleagues (Foa & Jaycox, 1999; Foa & Riggs, 1993; Foa et al., 1989; Foa & Rothbaum, 1998) later built on emotional processing theory to explain impeded natural recovery among those who develop PTSD. In the natural course of recovery, trauma survivors think often about their trauma and repeatedly encounter reminders of it. In doing so, they learn that although thinking about the trauma or being in situations that remind them of it may be initially distressing, they are not dangerous, and the anxiety associated with these experiences diminishes over time. Repeated confrontation with the trauma memory also serves to organize and make sense of the experience, which facilitates its integration. Recovery is hampered by cognitive and behavioral avoidance that precludes such learning and hinders the integration of corrective information into the fear structure. For example, by avoiding trauma reminders that are safe, the person does not have the opportunity to learn that his or her anxiety will not last indefinitely, nor that the feared consequence will not occur. Encountering "safe" or low-risk trauma-related situations and thus having an opportunity to disconfirm trauma-induced expectations of harm or inability to cope are integral to natural recovery from trauma, as well as treatment-facilitated recovery from PTSD.

In several publications, Foa and colleagues (e.g., Foa & Riggs, 1993; Foa & Rothbaum, 1998) have theorized that exaggerated interpretations of the world as dangerous and the self as incompetent (including the perception that PTSD symptoms themselves signify weakness) are the core dysfunctional cognitions that underlie PTSD. Indeed, it has been found that elevated perceptions about the dangerousness of the world and negative thoughts about the self discriminated individuals with PTSD from trauma survivors without PTSD and from nontraumatized individuals (Foa, Ehlers, Clark, Tolin, & Orsillo, 1999). Accordingly, emotional processing theory suggests that successful treatment for PTSD should not only encourage emotional engagement with trauma memories and promote reduction of trauma-related fear but must also alter the dysfunctional beliefs that contribute to persistent PTSD.

In a related vein, Ehlers and colleagues (e.g., Ehlers & Clark, 2000) have highlighted the importance of unhelpful interpretations of PTSD symptoms themselves (e.g., flashbacks and intrusive thoughts) and have hypothesized that these symptom interpretations contribute substantively to the persistence of the disorder. They suggest that the negative meanings (e.g., "these thoughts mean I'm losing control") intensify the distress related to the intrusions, maintain a perception of threat, and thus influence the degree of behavioral and cognitive avoidance. Evidence for this notion comes from findings that dysfunctional interpretations of intrusive thoughts are predictive of PTSD severity above and beyond the frequency of intrusions themselves and the use of avoidance strategies (Steil & Ehlers, 2000). These results are in line with emotional processing theory, as well, and similarly suggest that interventions for PTSD include a focus on trauma-related dysfunctional interpretations, including PTSD symptoms, the self, others, and the world.

COGNITIVE-BEHAVIORAL APPROACHES
TO TREATMENT OF PTSD

Influenced by theoretical conceptualizations of PTSD, several cognitive-behavioral therapies have been developed and tested. Studies of treatment for

PTSD have investigated four different forms of cognitive-behavioral therapy (CBT): exposure therapy, stress inoculation training (SIT), cognitive therapy (CT), and eye movement desensitization and reprocessing (EMDR). In various studies, these treatment approaches have been compared with control conditions (e.g., wait list and active control, such as supportive counseling or relaxation training) and with one another, either individually or in combination (e.g., exposure combined with CT or SIT). We first describe each CBT approach and then briefly summarize the current empirical support for these treatments.

Exposure Therapy

As described elsewhere in this volume, exposure therapy has been extensively applied as a treatment for persistent, pathological anxiety. The chief aim of this form of treatment is to help patients approach feared and avoided objects, situations, memories, and images until anxiety attenuates. One of the first cognitive-behavioral interventions utilized to treat PTSD, exposure therapy for trauma survivors is based on the idea that avoidance of trauma-related memories and external reminders, although common and part of PTSD, interferes with recovery from the traumatic event by preventing opportunities to habituate to harmless trauma-related stimuli and to disconfirm erroneous cognitions, thus maintaining unrealistic fear. This concept is central to emotional processing theory, as described earlier, and is discussed extensively by Foa, Huppert, and Cahill in Chapter 1 of this volume.

Exposure therapy programs for PTSD patients usually include two forms of exposure that aim to help the person emotionally process the trauma: imaginal exposure, which involves repeatedly visualizing or reliving a traumatic memory in imagination, and *in vivo* exposure, which involves repeatedly approaching safe or low-risk situations or objects that remind one of the trauma and evoke excessive or unrealistic anxiety. Imaginal exposures are typically conducted across multiple treatment sessions and between them in the form of homework. In this procedure, the patient is asked to vividly imagine the traumatic event and to describe it aloud, along with the thoughts and feelings that occurred during the event. *In vivo* exposures are typically done outside treatment sessions as homework and involve systematic, prolonged, and repeated confrontation with external situations, places, or activities that trigger trauma-related fear and anxiety. With *in vivo* exposure, the patient is encouraged to remain in the anxiety-provoking situation until his or her fear declines (i.e., habituates) by a significant amount.

Stress Inoculation Training

SIT (Meichenbaum, 1975) was also one of the first cognitive-behavioral treatments applied with patients with PTSD. One of the most common anxiety management treatment approaches, SIT was primarily used in early research on female crime victims (e.g., Veronen & Kilpatrick, 1982; Foa, Rothbaum, Riggs, & Murdock, 1991; Foa, Dancu, Hembree, et al., 1999). A fundamental concept underlying this approach is the idea that stress results from the interaction of the person and the environment. Stress occurs when the person experiences environmental events as taxing or exceeding coping resources and thereby threatening safety or welfare. It is an inevitable part of life. Anxiety is a normal response to stress and signals the person to increase efforts to cope with or somehow manage the eliciting situation. In the case of individuals with PTSD (or other anxiety disorders), anxiety has reached an intensity and/or frequency that is excessive and disruptive.

SIT therefore involves the acquisition and repeated practice of specific coping skills, with the goal of helping patients to develop or enhance their ability to manage stress effectively and to reduce anxiety. Coping skills typically include tools such as breathing and relaxation training, guided self-dialogue, assertiveness training, role playing, covert modeling, and cognitive restructuring. PTSD patients are taught the skills in treatment sessions and are instructed to repeatedly practice them between sessions to manage anxiety and fear brought on by trauma-related cues or situations. In some PTSD treatment programs, SIT skills have been specifically paired with *in vivo* exposure exercises (e.g., Veronen & Kilpatrick, 1982).

Cognitive Therapy

As noted previously, the early, purely behavioral conceptualizations of PTSD quickly gave way to theories that acknowledged the role of cognitive mediation in explaining the development and maintenance of this disorder. This led to a corresponding increase in studies investigating the efficacy of cognitive intervention as a treatment for PTSD. In classic cognitive theory (e.g., Beck, 1976), it is the interpretation of events, rather than events per se, that leads to specific emotional responses. Accordingly, when "safe" or harmless events are viewed as threatening, unrealistic or excessive anxiety results. This is a core aspect of the theoretical accounts of PTSD offered by Foa and colleagues (e.g., Foa et al., 1989; Foa & Rothbaum, 1998), Ehlers and Clark (2000), and others.

The aim of cognitive therapy for PTSD is to help the patient to understand the role of his beliefs and interpretations in influencing emotional reactions, to identify trauma-related irrational thoughts or beliefs that trigger avoidance and/or excessive negative emotions (e.g., fear, shame, rage), and to learn to challenge these beliefs and expectations in a rational, evidence-based manner. In challenging these beliefs, evidence is weighed and alternative ways of viewing the situation are evaluated. In treatment sessions and in daily life situations as homework between sessions, the patient practices responding to automatic thoughts and interpretations by reviewing the facts, considering alternative explanations, and sometimes experimenting with different ways of behaving in response to situations or events that trigger anxiety and other negative emotions. As a consequence, the patient learns whether or not his trauma-related beliefs and expectations accurately reflect reality and are appropriate or helpful and modifies them accordingly. An example of such treatment is cognitive processing therapy (CPT; Resick, Nishith, Weaver, Astin, & Feuer, 2002; Resick & Schnicke, 1992), an intervention developed specifically for use with sexual assault victims but also implemented with other trauma survivors.

Eye Movement Desensitization and Reprocessing

EMDR (Shapiro, 1989, 1995) emerged as a treatment for PTSD in the early 1990s, and an increasing number of studies have investigated its efficacy in the past decade. A core component of this intervention is the therapist's repeated elicitation of rapid, saccadic eye movements (or elicitation of some form of laterally alternating stimulation) in the patient during the processing of traumatic memories. Shapiro theorized that the rapid eye movements in some way override or reverse neural blockage or obstruction induced by the traumatic event(s).

During EMDR treatment sessions, the patient is asked to generate images of the trauma or focus on trauma-related thoughts, feelings, and/or sensations, while the therapist elicits the saccadic eye movements by having the patient visually track a finger rapidly waved back and forth in front of his or her face. Other forms of laterally alternating stimuli (e.g., tapping, flashing lights) are sometimes used rather than the original finger tracking. The patient is asked to evaluate the cognitions associated with these images and experiences and to generate alternative cognitive appraisals of the trauma or of his or her behavior during it. As the patient focuses on the distressing images and thoughts and later focuses on the alternative cognition, the saccadic eye movements (or whatever form of alternating stimulation used) are intermittently generated.

SUMMARY OF MAJOR FINDINGS
OF CBT OUTCOME STUDIES

Randomized controlled trials (RCTs) of CBT interventions have included patients with chronic PTSD resulting from a variety of traumas: combat veterans; survivors of rape, physical assault, childhood sexual abuse, and domestic violence; survivors of motor vehicle accidents or disasters; and refugees from war-torn countries. A thorough review of these outcome studies is beyond the scope of this chapter, but we briefly summarize some of the major findings. For a more detailed review of the treatment outcome literature, see Rothbaum, Meadows, Resick, and Foy (2000) or Harvey, Bryant, and Tarrier (2003).

Numerous studies have found CBT effective in reducing PTSD and associated symptoms, making it the most empirically validated approach among the psychosocial treatments for PTSD. In general, comparative treatment studies have shown that patients treated with exposure therapy, SIT, cognitive therapy, and combinations of these three (e.g., exposure with SIT, exposure with cognitive therapy) achieve comparable and highly significant reductions in target symptoms, including PTSD, depression, and anxiety (e.g., Foa, Rothbaum, Riggs, & Murdock, 1991; Foa, Dancu, et al., 1999; Foa et al., in press; Marks, Lovell, Noshirvani, Livanou, & Thrasher et al., 1998; Resick et al., 2002). These interventions are also quite efficient; treatment is usually completed in 12 sessions or less. Follow-up evaluations of up to 1 year generally indicate excellent maintenance of treatment gains. The outcome studies on EMDR to date suggest that this treatment is also effective at reducing chronic PTSD and associated trauma-related pathology. Overall, studies comparing the outcome of patients treated with EMDR with those treated with exposure therapy or CBT combinations (e.g., PE and SIT) have shown comparable reductions in symptoms at posttreatment (e.g., Lee, Gavriel, Drummond, Richards, & Greenwald, 2002; Power et al., 2002; Rothbaum, 2002; Taylor et al., 2003). However, assertions about the integral role of eye movements or any other laterally alternating stimuli on treatment outcome (i.e., reductions in PTSD symptoms) have not been supported by dismantling studies (see Cahill, Carrigan, & Frueh, 1999, for a review) or meta-analyses (Davidson & Parker, 2001).

There are more studies demonstrating the efficacy of exposure therapy than any other CBT for PTSD, and thus Rothbaum et al. (2000) recommended that exposure therapy be considered as the first-line CBT intervention unless reasons exist for ruling it out. The exposure therapy program that has been most frequently studied in randomized controlled trials is PE (Foa & Rothbaum, 1998). PE, rooted in emotional processing theory, has been shown highly effective in treating PTSD associated with a variety of traumas.

Cognitive therapy has also been shown highly effective, although only two studies to date (Marks et al., 1998; Tarrier et al., 1999) have evaluated the efficacy of cognitive therapy alone against exposure therapy or other CBTs. The cognitive therapy protocols utilized in most studies have included varying degrees of exposure. For example, the core intervention in CPT (Resick et al., 2002) is clearly cognitive, but exposure in the form of writing and rereading the trauma narrative is included in several sessions. CPT has been shown to be an efficacious intervention for the treatment of PTSD, with long-term maintenance of gains. In general, the CBT interventions that have been studied in RCTs often include both cognitive and exposure components, rendering it difficult if not impossible to assess their relative contribution to outcome. Of note, the addition of cognitive restructuring to exposure has not enhanced outcomes achieved by exposure alone (e.g., Foa et al., in press; Marks et al., 1998).

SIT has also been found effective, but there have been few studies, and the generalizability of the results to populations other than female assault victims is unknown. As noted earlier, EMDR is an effective treatment for PTSD, and the number of controlled trials supporting its efficacy has increased significantly in the past 5 years.

PROLONGED EXPOSURE THERAPY

Given the amount of empirical support for the efficacy of PE, we now present an overview of the PE program that has been utilized with hundreds of patients in studies and in routine clinical care and illustrate the treatment with a brief case description of a man with chronic PTSD resulting from an industrial accident. For a detailed description of the treatment program, please see Foa and Rothbaum (1998).

PE typically consists of 9 to 12 individual therapy sessions that are 90–120 minutes in length. The number of sessions is determined by the patient's response to treatment: Self-reported PTSD symptoms are monitored throughout treatment, and therapy ends when the patient achieves a substantial reduction in symptom severity (in studies, this is at least 70% reduction). The core components of PE include: education about common reactions to trauma and PTSD symptoms, breathing retraining, *in vivo* exposure, and imaginal exposure.

The cornerstones of PE are a strong therapeutic alliance and providing a clear and compelling rationale for the treatment program. In Session 1, the therapist thoroughly explains the idea that avoidance and the presence of trauma-related thoughts and beliefs serve to maintain posttrauma reactions and why confronting rather than avoiding trauma memories and reminders is helpful. The remainder of the session is devoted to gathering relevant information and, at the end of the session, brief instruction in slow, paced breathing. This session and all subsequent sessions are audiotaped, and the patient is asked to listen to the session tape once before the next session.

In Session 2, education about trauma reactions and a discussion of the patient's own experience of these reactions are intended to help the patient to understand that symptoms of PTSD and trauma-related problems are common. The goal of this discussion is to normalize these symptoms and problems in the context of PTSD and, in doing so, to reduce negative appraisal of symptoms and set the focus of treatment on PTSD. The rationale for exposure is presented again in Session 2 with emphasis on *in vivo* exposure, and situations or activities that trigger trauma-related anxiety are identified. A hierarchy of safe or low-risk but avoided situations is constructed, with rankings based on the patient's anticipated distress level when imagining him- or herself in each situation. Beginning in this session and continuing throughout treatment, the patient chooses *in vivo* exposures to confront for homework each week, starting with the relatively low items on the hierarchy. The patient is instructed to stay in each situation for 30 to 45 minutes or until his or her anxiety drops considerably, if possible. By the end of treatment, patients are generally able to comfortably confront most of the situations.

Imaginal exposure is initiated in Session 3. The detailed rationale for exposure is discussed yet again, with the therapist explaining how imaginal reliving of the trauma will help to emotionally process and organize the memory. During imaginal exposure, the patient is instructed to describe aloud what happened during the trauma while visualizing it as vividly as possible. With eyes closed, and using the present tense, the patient also includes the thoughts, emotions, and sensory experiences that occurred during the traumatic event. Throughout the imaginal reliving, the therapist monitors the patient's distress level. Imaginal exposure is continued for 45 to 60 minutes and includes multiple repetitions of the memory if necessary. The aim in this reliving of the trauma is to help the patient access and emotionally engage in the memory. Accordingly, the therapist talks as little as possible during the reliving, usually only speaking to offer support or encouragement, to prompt for distress level, or to ask for more detail. Immediately after the reliving, the patient and therapist discuss the experience, any thoughts or feelings the patient has about it or new understanding that may have emerged, and patterns of habituation that may have occurred. In addition to the *in vivo* exposure homework, the patient is also asked to listen to an audiotape of that session's imaginal exposure once per day until the next session. With these two forms of exposure homework, the patient continues the work of emotionally processing the trauma.

Sessions 4 to 10 (or final) begin with a review of the preceding week's homework. The therapist and patient discuss patterns of habituation, any learning that has occurred, and changes in the way the patient is viewing the trauma or other situations in life. Decisions are made about where to focus exposures next. Then imaginal reliving is conducted for 30–45 minutes. This is followed by a postimaginal "processing" of the experience, in which the therapist provides support as necessary, elicits the patient's thoughts and feelings, and sometimes shares his or her own observations of changes or shifts in the patient's reliving. As therapy progresses, the therapist directs the patient to focus imaginal exposure on the most distressing parts of the trauma memory, or "hot spots." The hot spot work is designed to facilitate processing of these most distressing and often painful memories.

During imaginal exposures, the therapist tries to remain aware of the patient's degree of emotional engagement and distress level. In addition to providing ample support, encouragement, and reinforcement, the therapist may need to direct the patient's reliving to titrate emotional engagement: prompting for more detail and feelings if the patient is not emotionally engaged with the memory or helping him or her to decrease detail and engagement if the distress feels overwhelming. *In vivo* and imaginal exposure homework, assigned at the end of each session, is an integral part of the treatment.

In the final PE session, after reviewing homework, imaginal exposure is conducted, but usually for only 20–30 minutes. The remainder of the session is spent reviewing progress, changes in symptoms, and what the patient has learned from the therapy. Typically, the patient has adopted a new orientation to the PTSD symptoms: avoidance maintains fear, whereas confronting trauma memories and reminders reduces fear and promotes recovery and mastery.

The following is a case vignette of a man treated with PE for accident-related chronic PTSD. Details of the case have been altered to protect confidentiality.

Case Vignette: "Sam"

"Sam," age 36, was referred for treatment by his company's employee assistance department. An assembly line operator, Sam was severely injured while at work about 2 years prior. His hand and forearm became caught in the teeth of a large and powerful machine. He fought very hard to extricate his arm, all the while terrified that he would lose the limb entirely. Sam was finally able to free himself, but not before the machine removed a large area of skin and tissue and broke his arm. Over the months following the accident, he endured several surgeries, including painful skin grafts. Sam tried to return to work about 1 year after the accident, but he did not last more than several months, due to intolerable anxiety and extensive avoidance that interfered with his ability to perform his job. Initial evaluation found Sam to be suffering moderately severe PTSD, major depressive disorder, and social anxiety. He had been receiving ongoing pharmacotherapy since shortly after the accident

Sam accepted the recommendation for a course of PE, although he expressed worry about being able to engage in the imaginal exposure. He reported that a previous therapist had tried to get him to talk about the trauma and that he did it one time but found it very upsetting. Over the first few treatment sessions, the therapist made certain to explain the rationale for exposure carefully and thoroughly, emphasizing that avoidance of this painful memory, although understandable, was preventing Sam from recovering and taking back his life.

Items on Sam's *in vivo* hierarchy included watching crime and medical shows on TV, where he might see blood and injuries; going out with friends from his job with whom he used to socialize; talking about his accident with his friends; going into the building where he worked; gradually approaching the area where he was injured; and going out to crowded stores and shopping malls. Some of these exposures had dual purpose, as is often the case: in addition to engaging in activities that would elicit trauma-related anxiety, Sam's exposure homework functioned as behavioral activation exercises aimed at getting him out of the house and interacting with friends and family members.

Imaginal exposure was begun in the third session and continued for eight consecutive sessions. Sam was able to emotionally engage well in the reliving, and although he found it distressing, he said that it also made sense to him that it could be helpful. He listened to his imaginal exposure tape a few times before the next session and practiced the *in vivo* exposures that he had selected. Subsequent sessions included discussion of homework, planning and progressing through *in vivo* exposures, imaginal exposure, and processing the reliving. Sam worked hard in the treatment and reported that it was progressively easier to do the imaginal exposures in sessions. His self-reported distress levels (subjective units of discomfort scale; SUDS; range of 0 to 100) reflected this habituation: In the first session of imaginal exposure, Sam's SUDS ranged from 30 to 100, with a mean SUDS of 55. In the fourth imaginal, his SUDS ranged from 15 to 80, with a mean of 38. In his eighth and final imaginal exposure, Sam's SUDS ranged from 5 to 35, with a mean of 10.

Midway through treatment, Sam began doing odd jobs for other people who needed help or work done on their houses. He enjoyed working with his hands and found these jobs very satisfying. His confidence increased, visits to the work plant became longer, and he began making arrangements to return to work in his former job. By the end of PE, Sam's assessor-rated PTSD severity had decreased by 80%. His depression was significantly reduced, and he felt more optimistic about his future.

CONCLUSION

Since the introduction of PTSD into the diagnostic nomenclature in 1980, we have learned a great deal about natural recovery following trauma, factors that influence the development and maintenance of PTSD, and of how to effectively treat chronic PTSD. Emotional processing theory (Foa & Kozak, 1986) shaped conceptualizations of the development and maintenance of PTSD and how to effectively intervene with those who had persistent PTSD (e.g., Foa & Jaycox, 1999; Foa & Riggs, 1993; Foa et al., 1989; Foa & Rothbaum, 1998). A series of RCTs conducted in various treatment research clinics around the world have provided strong empirical support for the efficacy of exposure therapy and other forms of CBT in treating PTSD and associated psychopathology. Recent and ongoing studies have begun to investigate the dissemination of efficacious treatments for PTSD (Foa et al., in press). At this time there are several well-validated CBT treatments for PTSD (i.e., SIT, CT/CPT, PE, EMDR); unfortunately, most individuals do not receive such intervention. As such, dissemination is one of the most important clinical and research issues to face our field today. Systematic PTSD effectiveness research is needed that extends efficacy findings beyond academic centers and examines the utility of validated treatments in the hands of nonexperts.

REFERENCES

American Psychiatric Association. (1980). *Diagnostic and statistical manual of mental disorders* (2nd ed.). Washington, DC: American Psychiatric Press.

American Psychiatric Association. (1994). *Diagnostic and statistical manual of mental disorders* (4th ed.). Washington, DC: Author.

Beck, A. T. (1976). *Cognitive therapy and the emotional disorders.* New York: International Universities Press.

Breslau, N., Davis, G. C., Andreski, P., & Peterson, E. (1991). Traumatic events and posttraumatic stress disorder in an urban population of young adults. *Archives of General Psychiatry, 48*, 218–228.

Breslau, N., Kessler, R. C., Chilcoat, H. D., Schultz, L. R., Davis, G., & Andreski, P. (1998). Trauma and posttraumatic stress disorder: The 1996 Detroit area survey of trauma. *Archives of General Psychiatry, 55*, 626–632.

Cahill, S. P., Carrigan, M. H., & Frueh, B. C. (1999). Does EMDR work? And if so, why? A critical review of controlled outcome and dismantling research. *Journal of Anxiety Disorders, 13*, 5–33.

Davidson, P. R., & Parker, K. C. H. (2001). Eye movement desensitization and reprocessing (EMDR): A meta-analysis. *Journal of Consulting and Clinical Psychology, 69*, 305–319.

Ehlers, A., & Clark, D. M. (2000). A cognitive model of persistent posttraumatic stress disorder. *Behaviour Research and Therapy, 38*, 319–345.

Foa, E. B., Dancu, C. V., Hembree, E., Jaycox, L. H., Meadows, E. A., & Street, G. P. (1999). The efficacy of exposure therapy, stress inoculation training and their combination in ameliorating PTSD for female victims of assault. *Journal of Consulting and Clinical Psychology, 67*, 194–200.

Foa, E. B., Ehlers, A., Clark, D., Tolin, D. F, & Orsillo, S. (1999). Posttraumatic cognitions inventory (PTCI): Development and comparison with other measures. *Psychological Assessment, 11*, 303–314.

Foa, E. B., Hembree, E. A., Cahill, S. P., Rauch, S. A., Riggs, D. S., & Feeny, N. C. (in press). Prolonged exposure for PTSD with and without cognitive restructuring: Outcome at academic and community clinics. *Journal of Consulting and Clinical Psychology.*

Foa, E. B., & Jaycox, L. H. (1999). Cognitive-behavioral theory and treatment of posttraumatic stress disorder. In D. Spiegel (Ed.), *Efficacy and cost-effectiveness of psychotherapy* (pp. 23–61). Washington, DC: American Psychiatric Press.

Foa, E. B., & Kozak, M. J. (1986). Emotional processing of fear: Exposure to corrective information. *Psychological Bulletin, 99*, 20–35.

Foa, E. B., & Riggs, D. S. (1993). Post-traumatic stress disorder in rape victims. In J. Oldham, M. B. Riba, & A. Tasman (Eds.), *American Psychiatric Press review of psychiatry* (Vol. 12, pp. 273–303). Washington, DC: American Psychiatric Press.

Foa, E. B., & Rothbaum, B. O. (1998). *Treating the trauma of rape*. New York: Guilford Press.

Foa, E. B., Rothbaum, B. O., Riggs, D., & Murdock, T. (1991). Treatment of PTSD in rape victims: A comparison between cognitive-behavioral procedures and counseling. *Journal of Consulting and Clinical Psychology, 59*, 715–723.

Foa, E. B., Steketee, G., & Rothbaum, B. (1989). Behavioral/cognitive conceptualizations of post-traumatic stress disorder. *Behavior Therapy, 20*, 155–176.

Harvey, A. G., Bryant, R. A., & Tarrier, N. (2003). Cognitive behaviour therapy for posttraumatic stress disorder. *Clinical Psychology Review, 3*, 501–522.

Janoff-Bulman, R. (1992). *Shattered assumptions: Towards a new psychology of trauma*. New York: Free Press.

Kessler, R. C., Sonnega, A., Bromet, E., Hughes, M., & Nelson, C. B. (1995). Posttraumatic stress disorder in the National Comorbidity Survey. *Archives of General Psychiatry, 52*, 1048–1060.

Kulka, R. A., Schlenger, W. E., Fairbank, J. A., Hough, R. L., Jordan, B. K., Marmar, C. R., & Weiss, D. S. (1990). *Trauma and the Vietnam war generation*. New York: Brunner/Mazel.

Lang, P. J. (1977). Imagery in therapy: An information processing analysis of fear. *Behavior Therapy, 8*, 862–886.

Lang, P. J. (1979). A bio-informational theory of emotional imagery. *Psychophysiology, 16*, 495–512.

Lee, C., Gavriel, H., Drummond, P., Richards, J., & Greenwald, R. (2002). Treatment of PTSD: Stress inoculation training with prolonged exposure compared to EMDR. *Journal of Clinical Psychology, 58*, 1071–1089.

Marks, I., Lovell, K., Noshirvani, H., Livanou, M., & Thrasher, S. (1998). Treatment of posttraumatic stress disorder by exposure and/or cognitive restructuring. *Archives of General Psychiatry, 55*, 317–325.

Meichenbaum, D. (1975). Self-instructional methods. In F. H. Kanfer & A. P. Goldstein (Eds.), *Helping people change* (pp. 357–391). New York: Pergamon.

Mowrer, O. A. (1960). *Learning theory and behavior*. New York: Wiley.

Norris, F. H., Murphy, A. D., Baker, C. K., Perilla, J. L., Rodriguez, F. G., & Rodriguez, J. J. G. (2003). Epidemiology of trauma and posttraumatic stress disorder in Mexico. *Journal of Abnormal Psychology, 112*, 646–656.

Pham, P. N., Weinstein, H. M., & Longman, T. (2004). Trauma and PTSD symptoms in Rwanda: Implications for attitudes toward justice and reconciliation. *Journal of the American Medical Association, 292*, 602–612.

Power, K., McGoldrick, T., Brown, K., Buchanan, R., Sharp, D., Swanson, V., & Karatzias, A. (2002). A controlled comparison of eye movement desensitization and reprocessing versus exposure plus cognitive restructuring versus waiting list in the treatment of posttraumatic stress disorder. *Clinical Psychology and Psychotherapy, 9*, 299–318.

Rachman, S. (1980). Emotional processing. *Behaviour Research and Therapy, 18*, 51–60.

Resick, P. A., Nishith, P., Weaver, T., Astin, M. C., & Feuer, C. A. (2002). A comparison of cognitive processing therapy, prolonged exposure, and a waiting condition for the treatment of posttraumatic stress disorder in female rape victims. *Journal of Consulting and Clinical Psychology, 70*, 867–879.

Resick, P. A., & Schnicke, M. K. (1992). Cognitive processing therapy for sexual assault victims. *Journal of Consulting and Clinical Psychology, 60*, 748–756.

Resnick, H. S., Kilpatrick, D. G., Dansky, B. S., Saunders, B. E., & Best, C. L. (1993). Prevalence of civilian trauma and posttraumatic stress disorder in a representative national sample of women. *Journal of Consulting and Clinical Psychology, 61*, 984–991.

Riggs, D. S., Rothbaum, B. O., & Foa, E. B. (1995). A prospective examination of symptoms of posttraumatic stress disorder in victims of nonsexual assault. *Journal of Interpersonal Violence, 2*, 201–214.

Rothbaum, B. O. (2002, March). A controlled study of PE versus EMDR for PTSD in rape victims. In L. A. Zoellner (Chair), *Recent innovations in posttraumatic stress disorder treatment*. Symposium conducted at the annual convention of the Anxiety Disorders Association of America, Austin, TX.

Rothbaum, B. O., Foa, E. B., Riggs, D. S., Murdock, T., & Walsh, W. (1992). A prospective examination of post-traumatic stress disorder in rape victims. *Journal of Traumatic Stress, 5*, 455–475.

Rothbaum, B. O., Meadows, E. A., Resick, P., & Foy, D. (2000). Cognitive-behavioral therapy. In E. B. Foa, T. M. Keane, & M. J. Friedman (Eds.), *Effective treatments for PTSD: Practice guidelines from the International Society for Traumatic Stress Studies* (pp. 320–325). New York: Guilford Press.

Shapiro, F. (1989). Efficacy of the eye movement desensitization procedure in the treatment of traumatic memories. *Journal of Traumatic Stress, 2*(2), 199–223.

Shapiro, F. (1995). *Eye movement desensitization and reprocessing: Basic principles, protocols, and procedures*. New York: Guilford Press.

Steil, R., & Ehlers, A. (2000). Dysfunctional meaning of posttraumatic intrusions in chronic PTSD. *Behaviour Research and Therapy, 38*, 537–558.

Tarrier, N., Pilgrim, H., Sommerfield, C., Faragher, B., Reynolds, M., Graham, E., et al. (1999). A randomized trial of cognitive therapy and imaginal exposure in the treatment of chronic posttraumatic stress disorder. *Journal of Consulting and Clinical Psychology, 67*, 13–18.

Taylor, S., & Koch, W. J. (1995). Anxiety disorders due to motor vehicle accidents: Nature and treatment. *Clinical Psychology Review, 15*, 721–738.

Taylor, S., Thordarson, D. S., Maxfield, L., Fedoroff, I. C., Lovell, K., & Ogrodniczuk, J. (2003). Comparative efficacy, speed, and adverse effects of three PTSD treatments: Exposure therapy, EMDR, and relaxation training. *Journal of Consulting and Clinical Psychology, 71*, 330–338.

Veronen, L. J., & Kilpatrick, D. G. (1982) Stress inoculation training for victims of rape: Efficacy and differential findings. In *Sexual violence and harassment*. Symposium conducted at the 16th annual convention of the Association for the Advancement of Behavior Therapy, Los Angeles, CA.

PART III

Innovative Treatment Applications and Future Directions

13

Adapting Imaginal Exposure to the Treatment of Complicated Grief

KATHERINE SHEAR

Complicated grief (CG) is a newly recognized, chronic, debilitating psychiatric condition. CG comprises symptoms of separation distress, along with prominent symptoms of traumatic stress. We recently undertook the task of devising a treatment for CG. As we considered how best to address symptoms of traumatic distress, we sought consultation from Edna Foa. Foa's work in anxiety disorders has had a far-reaching impact on the field. Her strong theoretical grounding, combined with a notable capacity for highly empathic and intuitive clinical work, have led her to develop some of the most innovative and effective psychosocial interventions in the world. We believed that incorporating her efficacious techniques for treating post-traumatic stress disorder (PTSD), as well as gaining her participation as a consultant, would optimize our chances of producing a useful treatment. This chapter outlines the process of incorporating and modifying Foa's exposure techniques, imaginal exposure in particular, as a component of a treatment for CG.

CG, described in more detail later, shares features of both mood and anxiety disorders. Grief is accompanied by a depressed mood and other dysphoric affect. Sleep and appetite disturbance is common in the wake of a difficult loss, as is guilt, hopelessness, and suicidal ideation. CG also includes prominent symptoms of traumatic distress, bearing some resemblance to PTSD. Often the sufferer experiences recurrent intrusive images of the person who died, accompanied by a sense of horror or helplessness. Fear of experiencing intense uncontrollable emotions or of sinking into a state of hopeless despair drives a broad range of avoidance behaviors. This avoidance is accompanied by a sense of estrangement from others, who are seen as unable to understand and as creatures existing on the other side of a deep chasm. These trauma symptoms constrict the lives of complicated grievers, impeding their ability to derive joy and satisfaction from their lives.

Given the amalgam of depressive and trauma-like symptoms, we decided to develop a treatment that integrates techniques found helpful for depression with those used for PTSD. Edna Foa's PTSD treatment was highly effective and carefully studied. We consulted with her to develop the trauma-focused component of CG treatment. In the remainder of this chapter, we (1) describe the syndrome of CG and review treatments for bereavement-related distress, (2) explain the process we used to develop CG treatment (CGT), (3) present techniques we use to train therapists, and (4) give an overview of data from our studies of this condition.

THE SYNDROME OF CG

The suffering imposed by chronic grief has been observed by authors as diverse as Freud (1917) Lindemann (1979), Bowlby (1973, 1980), Parkes (1986, 1998), Raphael (1975, 1983a, 1983b), Horowitz (Horowitz et al., 1993; Horowitz, Wilner, Marmar, & Krupnick, 1980) and Jacobs (Jacobs, Kasl, Ostfeld, Berkman, & Charpentier, 1986; Jacobs, Kasl, Ostfeld, Berkman, Kosten, & Charpentier, 1986). Within this literature there is general agreement about the type of symptoms that would constitute a disorder of grief. For decades, clinicians and researchers interested in helping the bereaved have expressed frustration over the lack of standardized diagnostic criteria. Recently this problem has been addressed. Two groups independently proposed specific criteria that are very similar. Horowitz et al. (1997) were the first to suggest criteria. This group has been studying grief for a number of years, and results of their empirical studies indicated that a putative complicated grief disorder includes intrusive thoughts, strong pangs of severe emotions, strong yearnings, feeling alone and empty, avoidance of people and places that act as reminders of the loss, and loss of interest in personal activities. Working independently, our group found a similar criteria set for the syndrome we called at the time "traumatic grief" (Prigerson et al., 1999), drawing on our own research findings and developed by a strategy of consensus of experts in the field. The similarity of these independently derived criteria sets provides some support for the validity of the syndrome. Also supportive is the fact that the syndrome of CG meets several of the criteria outlined by Robins and Guze (Robins & Guze, 1970) that are needed to confirm validity of a new diagnostic entity.

First, there is a replicable, identifiable clinical description. Symptoms reflect separation distress (e.g. inability to accept the death, with yearning and longing and persistent intense grief and preoccupation with thoughts of the deceased, including a tendency to enter states of reverie) and traumatic distress (e.g., intrusive images of the death, often accompanied by feelings of guilt; being upset by memories of the deceased, with avoidance of situations that trigger these memories; difficulty trusting and/or caring about others, sometimes accompanied by feelings of unfairness, bitterness, envy of others, and feeling very lonely and estranged from others). Symptoms of separation distress and traumatic distress load together on factor analysis of the Inventory of Complicated Grief (ICG), supporting their close relationship.

It is also possible to clearly discriminate CG from other disorders. There is good evidence that CG is distinguishable from both major depressive disorder (MDD) and PTSD. CG and MDD have different risk factors, clinical correlates, temporal course, and response to antidepressant medication and to interpersonal psychotherapy. In a community sample of widows and widowers, 46% of participants who have syndromal-level CG did *not* meet criteria for a diagnosis of MDD. In our ongoing study, only 60% meet criteria on the Structured Clinical Interview for DSM-IV Axis I Disorders (SCID) for current MDD. CG also differs from PTSD. CG occurs following loss of an important relationship rather than exposure to a life-threatening event. PTSD does not include yearning or searching, and the primary emotional reaction is fear, not the sadness and anguish of grief. Many people with CG do not meet criteria for PTSD. In our current treatment study, only about 30% meet SCID criteria for PTSD. Additionally, CG can be distinguished from adjustment disorder, as criteria for this disorder explicitly state that the symptoms cannot be a consequence of bereavement.

Follow-up studies provide further support for the validity of the syndrome. CG symptoms predict onset of cancer, heart trouble, high blood pressure, substance abuse, and suicidal ideation in the aftermath of the loss (Chen et al., 1999). Suicidality, a growing public health problem among the elderly, is twice as common in bereaved spouses over the age of 50 with CG as opposed to those without CG.

Considering the importance of the problem, the existing literature on grief interventions is remarkably small. Reported interventions include two main strategies. The first is preventative and based on observations that greater social support predicts better adjustment to spousal loss. Supportive psychotherapy, self-help groups, and widow-to-widow programs show moderate success (Marmar, Horowitz, Weiss, Wilner, & Kaltreider, 1988; Shuchter & Zisook, 1986; Windholz, Marmar, & Horowitz, 1985). However, a recent meta-analysis showed a strikingly low effect size (0.15) for grief interventions that have been tested, and a minority of individuals actually worsened with intervention. More directly pertinent to our work are reports describing treatments that target pathological grief (Gauthier & Marshall, 1977; Lieberman, 1997; Ramsay, 1977a, 1977b; Rando, 1993; Raphael, 1975; Volkan, 1971). These authors consistently recommend focus on the loss, as does CGT. However, we could locate only three controlled studies, none of which used reliable methods of identification of study participants or psychometrically sound grief assessment. Two studies of "guided mourning" (Mawson, Marks, Ramm, & Stern, 1981; Sireling, Cohen, & Marks, 1988) compared a brief exposure intervention with an antiexposure treatment, in which patients were encouraged to avoid thinking about the deceased and avoid doing anything upsetting. These showed a significant treatment effect of exposure on only a few measures, none of which was a measure of CG. The third study compared psychodynamic psychotherapy with a self-help support group and found no difference (Horowitz, Marmar, Weiss, Kaltreider, & Wilner, 1986). There is clearly a need to find efficacious treatments for CG. Such treatment needs to target both separation distress and traumatic distress.

OVERVIEW OF OUR PROCESS IN DEVELOPING CGT

We began our CGT project by reviewing effects of treatments for depression on these symptoms. A study from our late-life-depression group targeted bereavement-related depression and included the ICG (Prigerson et al., 1995) in a subset of patients. Results showed little effect of nortriptyline or interpersonal psychotherapy (IPT) for symptoms of CG (Reynolds et al., 1999). Subsequently a study of bupropion showed a similar small effect (Zisook, Shuchter, Pedrelli, Sable, & Deaciue, 2001). Because complicated grief bears some resemblance to depression and because IPT includes grief as a possible focus, we began by attempting to augment IPT. The advantage of using IPT includes the fact that it has been shown to be an excellent treatment for MDD in a number of studies (Frank, 1991). It is a practical, innovative approach that is relatively easy for most practicing therapists to learn. In a dramatic example of the ease of dissemination, IPT was used to treat depression in a village in Africa (Bolton et al., 2003). IPT fosters a strong therapeutic alliance, and dropout rates are among the lowest observed for any psychotherapy.

Our initial work, published as a combination study with paroxetine (Zygmont et al., 1998) showed some promise. However, we found that a number of patients appeared to be only moderately responsive. At this point, given the prominence of trauma-like symptoms, we enlisted the assistance of Edna Foa. She provided important consultation to the developers and therapists in this project by introducing the use of prolonged exposure, as well as *in vivo* exposure techniques for this condition. We began using an imaginal exposure strategy modeled on the techniques used to treat PTSD (Foa & Rothbaum, 1998).

The integration of exposure and other cognitive-behavioral techniques into IPT bears some discussion. Our experience integrating cognitive and behavioral techniques into IPT has been very positive. We have done this successfully in CGT and also in a NIMH funded treatment development project targeting panic and other anxiety symptoms in treatment for depression. IPT, like CBT, is a short-term treatment with a clear focus. The work is present-oriented and practical. IPT differs from CBT in its focus on interpersonal relationships. However, the techniques used to effect change in relationships include engaging in behavioral exercises to effect change in a targeted relationship or to accomplish a new task in a role transition, analyzing communication in interpersonal relationships to uncover distorted thinking and thinking through options for dealing with interpersonal problems. Direct advice and role play are standard techniques in IPT, as they are in CBT. Many IPT therapists ask their patients to do some kind of homework, though IPT generally refrains from regular symptom monitoring or any highly structured homework assignments. The similarities between CBT and IPT were documented in a recent a study in which marked similarities were found in the nature of the interaction between the patient and therapist in IPT and CBT (Ablon & Jones, 2002). These authors conclude that there are more similarities than differences in these two forms of therapy. Our experience is congruent with these observations. In CGT we began with standard grief-focused IPT and augmented the treatment with exposure-based techniques and later some additional CBT-based modifications. We found that integration of these techniques was straightforward and, with the possible exception of some different therapist training techniques (described later), required little modification of the underlying IPT structure.

The use of prolonged exposure and planned *in vivo* exposures further strengthened our treatment. However, several problems emerged. First, there were often numerous challenging "traumatic" experiences in the course of a serious medical illness, leaving open many possible foci for imaginal exposure exercises. At Foa's suggestion, we originally handled this by asking the patient about the most difficult time. After working in this way for awhile, we began to notice that patients often omitted the death of their loved one as one of the most difficult times. However, when we conducted imaginal exposure targeting other traumatic moments (e.g. diagnosis of a terminal illness, an emergency hospitalization, a cardiac arrest), CG scores remained high. We thus decided to introduce an imaginal exercise focused on the death in every case. When we did this, grief symptoms abated well.

A second problem we faced was that the story of the death regularly evoked extremely high levels of emotion, and patients who underwent this exercise began either refusing to continue or expressing markedly increased distress and occasionally increased suicidal ideation or the onset of self-destructive behaviors. For example, one patient spent the night drinking at the graveside of his loved one. Similarly, patients were refusing to participate in some of the *in vivo* exercises, especially ones that had no potential benefit to them (e.g., going to the hospital or emergency room where the patient died; going to the site of an accident). Around the same time, in conjunction with extensive discussions and further review of the grief literature, we came to the conclusion that the treatment should follow Stroebe and Schut's "dual process model" of coping (Stroebe & Schut, 1999). According to these experienced grief researchers, adaptive grief proceeds in an oscillating manner on two fronts. One they refer to as "loss oriented," and the other "restoration oriented." Although IPT has some focus on restoration orientation, we decided this needed to be enhanced and introduced early in the treatment. In addition, the use of exposure techniques was greatly helpful in targeting a part of the loss response, but more was needed to address separation distress.

At this point we made several more modifications to the treatment to construct the approach that was used in our randomized controlled trial. First, we added a focus on personal goals. To do this, we modified a technique used in motivational enhancement therapy. In our personal goals work, the therapist asks the patients to envision what they would want for themselves if their grief could be magically removed. The therapist works with the patient to articulate one or more life goals. This can be something the person has always wanted to do and has not had the chance, something he or she had wanted to do with the person who died, or something that he or she could not do because of the relationship with this person. Sometimes this goal is something altogether new. For example, one patient who had worked as a white-collar worker in a corporate environment for many years had a long-standing wish to open a retail store. The therapist helped her identify this goal and then to work with it through the period of the treatment. By the end of the treatment, she had rented a store, and opening day was set. This work on personal goals was complemented by standard strategies in IPT used to improve current relationships. Working to enhance satisfaction with ongoing relationships also forms a component of the restoration focus.

To further develop the loss focus of the treatment, we modified the exposure techniques and added two new strategies to target separation distress. The modifications of imaginal exposure entailed changing the name to "revisiting" and shortening the exercises. The two strategies we added were an imaginal conversation with the deceased and a series of sequential-memories forms that tapped positive, then negative, then both positive and negative memories. The imaginal conversation was derived from a psychodrama technique frequently used by one of our therapists in which patients imagine they can talk with their deceased loved ones and that the loved ones can hear and respond. In this exercise, the patient both talks to the deceased and then responds for the deceased. This has proved to be a very powerful component of the treatment. However, we learned that it cannot be done until the imaginal revisiting work has sufficiently reduced the intensity of emotion surrounding the death.

The reason for changing the terminology "exposure" to "revisiting" was to reduce the degree of fear engendered in patients on description of the treatment and to reflect the goal of reprocessing the death in a way that can help the bereaved person better accept the death. We shortened the discussion of the death because we found that the shorter period successfully activated highly emotional memories of the death that could then be discussed. We modified the *in vivo* exposures in a similar manner, calling this "revisiting situations and activities." We further encouraged patients to identify those situations and activities that they would like to do. Each of these modifications appeared to be successful.

In summary, Edna Foa's consultation on the development of CGT led to incorporation of an imaginal revisiting strategy that we believe markedly improved the effectiveness of the treatment. This technique contributed importantly to work on the loss, one of the two processes that need attention in the aftermath of the death of an attachment figure. However, we believe that prolonged exposure (PE) in the context of CG is better administered in a somewhat modified way. First, we consider it important to focus the exercise on the death itself, even in the context of a prolonged illness with numerous traumatic episodes. The rationale for this is both practical and theoretical. From a practical standpoint, we found that several patients failed to show reduction in CG scores after effectively addressing other traumatic events related to prolonged illness. This lack of response occurred even though they stated that the death itself "wasn't that bad." Moreover, scores decreased immediately following an exercise focused on the death. Theoretically, we believe this makes sense because we consider the traumatic distress to be linked to the separation from a close attachment. Thus it is the loss of the person, rather than exposure to a horrifying event or events, that is experienced as a trauma.

TRAINING OF THERAPISTS

Training therapists is important for any psychotherapy study. A range of techniques have been devised to accomplish this goal, and Foa has again been a leader in training therapists to provide difficult anxiety disorder treatments. Exposure interventions typically evoke intense emotions in patients, and this can be quite difficult for therapists. Foa utilizes didactic training with heuristic models, videotape examples, in-person demonstrations, and therapist role plays in an artful manner to help therapists learn how to combine gentle, empathic support with confident unambivalent exposure instructions. She has successfully trained inexperienced students, experienced therapists, and community counselors to use her highly effective PTSD approach.

We began our training procedures using Foa's model. We provided a 2-day didactic seminar for new therapists, including presentation of characteristics of normal and complicated grief; an overview of the treatment, including its central goals of addressing loss and restoration-oriented problems; a review of the strategies used to address traumatic and separation distress, as well as those focused on restoration goals; and a detailed review of the specific techniques used for each strategy. We obtained permission from patients and utilized videotaped examples of actual treatment cases. We conducted demonstrations and assisted therapists in role play of the various techniques. This method appeared to be successful in training a cadre of new therapists. However, as work with CGT got under way, we began to see a phenomenon we had not seen previously in conducting different mood and anxiety studies over a 20-year period. We had a high rate of therapist dropout, and several therapists stipulated certain types of patients they would not agree to see. For this reason we rethought our training procedures.

We understood that therapists were being triggered emotionally by confronting the universal experience of loss. Virtually all of the therapists we trained had experienced a loss of an important person themselves. Working with these patients was evoking painful reminders of their own experience, sometimes only partially resolved.

We therefore initiated experiential exercises for therapists as part of their training. These exercises had two purposes: to practice learning the procedures for revisiting and imaginal conversation and to activate the therapists' own emotions related to grief. This activation gives the therapists a chance to become aware of the intensity of their own feelings, to know more about the nature of these feelings, and to work with the feelings if they wish to do so. The exercise also helps the therapist better understand and prepare for the emotional intensity evoked by the revisiting exercise. Under some circumstances, it is also useful for the therapists to share their own experiences doing this exercise.

The imaginal conversation is similarly powerful and helpful for most therapists. This technique entails both speaking to and speaking for the deceased loved one, imagining that they can hear and respond. Most patients who do this exercise tell us it is extremely powerful, and therapists in training have reported this as well. This conversation provides the training therapist with a very helpful opportunity to work with any nagging problems related to the death of a close loved one. Several therapists have told us this is a unique and extremely interesting and helpful part of the training.

TREATMENT OUTCOME

During the process of our treatment development we undertook several outcome projects. The first entailed our earliest efforts at integrating IPT and behavioral techniques. This was done in the context of an ongoing open pharmacotherapy study (Zygmont et al., 1998) in which some patients received nortriptyline and some paroxetine. Although we found nortriptyline without psychotherapy ineffective for CG (Reynolds et al., 1999), when combined with our initial grief-focused psychotherapy, results were better. Paroxetine showed similar positive effects when combined with the psychotherapy. During this early period of work, we observed that talking about the death seemed to be a helpful component of the treatment. However, we further noted that intrusive images persisted for many people and that treatment results were still only moderate. For this reason we contacted Foa, who provided a 2-day seminar on treatment for PTSD.

Our CG therapists attended this seminar and learned techniques of PE and *in vivo* exposure. We began implementing these techniques, again with Foa's help, and found that we could produce much greater results, as documented in an open pilot study of 21 individuals, including 13 completers. Mean ICG score was 40.3 ± 9.0 at baseline, and this decreased to 23.4 ± 14.4 in the full group of 21 patients. Among the 13 who completed the treatment, mean baseline score was 38.9 ± 9.9, and posttreatment mean ICG score was 18.1 ± 10.9. These results (-16.9 ± 15.0 in the intent-to-treat group and 22.8 ± 13.1 in the completers) compared to a mean change in ICG score of -8.75, SD 14.1, with IPT alone.

We found similar results for the Beck Anxiety Inventory (BAI) and Beck Depression Inventory (BDI). On these, symptoms were reduced from 19.4 ± 13.3 to 6.62 ± 10.25, and from 22.06 ± 8.68 to 11.67 ± 10.17, respectively. These results consist of large effect sizes for ICG of 2.19 and 1.45 for completers and intent-to-treat, respectively; for BAI, of 2.04 and 1.08, and for BDI, of 1.80 and 1.16. Based upon these results, we obtained NIMH funding for a randomized controlled trial comparing CGT to IPT.

We have now completed the randomized trial, in which 95 individuals participated (Shear et al., 2005). We used a further refined version of the treatment in this study, as described earlier in the chapter. Foa continued to consult with us, especially the component related to imaginal revisiting. This study succeeded in confirming significant differences between IPT and CGT, more pronounced in those who completed the treatment. Response rates were determined by the judgment of an independent evaluator, using the Clinical Global Improvement scale (Guy, 1976). CGT produced significantly greater response (i.e., a rating of 2 [much] or 1 [very much] improved) than IPT. This was true for treatment completers, 66% versus 32% ($p = 0.006$) and for all randomized participants; 51% for CGT versus 28% for IPT ($p = 0.024$). A survival analysis also showed median time to response on the Inventory of Complicated Grief (Prigerson et al., 1995) was shorter for CGT than for IPT ($p = 0.017$). Mean reduction in dimensional measures of depression and functional impairment were also greater for CGT patients, especially completers. For example, the Beck Depression Inventory (Beck et al., 1988) scores showed a mean decrease of 12.7 ± 9.8 for CGT and 7.3 ± 5.6 for IPT ($p = 0.02$) in completers, and 10.4 ± 9.6 for CGT versus 7.2 ± 7.2 for IPT; ($p = 0.10$) in all randomized participants. The mean decrease in the Work and Social Adjustment Scale (Mundt et al., 2002) was 10.4 ± 11.2 for CGT versus 5.0 ± 9.9 for IPT ($p = 0.04$) among completers, and 7.8 ± 11.3 for CGT versus 4.2 ± 9.5 for IPT ($p = 0.006$) among all randomized participants.

We further succeeded in reducing the dropout rate from 13 out of 21 (62%) in the pilot study to 13 out of 49 (27%) in the randomized trial. Dropout from IPT was 12 out of 46 (26%). We tape-recorded all therapy sessions, and we collected data on grief diary levels and revisiting subjective units of disturbance (SUDS) levels during the treatment. Work is under way to examine hypotheses related to treatment effects.

In summary, we have described a new application of Foa's prolonged exposure and *in vivo* exposure strategies. We modified these techniques in order to apply them to patients who present with the condition of CG. We consider this work further evidence of the major impact of Edna Foa's work in helping people suffering from a wide range of psychiatric conditions. We join our colleagues in expressing deep admiration and heartfelt thanks for her energy, her intelligence, and her wonderful good heart.

ACKNOWLEDGMENTS

This work was supported by National Institute of Mental Health Grant Nos. MH-60783, 30915, and 52247.

REFERENCES

Ablon, J. S., & Jones, E. E. (2002). Validity of controlled clinical trials of psychotherapy: Findings from the NIMH Treatment of Depression Collaborative Research Program. *American Journal of Psychiatry, 159,* 775–783.

Beck, A. T., Epstein, N., Brown, G., & Steer, R. A. (1988). An inventory for measuring clinical anxiety: Psychometric properties. *Journal of Consulting and Clinical Psychology, 56*(6), 893–897.

Bolton, P., Bass, J., Neugebauer, R., Verdeli, H., Clougherty, K. F., Wickramaratne, et al. (2003). Group interpersonal psychotherapy for depression in rural Uganda: A randomized controlled trial. *Journal of the American Medical Association, 289,* 3117–3124.

Bowlby, J. (1973). *Attachment and loss: Vol. II. Separation, anxiety and anger.* London: Hogarth Press.

Bowlby, J. (1980). *Attachment and loss: Vol. III. Loss.* New York: Basic Books.

Chen, J. H., Bierhals, A. J., Prigerson, H. G., Kasl, S. V., Mazure, C. M., Reynolds, C. F., et al. (in press). Gender differences in the effects of bereavement-related psychological distress on health outcomes. *Psychological Medicine, 29,* 367–380.

Foa, E. B., & Rothbaum, B. O. (1998). Treating the trauma of rape: Cognitive-behavioral therapy for PTSD. In E. B. Foa & B. O. Rothbaum (Eds.), *Treatment manuals for practitioners* (p. 286) New York: Guilford Press.

Frank, E. (1991). Interpersonal psychotherapy as a maintenance treatment for patients with recurrent depression. *Psychotherapy, 28,* 259–266.

Freud, S. (1917). Mourning and melancholia. *Internationale Zeitschrift für arzliche Psychoanalyse, 4,* 288–301.

Gauthier, J., & Marshall, W. L. (1977). Grief: A cognitive-behavioral analysis. *Cognitive Therapy and Research, 1,* 39–44.

Guy, W. (1976). *Clinical global impressions: ECDEU assessment manual for psychopharmacology, revised.* Washington, DC: National Institute of Mental Health.

Horowitz, M., Stinson, C., Fridhandler, B., Milbrath, C., Redington, D., & Ewert, M. (1993). Pathological grief: An intensive case study. *Psychiatry, 56,* 356–374.

Horowitz, M. J., Marmar, C. R., Weiss, D. S., Kaltreider, N. B., & Wilner, N. R. (1986). Comprehensive analysis of change after brief dynamic psychotherapy. *American Journal of Psychiatry, 143,* 582–589.

Horowitz, M. J., Siegel, B., Holen, A., Bonanno, G. A., Milbrath, C., & Stinson, C. H. (1997). Diagnostic criteria for complicated grief disorder. *American Journal of Psychiatry, 154,* 904–910.

Horowitz, M. J., Wilner, N., Marmar, C., & Krupnick, J. (1980). Pathological grief and the activation of latent self-images. *American Journal of Psychiatry, 137,* 1152–1157.

Jacobs, S. C., Kasl, S., Ostfeld, A. M., Berkman, L., & Charpentier, P. (1986). The measurement of grief: Age and sex variation. *British Journal of Medical Psychology, 59,* 305–310.

Jacobs, S. C., Kasl, S. V., Ostfeld, A. M., Berkman, L., Kosten, T. R., & Charpentier, P. (1986). The measurement of grief: Bereaved versus non-bereaved. *Hospice Journal, 2,* 21–36.

Lieberman, M. A. (1997). Bereavement self-help groups: A review of conceptual and methodological issues. In M. S. Stroebe, W. Stroebe, & R. O. Hansson (Eds.), *Handbook of bereavement: Theory, research and intervention* (pp. 411–426). New York: Cambridge University Press.

Lindemann, E. (1979). *Beyond grief: Studies in crisis intervention.* New York: Aronson.

Marmar, C. R., Horowitz, M. J., Weiss, D. S., Wilner, N. R., & Kaltreider, N. B. (1988). A controlled trial of brief psychotherapy and mutual-help group treatment of conjugal bereavement. *American Journal of Psychiatry, 145,* 203–209.

Mawson, D., Marks, I. M., Ramm, L., & Stern, R. S. (1981). Guided mourning for morbid grief: A controlled study. *British Journal of Psychiatry, 138,* 185–193.

Mundt, J. C., Marks, I. M., Shear, M. K., & Greist, J. H. (2002). The work and social adjustment scale: A simple measure of impairment in functioning. *British Journal of Psychiatry, 180,* 461–464.

Parkes, C. M. (1986). *Bereavement: Studies of grief in adult life* (2nd ed.). Madison, CT: International Universities Press.

Parkes, C. M. (1998). Bereavement in adult life [Review]. *British Medical Journal, 316,* 856–859.

Prigerson, H. G., Maciejewski, P. K., Reynolds, C. F., Bierhals, A. J., Newsom, J. T., Fasiczka, A., et al. (1995). Inventory of Complicated Grief: A scale to measure maladaptive symptoms of loss. *Psychiatry Research, 59,* 65–79.

Prigerson, H. G., Shear, M. K., Jacobs, S. C., Reynolds, C. F., Maciejewski, P. K., Rosenheck, R., et al. (1999). Consensus criteria for traumatic grief: A rationale and preliminary empirical test. *British Journal of Psychiatry, 174,* 67–73.

Ramsay, R. W. (1977a). Behavioural approaches to bereavement. *Behaviour Research and Therapy, 15,* 131–135.

Ramsay, R. W. (1977b). *Bereavement: A behavioral treatment of pathological grief.* Unpublished manuscript.

Rando, T. A. (1993). *Treatment of complicated mourning.* Champaign, IL: Research Press.

Raphael, B. (1975). The management of pathological grief. *Australian and New Zealand Journal of Psychiatry, 9,* 173–180.

Raphael, B. (1983a). Caring for the bereaved. In B. Raphael (Ed.), *The anatomy of bereavement* (pp. 352–401). New York: Basic Books.

Raphael, B. (1983b). The experience of bereavement: Separation and mourning. In B. Raphael (Ed.), *The anatomy of bereavement* (pp. 33–73). New York: Basic Books.

Reynolds, C. F., Miller, M. D., Pasternak, R. E., Frank, E., Perel, J. M., Cornes, C., et al. (1999). Treatment of bereavement-related major depressive episodes in later life: A randomized, double-blind, placebo-controlled study of acute and continuation treatment with nortriptyline and interpersonal psychotherapy. *American Journal of Psychiatry, 156,* 202–208.

Robins, E., & Guze, S. B. (1970). Establishment of diagnostic validity in psychiatric illness: Its application to schizophrenia. *American Journal of Psychiatry, 126,* 983–987.

Shear, K., Frank, E., Reynolds, C., & Houck, P. (2005). Treatment of complicated grief: A randomized controlled trial. *Journal of the American Medical Association, 293,* 2601–2608.

Shuchter, S. R., & Zisook, S. (1986). Treatment of spousal bereavement: A multidimensional approach. *Psychiatric Annals, 16,* 295–305.

Sireling, L., Cohen, D., & Marks, I. (1988). Guided mourning for morbid grief: A controlled replication. *Behavior Therapy, 19,* 121–132.

Stroebe, M., & Schut, H. (1999). The Dual Process Model of coping with bereavement: Rationale and description. *Death Studies, 23,* 197–224.

Volkan, V. (1971). A study of a patient's "re-grief work": Through dreams, psychological tests and psychoanalysis. *Psychiatric Quarterly, 45,* 255–273.

Windholz, M. J., Marmar, C. R., & Horowitz, M. J. (1985). A review of the research on conjugal bereavement: Impact on health and efficacy of intervention. *Comprehensive Psychiatry, 26,* 433–447.

Zisook, S., Shuchter, S. R., Pedrelli, P., Sable, J., & Deaciue, S. C. (2001). Acute, open-trial of bupropion SR therapy in bereavement. *Journal of Clinical Psychiatry, 62,* 227–230.

Zygmont, M., Prigerson, H. G., Houck, P. R., Miller, M. D., Shear, M. K., Jacobs, S., & Reynolds, C. F. (1998). A post hoc comparison of paroxetine and nortriptyline for symptoms of traumatic grief. *Journal of Clinical Psychiatry, 59,* 241–245.

14

Virtual Reality Exposure Therapy

BARBARA OLASOV ROTHBAUM

Virtual reality (VR) allows individuals to become active participants within a computer-generated three-dimensional world that changes in a natural way with head and body motion. Emotional processing theory as applied to anxiety disorders purports that fear memories include information about stimuli, responses, and meaning (Foa & Kozak, 1986; Foa, Steketee, & Rothbaum, 1989). Therapy is aimed at facilitating emotional processing and modifying the fear structure. Foa and Kozak (1986) suggested that two conditions are required for the reduction of fear. First, the fear memory must be activated. Second, new information must be provided to change the fear structure. Any method capable of activating the fear structure and modifying it would be predicted to improve symptoms of anxiety. Thus virtual reality is a potential tool for the treatment of anxiety disorders; if an individual becomes immersed in a feared virtual environment, activation and modification of the fear structure is possible. Although this technology is still in its infancy, a number of research reports have indicated that virtual reality exposure therapy (VRE) can help patients overcome a number of anxiety disorders. This chapter provides an overview of research supporting the use of VR to help treat anxiety disorders, the rationale for its use, and future directions for the field. In this chapter, I will present data on the use of VRE in the treatment of the fear of heights, the fear of flying, social phobia, and posttraumatic stress disorder (PTSD). In general, these data support Foa and Kozak's propositions about emotional processing and therapy.

VIRTUAL REALITY

VR is a relatively new medium of human–computer interactions in which the user becomes an active participant in a three-dimensional computer-generated virtual world. The user experiences visual, auditory, and often tactile stimuli that serve to immerse him or her in the computer-generated environment and create a sense of presence or immersion within the environment.

In our applications, the user wears a head-mounted display that consists of video display screens for each eye, earphones, and a head-tracking device. The tracker allows the individual's views to change in the virtual world in real time with the head movements made in the real world. Many virtual environments also allow for other input devices, such as joysticks, that allow movement within the virtual world or interaction within the virtual environment, such as pushing the "up" button in the virtual elevator. The combination of these technologies with other types of stimuli, such as realistic sounds (e.g., the airplane engine) and tactile information (e.g., feeling the vibrations on the virtual airplane), combine to create a sense of presence or immersion by having the environment change in real time with the users' movements, thus making the user feel like an active participant within this new world (Rothbaum, Hodges, & Kooper, 1997). For many of our applications, the user's chair sits on a raised platform with a bass shaker underneath. This allows vibrations to be felt that correspond with sounds and events presented in the virtual environment, such as bomb blasts in the Virtual Vietnam or the raising of the landing gear in the virtual airplane.

THEORETICAL BASIS FOR THE USE OF VR IN THE TREATMENT OF ANXIETY DISORDERS

Emotional processing theory as applied to anxiety disorders (Foa & Kozak, 1986; Foa et al., 1989) purports that fear memories can be construed as structures that contain information regarding stimuli (e.g., airplanes), responses (e.g., heart pounding), and meaning (e.g., crashing danger). It has been proposed that exposure therapy purportedly facilitates emotional processing by first activating this fear structure through presenting to the patient stimuli that elicit fearful responses. With prolonged exposure to the feared stimuli in the absence of the feared consequences, habituation and extinction—in which the feared stimuli no longer elicit anxiety—help modify the fear structure by making its meaning less threatening, and thereby changing the fear structure. Therefore, if VR can activate this fear structure just as traditional exposure does and allow for repeated prolonged exposure, and if patients' anxiety decreases during exposure to this stimuli, then it should be effective as a tool in reducing anxiety. Standard exposure therapy has been very effective in treating many of the anxiety disorders; however, there are often logistical barriers to its use that have daunted many clinicians, such as having to leave the office to expose the patient to the feared stimuli.

VRE AS APPLIED TO ANXIETY DISORDERS

VR overcomes many of these logistical obstacles by bringing the real-world stimuli into the therapist's office. It has been our experience that the sense of presence felt by individuals within the virtual environment can elicit fears similar to what one would experience in the real world. In addition to subjective units of discomfort scale (SUDS) ratings, we also recorded the number and type of physical symptoms of anxiety that were described by participants during exposure in the first fear of heights study (described in the next subsection). Physical symptoms of anxiety described by the participants while in virtual height situations included sweating, abdominal discomfort usually described as "butterflies," loss of balance or light-headedness, heart palpitations, pacing, tremors or shaking, feeling "nervous" or "scared," weakness in the knees, tightness in the chest, and feeling "tense." In addition to these classic anxiety symptoms, some participants also reported feeling physical motion sensations such as impact in their knees when the elevator stopped going down (Hodges et al., 1995).

VR has been found helpful as a tool for exposure therapy (Rothbaum et al., 1997; Rothbaum & Hodges, 1999), particularly for anxiety disorders (Rothbaum, Hodges, Alarcon, et al., 1999; Rothbaum, Hodges, Smith, Lee, & Price, 2000; Rothbaum et al., 1995a). Generally, the research has been characterized by testing in a case study and then a controlled clinical trial. VRE has been found helpful for a number of anxiety disorders, including specific phobia, PTSD, and social phobia. Several of these reports are reviewed here.

Specific Phobia

Acrophobia

The first specific phobia that was treated successfully with VRE was the fear of heights (acrophobia). VRE was used to treat a 19-year-old student with a fear of heights using a virtual elevator program (Rothbaum et al., 1995b). Exposure therapy sessions were conducted twice weekly for a total of five sessions. Responses on self-report measures indicated decreases in anxiety, avoidance, and distress in the real world and improvements in attitudes about heights. A real-world behavioral avoidance test in an actual elevator following treatment indicated that VR was an effective tool for exposure therapy for this individual.

In the first published controlled study of VRE in the treatment of a psychiatric disorder, 20 individuals who met criteria for acrophobia were randomly assigned to VRE treatment or wait-list (WL) control, and 17 completed treatment (Rothbaum et al., 1995a). Following a group pretreatment assessment and an orientation to the VR equipment and environments, the treatment group received seven weekly individual treatment sessions consisting of exposure to virtual footbridges, virtual balconies, and a virtual elevator. The environments were presented in the order determined by each participant's self-rated hierarchy completed at the pretreatment assessment. As in standard exposure, patients were allowed to progress at their own pace, but they were encouraged to spend as much time in each situation as needed for their anxiety to decrease. In order to create a greater sense of realism, participants stood on a 4-foot × 4-foot square platform raised approximately 6 inches off the ground, surrounded with actual railings corresponding to computer-generated railings in the virtual environments, giving the participants something to hold and an edge to approach. As always, what the patient viewed in the head-mounted display was visible on the computer monitor to allow appropriate comments by the therapist. Therapist comments were exactly analogous to comments in standard exposure therapy, such as "Can you approach the edge now?" "Can you look over the railing now?" and "Are you ready to let go of the railing now?".

Results indicated significant decreases in anxiety, avoidance, and distress from pre- to posttreatment for the VRE group but not for the control group (see Figure 14.1). At posttreatment, the VRE group reported more positive attitudes toward heights than the control group, indicating a change in the meaning of the stimuli (see Figure 14.2). In addition, 7 of the 10 VRE treatment completers exposed themselves to real-life height situations by the end of treatment, indicating a generalization of treatment effects to real-world stimuli. In summary, VRE for fear of heights was very effective in reducing self-reported anxiety and avoidance of heights and improving attitudes toward heights, whereas the WL control group did not evidence any change. This well-controlled but small study represented the first finding that fear could be experienced and overcome in the virtual world and that this experience would translate to changed feelings and behavior in the real world.

Fear of Flying

As mentioned earlier, despite the fact that *in vivo* exposure is very effective in treating specific phobias, many clinicians are reluctant to engage in it due to logistical constraints. Standard exposure therapy on an airplane to treat

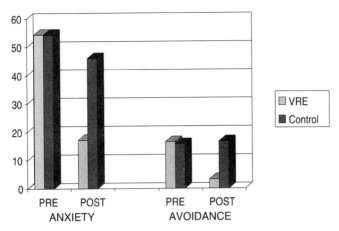

FIGURE 14.1. Anxiety and avoidance means for VRE (lighter) versus controls (darker) pre- and posttreatment. From Rothbaum et al. (1995a). Copyright 1995 by the American Psychiatric Association; www.ajp.psychiatryonline.org. Reprinted by permission.

fear of flying (FOF) is often inconvenient and cumbersome for therapists, as well as extremely expensive for patients, especially if therapists must accompany patients to the airport and on real airplanes. There are a number of uncontrollable elements in standard exposure for FOF, such as weather, turbulence, and the occurrence of only one takeoff and landing per flight.

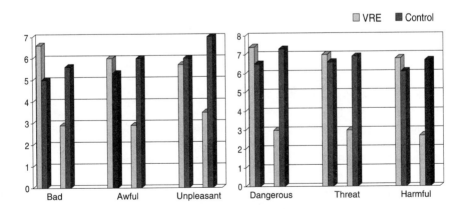

FIGURE 14.2. Results on Attitudes Toward Heights Questionnaire means for VRE (lighter) versus controls (darker) pre- and posttreatment. From Rothbaum et al. (1995a). Copyright 1995 by the American Psychiatric Association; www.ajp.psychiatryonline.org. Reprinted by permission.

For these reasons, clinical researchers developed and tested a virtual airplane for FOF.

The efficacy of VRE for FOF has been reported in several case studies, as well as a controlled trial. The first was a fearful flier who was treated with VRE over 13 sessions, with 7 sessions devoted to anxiety management training and 6 exposure sessions using a virtual airplane (Rothbaum, Hodges, Watson, Kessler, & Opdyke, 1996). Results indicated posttreatment decreases in self-reported anxiety and fearful attitudes toward flying, as well as taking an actual cross-country flight in relative comfort. Another case study by the same research group (Smith, Rothbaum, & Hodges, 1999) involved a shorter course of treatment (4 anxiety management sessions and 4 exposure sessions using a virtual airplane), and therapy was conducted according to a standard treatment manual (Rothbaum, Hodges, & Smith, 1999). Similar to the first case study, treatment resulted in decreases in self-reported anxiety and fearful attitudes toward flying, as well as relatively low levels of self-reported anxiety (SUDs = 15–35) on an actual posttreatment flight. Furthermore, 6-month follow-up data indicated maintenance of the gains made in treatment, as measured by self-report questionnaires and by two subsequent flights.

A recently published controlled treatment-outcome study expanded on these case studies. In a controlled study, VRE was compared with standard exposure (SE) therapy and with a WL control in the treatment of FOF (Rothbaum, Hodges, et al., 2000). Forty-nine participants who met DSM-IV criteria for either agoraphobia in which flying was the primary feared stimuli or specific phobia of flying were randomly assigned to one of the three conditions, with 45 participants, or 15 per group, completing the study.

Treatment consisted of eight individual therapy sessions conducted over 6 weeks. The first four sessions consisted of anxiety-management training, including breathing retraining, cognitive restructuring for irrational beliefs, and hyperventilation exposure for panic attacks, if present. Anxiety-management training sessions were followed by exposure to a virtual airplane (for VRE participants; see Figures 14.3 and 14.4) or exposure to an actual airplane at the airport (for SE participants). VRE sessions were conducted twice weekly in the therapist's office according to a treatment manual (Rothbaum et al., 1999b). These sessions included such stimuli as sitting in the virtual airplane, taxiing, taking off, landing, and flying in both calm and turbulent weather. During VRE sessions, a head-mounted display with stereo earphones provided visual and audio cues consistent with being a passenger on a commercial airplane flight, and a chair with a woofer under the seat provided consistent tactile cues (i.e., vibrations).

For SE sessions, *in vivo* exposure was conducted at the airport, exposing patients to preflight stimuli (e.g., ticketing, trains, planes, waiting area)

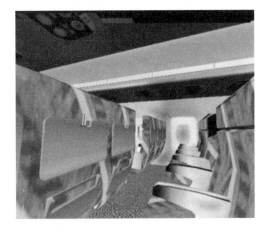

FIGURE 14.3. The passenger cabin of the virtual airplane. From www.virtuallybetter.com. Copyright by Virtually Better, Inc. Reprinted by permission.

and time on a stationary airplane habituating to airplane stimuli and conducting imaginal exposure (i.e., imagining takeoffs, cruising, landing, etc). Immediately following the treatment or WL period, all patients were asked to participate in a behavioral avoidance test consisting of an actual commercial round-trip flight. The therapist accompanied participants in a group on a round-trip flight that lasted about 1.5 hours each way.

The results indicated that both VRE and SE were superior to the WL condition on all measures (see Figure 14.5). For WL participants, no signif-

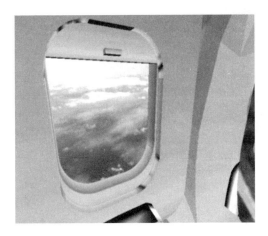

FIGURE 14.4. The view out of the window of the virtual airplane. From www.virtuallybetter.com. Copyright by Virtually Better, Inc. Reprinted by permission.

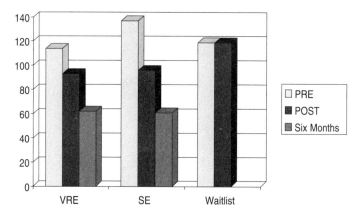

FIGURE 14.5. Fear of Flying Inventory means for VRE versus standard exposure therapy (SE) versus wait-list controls pre- (lighter) and post-(darker) treatment and at 6-month follow-up. From Rothbaum, Hodges, Smith, Lee, and Price (2000). Copyright 2000 by the American Psychological Association. Reprinted by permission.

icant differences were found between pre- and posttreatment self-report measures of anxiety and avoidance, and only one of the 15 WL participants completed the graduation flight (see Figure 14.6). In contrast, participants receiving VRE or SE showed substantial improvement, as measured by self-report questionnaires, willingness to participate in the graduation flight, self-report levels of anxiety on the flight, and self-ratings of improve-

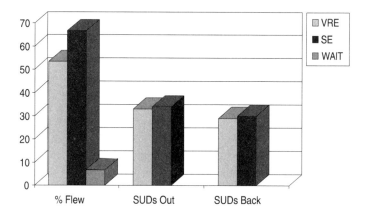

FIGURE 14.6. Actual flight data means for VRE (lighter) versus standard exposure therapy (SE) (darker) versus wait-list controls for percent who flew in the behavioral avoidance test posttreatment and their reported subjective units of discomfort (SUDs) on the flight out and back. From Rothbaum, Hodges, Smith, Lee, and Price (2000). Copyright 2000 by the American Psychological Association. Reprinted by permission.

ment, with no differences between the VRE and SE treatments on any of the measures. Participants receiving SE or VRE were approximately 3½ times more likely to take the commercial flight than the WL control group.

Follow-up data gathered 6 months posttreatment indicated that treated participants maintained their treatment gains. By the 6-month follow-up, 93% of the VRE and SE participants had flown since completing treatment. At 12 months post treatment, data were gathered on 24 of the 30 (80%) patients who were assigned to VRE or SE. Patients maintained their treatment gains, and 92% of VRE participants and 91% of SE participants had flown on a real airplane since the graduation flight (Rothbaum, Hodges, Anderson, Price, & Smith, 2002). This is the first year-long follow-up of patients who have been treated with VRE, and it indicates that short-term treatment can have lasting effects. These data represent the first controlled study to compare the use of VR in the treatment of a specific phobia with the current standard of care, standard exposure therapy. The findings indicate that VRE was as efficacious as SE on every outcome measure used and lend support to the contention that VRE can successfully treat FOF within the confines of a therapist's office.

In a replication of this study with a larger sample, 87 patients with FOF were randomly assigned to VRE, SE, or WL (Rothbaum, Hodges, Anderson, Ziman, & Wilson, in press). On all measures, VRE and SE were equally effective, and both were superior to WL. Follow-up assessments at 6 months (86% retention) and 12 months (80% retention) indicated that the treatment gains were maintained. The use of VRE in the treatment of FOF was unequivocally supported in this controlled study. This also represents the largest controlled study of VRE to date.

In an uncontrolled report, no group differences in treatment response were found among fearful fliers diagnosed with specific phobia, panic disorder, claustrophobia, or fear of heights (Kahan, Tanzer, Darvin, & Borer, 2000). In this sample, 68% of the treated participants flew after VRE treatment, regardless of diagnosis. This study provides further support for the efficacy of this technology for FOF as tested by a different research group.

Other Specific Phobias

There have been reports of case studies in the literature for the treatment of other specific phobias with VRE. A patient with spider phobia (Carlin, Hoffman, & Weghorst, 1997) and one with claustrophobia (Botclla et al., 1998) were both treated effectively with VRE.

Posttraumatic Stress Disorder

It is estimated that some 830,000 Vietnam veterans suffer from clinically significant symptoms of PTSD (Weiss et al., 1992). Evidence suggests that behavioral therapies with an imaginal exposure component have been more effective than most other types of treatment for combat-related PTSD (Rothbaum, Meadows, Resick, & Foy, 2000; van Etten & Taylor, 1998), although the effects are not robust in veterans. Obviously, *in vivo* exposure to combat situations is not a viable option. Thus a Virtual Vietnam environment was created to explore the efficacy of VRE with Vietnam combat veterans with PTSD. Two virtual environments, a virtual Huey helicopter (see Figure 14.7) and a virtual clearing surrounded by jungle (see Figure 14.8) were created. The therapist controls various visual and auditory effects, such as muzzle flashes, helicopters flying overhead and landing, low-flying fog, jungle sounds, gunfire, mine explosions, and men yelling. In the Virtual Helicopter, the participant flies over rice paddies, a jungle, and a river. Patients were exposed to their most traumatic Vietnam memories while immersed within the virtual environments following a standard treatment manual. The therapist attempts to match what the patient is describing for his imaginal exposure (e.g., "The chopper is landing now and I hear explosions all around me") with what the patient sees and hears and feels in the virtual reality (e.g., landing the helicopter amid explosions and gunfire). A difference between standard prolonged exposure (PE) for PTSD (Foa & Rothbaum, 1998) and virtual reality exposure for PTSD is that in VR patients' eyes are open to see the stimuli.

The first use of VRE for a Vietnam veteran with PTSD was reported in a case study (Rothbaum, Hodges, Alarcon, et al., 1999). The veteran was a 50-year-old European American male who met DSM-IV criteria for PTSD, major depressive disorder, and past alcohol abuse. He had served as a heli-

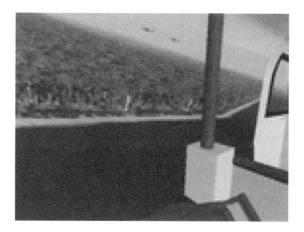

FIGURE 14.7. The view out of the virtual helicopter in the Virtual Vietnam. From www.virtuallybetter.com. Copyright by Virtually Better, Inc. Reprinted by permission.

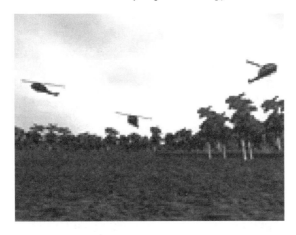

FIGURE 14.8. The landing zone (clearing) of the Virtual Vietnam. From www.virtuallybetter.com. Copyright by Virtually Better, Inc. Reprinted by permission.

copter pilot in Vietnam approximately 26 years prior to the study. Treatment consisted of fourteen 90-minute individual sessions conducted over a 7-week period. Results indicated posttreatment improvement on all measures of PTSD and maintenance of these gains at a 6-month follow-up.

This case study was followed by an open clinical trial of VRE for Vietnam veterans (Rothbaum, Hodges, Ready, Graap, & Alarcon, 2001). In this study, 16 male patients who met DSM-IV criteria for PTSD entered and 10 completed VRE. An average of ten 90-minute exposure therapy sessions delivered over 5 to 7 weeks resulted in a significant reduction in PTSD and related symptoms.

An interesting case report describes the treatment of a Vietnam veteran for PTSD related to his war experiences with exposure therapy using the Virtual Vietnam. There are two unique features of this particular treatment and case report. First, the nature of several of these traumatic memories included guilt over acts that the patient committed in Vietnam, a circumstance that oftentimes precludes a candidate from receiving exposure therapy. Second, psychophysiological monitoring occurred throughout the treatment, as well as at pre- and posttreatment. The patient's response to treatment in terms of guilt, anger, and anxiety, measured at pre- and posttreatment and follow-ups of 3 and 6 months, and his psychophysiological responding indicated a successful treatment (Rothbaum, Ruef, Litz, Han, & Hodges, 2003). This preliminary evidence suggests that VRE may be a promising component of a comprehensive treatment approach for veterans with combat-related PTSD. We are now working on a Virtual Iraq to use with returning military personnel from that conflict.

Social Phobia

Most recently, virtual environments have been developed for treatment of the fear of public speaking in which the therapist can control the reaction of virtual audiences while the patient practices a speech. There are both a small-group audience (5 people around a conference table; see Figure 14.9) and a large-group audience (approximately 30 people in a lecture hall; see Figure 14.10; Anderson, Rothbaum, & Hodges, 2003). In a report of two cases, VR for social anxiety was utilized in two different courses of individual treatment: weekly psychotherapy and a 3-day intensive course of therapy. Results indicated that treatment was successful, as measured by completion of a behavioral avoidance test at the end of treatment (giving an actual speech in front of a live audience), decreases in self-report measures of public speaking anxiety comparable with results of controlled clinical outcome trials for social phobia, and qualitative feedback.

In an open clinical trial, 10 participants meeting diagnostic criteria for social phobia with prominent public speaking fears or for panic disorder with agoraphobia in which speaking was the primary feared stimulus received eight individual therapy sessions, including four sessions of anxiety-management training and four sessions of VRE according to a standardized treatment manual. Participants completed self-report questionnaires at pretreatment, posttreatment, and 3-month follow-up and were asked to complete a behavioral avoidance test (BAT), which consisted of giving a speech to an actual audience at pre- and posttreatment. Results indicated that treatment was successful as measured by self-reported de-

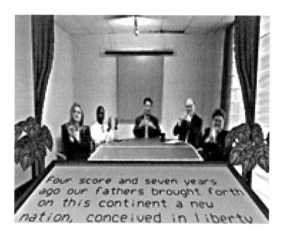

FIGURE 14.9. The small-group audience with podium with speech text of the Virtual Audiences. From www.virtuallybetter.com. Copyright by Virtually Better, Inc. Reprinted by permission.

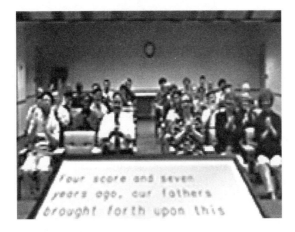

FIGURE 14.10. The large-group audience with podium with speech text of the Virtual Audiences. From www.virtuallybetter.com. Copyright by Virtually Better, Inc. Reprinted by permission.

creases in public speaking anxiety from pre- to posttreatment, by audience ratings of speakers' decreased anxiety and improved performance from the pre- to posttreatment BAT, and by qualitative feedback. Follow-up data, obtained at 3 months from 80% of participants, showed that treatment gains were maintained. These preliminary findings suggest that VR may be a useful tool for exposure therapy within a comprehensive treatment for social anxiety. We also found it interesting that the VR was able to elicit and help treat social, rather than just physical, fears, again indicating that if one is able to tap into the fear structure, it becomes amenable to change.

VRE Combined with Medication

Some very recent data suggest that medication may facilitate VRE (Rothbaum, Ressler, et al., 2003). D-Cycloserine (DCS, a partial agonist at the N-methyl-D-aspartate receptor, has previously been shown to improve extinction of fear in rodents. This study utilized a precisely controlled VRE paradigm to examine the ability of d-cycloserine to facilitate the emotional learning that occurs in behavioral exposure therapy. Twenty-eight patients who met DSM-IV criteria for acrophobia were enrolled in this randomized, double-blind placebo controlled study. After pretreatment measures of fear were obtained, patients were treated with two sessions of VRE to heights from a virtual glass elevator. Participants underwent two therapy sessions, considered a suboptimal amount of exposure therapy for acrophobia. These two therapy sessions were separated by 1–2 weeks. Participants were instructed to take a single pill of study medication (placebo, DCS 50 mg, or DCS 500 mg) 2–4 hours before each therapy session such that only two pills were taken for the entire study. Single doses of placebo or d-cycloserine were taken prior to each of the two sessions of VRE. Patients returned at 1 week and at 3 months for posttreatment measures to determine the presence and severity of acrophobia symptoms.

VRE resulted in significantly larger reductions of acrophobia symptoms within the virtual environment for those receiving d-cycloserine during therapy compared with those receiving placebo. The group receiving d-cycloserine during VRE demonstrated significantly greater improvements on general measures of real-world acrophobia symptoms that were evident early in treatment and were maintained at 3 months. Their scores on measures of anxiety, attitudes toward heights, clinical global improvement, and number of self-exposures to real-world heights also demonstrated improvement. There was also evidence of decreased physiological responding within the virtual environment. These data suggest that the improvement in extinction of fear achieved with DCS augmentation during exposure was evident in both subjective and objective physiological measures of fear. These data support the use of d-cycloserine, and potentially other cognitive enhancers, as adjuncts to psychotherapy to accelerate the learning processes that contribute to correcting psychopathology (Ressler et al., 2004). These data are extremely exciting: If a benign medication taken acutely immediately preceding a psychotherapy session can facilitate therapy, the broader implications for psychiatry are huge.

ADVANTAGES AND DISADVANTAGES OF VR

There are a number of advantages to using VR in treatment, particularly in exposure therapy for anxiety disorders. Recreating a situation for a patient is sometimes difficult or impossible in the real world. With VR, a therapist has the ability to control variables (e.g., turbulence) and to participate with the patient in a virtual scene. Additionally, the therapist can control the variables that might facilitate behavioral exposure for some patients. *In vivo* exposure therapies often require time-consuming and expensive efforts, such as planning, scheduling, and visiting locations outside the office. With VR, the therapist does not have to leave the office at all but instead can bring the world into his or her office, alleviating the need to travel, the loss of control, and the risks to client confidentiality.

Of course, there are some disadvantages to using VRE as well. Computer glitches can occur during exposure sessions. With some patients, the VR may not elicit the fear, particularly when the environment doesn't quite match the feared situation. The cost of the equipment and software may make the availability of such treatments prohibitive for some therapists. However, as the price of hardware continues to decline, the VR should become increasingly affordable.

A weakness in the strength of the data reported for VRE is that one research group conducted the majority of the studies, and work by other groups is just beginning to lend support to the initial results. As with many clinical procedures, there is a need for additional research groups to conduct controlled treatment outcome studies in the future. Such studies should provide the field with more convergent evidence for the efficacy of this treatment approach.

THE FUTURE OF VRE

Based on the studies to date, VRE for anxiety disorders seems promising. Future research should continue to push the envelope for using VR for exposure therapy. In considering VRE applications to treat other anxiety disorders, guiding principles include identifying types of exposure that are difficult to conduct *in vivo* and types of exposures that are difficult to control, repeat, or conduct for extended periods of time; all of these maximize the effectiveness of the exposure. Future research should examine predictors of treatment responders and the role of VR in therapy beyond exposure therapy and the combination of medication and therapy. Regarding the use of VR in clinical research, VR offers exact experimental control. One can exactly control the "dose" of exposure therapy within and between participants. It is also amenable to experimental designs that examine conditioning and extinction paradigms. We are exploring the use of VR for the treatment of substance use disorders and presented in a self-help format.

Edna Foa's work in emotional processing and exposure therapy for anxiety disorders laid the groundwork for our application of VR to exposure therapy. In general, my work using VR for exposure therapy has only offered support for Foa and Kozak's (1986) emotional processing theory. For example, interesting things happen once we tap into a patient's fear network. Although the virtual environments are limited to what we have built into them, we have found that patients tend to fill in gaps with other elements that are clearly present in their fear structures. For example, in the Virtual Vietnam, individual patients would report seeing tanks or the enemy, although we did not include tanks or people in that virtual environment. Also, an early question was whether a computer-generated environment could tap into a person's fear structure and elicit anxiety, clearly necessary for exposure therapy to be effective. We did find that if we were able to present enough of the salient cues, people did become anxious. So we found that (1) regarding *stimuli*, VR was able to act as a potent stimulus to elicit anxiety; the anxiety did decrease with prolonged and repeated exposure; and this effect generalized to the real world; (2) regarding *responses*, self-reported anxiety, standard symptom and impairment measures, and psychophysiological indices all improved with exposure to the VR stimuli (e.g., as seen in the DCS study; Ressler et al., 2004); and (3) regarding the *meaning*, the valence of the stimuli changed from negative to positive and less threatening after successful VR exposure therapy, as seen in the first fear-of-heights study (Rothbaum et al., 1995).

AUTHOR NOTE

Barbara Olasov Rothbaum receives research funding and is entitled to sales royalty from Virtually Better, Inc., which is developing products related to the research described in this chapter. In addition, she serves as a consultant to and owns equity in Virtually Better, Inc. The terms of this arrangement have been reviewed and approved by Emory University in accordance with its conflict of interest policies.

REFERENCES

Anderson, P., Rothbaum, B. O., & Hodges, L. F. (2003). Virtual reality exposure in the treatment of social anxiety: Two case reports. *Cognitive and Behavioral Practice, 10*, 240–247.

Botella, C., Banos, R. M., Perpina, C., Villa, H., Alcaniz, M., & Rey, A. (1998). Virtual reality treatment of claustrophobia: A case report. *Behaviour Research and Therapy, 36*(2), 239–246.

Carlin, A. S., Hoffman, H. G., & Weghorst, S. (1997). Virtual reality and tactile augmentation in the treatment of spider phobia: A case report. *Behaviour Research and Therapy, 35*(2), 153–158.

Foa, E. B., & Kozak, M. J. (1986). Emotional processing of fear: Exposure to corrective information. *Psychological Bulletin, 99*, 20–35.

Foa, E. B., & Rothbaum, B. O. (1998). *Treating the trauma of rape: Cognitive-behavioral therapy for PTSD*. New York: Guilford Press.

Foa, E. B., Steketee, G., & Rothbaum, B. O. (1989). Behavioral/cognitive conceptualizations of post-traumatic stress disorder. *Behavior Therapy, 20*, 155–176.

Hodges, L. F., Rothbaum, B. O., Kooper, R., Opdyke, D., Meyer, T., North, M., et al. (1995, July). Virtual environments for exposure therapy. *IEEE Computer Journal*, pp. 27–34.

Kahan, M., Tanzer, J., Darvin, D., & Borer, F. (2000). Virtual reality–assisted cognitive-behavioral treatment for fear of flying: Acute treatment and follow-up. *Cyberpsychology and Behavior, 3*(3), 387–392.

Ressler, K. J., Rothbaum, B. O., Tannenbaum, L., Anderson, P., Zimand, E., Hodges, L., & Davis, M. (2004). Facilitation of psychotherapy with D-cycloserine, a putative cognitive enhancer. *Archives of General Psychiatry, 61*, 1136–1144.

Rothbaum, B. O., & Hodges, L. F. (1999). The use of virtual reality exposure in the treatment of anxiety disorders. *Behavior Modification, 23*(4), 507–525.

Rothbaum, B. O., Hodges, L., Alarcon, R., Ready, D., Shahar, F., Graap, K., et al. (1999). Virtual reality exposure therapy for PTSD Vietnam veterans: A case study. *Journal of Traumatic Stress, 12*(2), 263–271.

Rothbaum, B. O., Hodges, L., Anderson, P. L., Price, L., & Smith, S. (2002). 12-month follow-up of virtual reality exposure therapy for the fear of flying. *Journal of Consulting and Clinical Psychology, 70*, 428–432.

Rothbaum, B. O., Hodges, L., Anderson, P., Zimand, E., Lang, D., & Wilson, J. (in press). Virtual reality exposure therapy and standard (*in vivo*) exposure therapy in the treatment of fear of flying. *Behavior Therapy.*

Rothbaum, B. O., Hodges, L., & Kooper, R. (1997). Virtual reality exposure therapy. *Journal of Psychotherapy Practice and Research, 6*(3), 219–226.

Rothbaum, B. O., Hodges, L. F., Kooper, R., Opdyke, D., Williford, J. S., & North, M. (1995a). Effectiveness of computer-generated (virtual reality) graded exposure in the treatment of acrophobia. *American Journal of Psychiatry, 152*(4), 626–628.

Rothbaum, B. O., Hodges, L. F., Kooper, R., Opdyke, D., Williford, J. S., & North, M. (1995b). Virtual reality graded exposure in the treatment of acrophobia: A case report. *Behavior Therapy, 26*, 547–554.

Rothbaum, B. O., Hodges, L., Ready, D., Graap, K., & Alarcon, R. (2001). Virtual reality exposure therapy for Vietnam veterans with posttraumatic stress disorder. *Journal of Clinical Psychiatry, 62*, 617–622.

Rothbaum, B. O., Hodges, L., & Smith, S. (1999). Virtual reality exposure therapy abbreviated treatment manual: Fear of flying application. *Cognitive and Behavioral Practice, 6*(3), 234–244.

Rothbaum, B. O., Hodges, L., Smith, S., Lee, J. H., & Price, L. (2000). A controlled study of virtual reality exposure therapy for the fear of flying. *Journal of Consulting and Clinical Psychology, 68*(6), 1020–1026.

Rothbaum, B. O., Hodges, L., Watson, B. A., Kessler, G. D., & Opdyke, D. (1996). Virtual reality exposure therapy in the treatment of fear of flying: A case report. *Behaviour Research and Therapy, 34*(5–6), 477–481.

Rothbaum, B. O., Meadows, E. A., Resick, P., & Foy, D. W. (2000). Cognitive-behavioral treatment position paper summary for the ISTSS Treatment Guidelines Committee. *Journal of Traumatic Stress, 13*, 558–563.

Rothbaum, B. O., Ressler, K. J., Tannenbaum, L., Anderson, P., Zimand, E., Hodges, L., & Davis, M. (2003, December). *Facilitation of psychotherapy with D-cycloserine, a putative cognitive enhancer.* Paper presented at the annual meeting of the American College of Neuropsychopharmacology, San Juan, PR.

Rothbaum, B. O., Ruef, A. M., Litz, B. T., Han, H., & Hodges, L. (2003). Virtual reality exposure therapy of combat-related PTSD: A case study using psychophysiological indicators of outcome. *Journal of Cognitive Psychotherapy: An International Quarterly, 17*, 163–178.

Smith, S., Rothbaum, B. O., & Hodges, L. F. (1999). Treatment of fear of flying using virtual reality exposure therapy: A single case study. *Behavior Therapist, 22*(8), 154–158.

van Etten, M., & Taylor, S. (1998). Comparative efficacy of treatments for post-traumatic stress disorder: A meta-analysis. *Clinical Psychology and Psychotherapy, 5*, 126–145.

Weiss, D. S., Marmar, C. R., Schlenger, W. E., Fairbank, J. A., Jordan, B. K., Hough, R. L., & Kulka, R. A. (1992). The prevalence of lifetime and partial post-traumatic stress disorder in Vietnam theater veterans. *Journal of Traumatic Stress, 5*, 365–376.

15

Pathological Anxiety
Where We Are and Where We Need to Go

SHAWN P. CAHILL
MARTIN E. FRANKLIN
NORAH C. FEENY

INTRODUCTION AND BRIEF HISTORY (PRE-DSM-III)

The contemporary cognitive-behavioral therapy (CBT) approaches to understanding and treating anxiety disorders described in the various chapters of this book have their roots in earlier behavioral approaches to the problem of pathological anxiety. In order to appraise where we are currently, it may be helpful to first briefly summarize from whence we came. We begin with two case studies conducted by John B. Watson, the early American proponent of *Psychology as the Behaviorist Views It* (J. B. Watson, 1913), and his colleagues. These case studies foreshadowed the development of what were to become the two foundational assumptions of the early behavioral models of the acquisition of treatment of pathological anxiety: that pathological anxiety was acquired through the process of Pavlovian conditioning and that such fears could in turn be unlearned or "deconditioned" through procedures analogous to counterconditioning or extinction.

Little Albert and Little Peter

In the first of these case studies, Watson and Rayner (1920) putatively established a phobia to a white rat in the human infant Little Albert by pairing presentations of the rat with a strong startle reaction induced by striking a metal bar. Testing conducted prior to the conditioning trial revealed that Albert showed no evidence of fear in response to a variety of stimuli, including the white rat, a rabbit, dog, fur coat, cotton wool, and wooden blocks. However, after the conditioning trials, he displayed a strong negative emotional reaction in response to the rat, such as crying and withdrawing from it, that generalized to other furry stimuli that had been tested prior to conditioning (i.e., the rabbit, dog, fur coat, and wool) but not to the wooden blocks. Watson and Rayner also proposed several potential methods to remove the conditioned fears, including trying to "recondition" Albert by feeding him in the presence of the feared stimuli, but they were not able to test their hypotheses about methods to eliminate the conditioned fears before the child was removed from the hospital.

In the second case study, Mary Cover Jones (1924), one of Watson's students, investigated methods to reduce a naturally occurring fear of a rabbit in another human infant, Little Peter. The different methods investigated included graduated *in vivo* exposure to the rabbit, feeding Peter in the presence of the rabbit, and exposure to the rabbit in the presence of other, nonfearful children. The case study also described two instances in which Peter's fear of the rabbit returned: once after he was frightened by a large dog and again when he received a scratch while carrying the rabbit to its cage. Additional treatment administered after each incident resulted in recovery of the previous gains and further improvement.

Systematic Desensitization and the Principle of Reciprocal Inhibition

The observations contained in the aforementioned case studies did not lead to any systematic development and evaluation of specific procedures to treat anxiety in humans until Joseph Wolpe, a South African psychiatrist who had been exposed to Hull's behavioral theory, began experimenting in 1947 with methods to eliminate "experimental neurosis" induced in cats by administering painful footshocks. Following administration of the shocks, Wolpe noted that the cats resisted being put back into the cage in which the shocks occurred and would not eat meat pellets and showed overt signs of emotional distress when placed in the cage. Wolpe also noticed that the neurotic behavior occurred not only in the room in which the original conditioning took place but also in a series of three other rooms that were similar to the original conditioning room. However, the strength of the cats' reactions was not equal across the different rooms but varied as a function of the similarity of each room to the original conditioning room.

Having established the experimental neurosis in his cats, Wolpe began investigating procedures to reduce or eliminate their anxious behavior.

Based on the observation that conditioned fear inhibited eating, he speculated that, given the right conditions, eating could inhibit fear. One procedure that worked particularly well took advantage of the fact that cats' feeding behavior was less disrupted in rooms other than the one in which the shock had been administered. Treatment began with feeding the cats in the least similar room. When feeding was no longer disrupted in that room, the cats were moved to the next room, where feeding continued, and so on until, over a series of sessions, feeding was no longer disrupted even when the cats were placed in the cage in which the shock had been administered. To explain his observations, Wolpe invoked Sherrington's (1961) concept of reciprocal inhibition and, in his seminal book *Psychotherapy by Reciprocal Inhibition* (Wolpe, 1958), proposed the following as a general therapeutic principle:

> If a response antagonistic to anxiety can be made to occur in the presence of anxiety-evoking stimuli so that it is accompanied by a complete or partial suppression of the anxiety response, the bond between these stimuli and the anxiety response will be weakened. (p. 71)

From this principle, Wolpe developed his now famous technique of systematic desensitization, in which relaxation induced through the methods described by Jacobson (1938) is used to inhibit anxiety evoked by mental images of feared stimuli. Because the relaxation induced by the Jacobsonian "tense and relax" procedure is weak relative to a strong fear response, a hierarchy of fear situations is created, and treatment begins with stimuli that elicit a weak fear response. As in Wolpe's experiment in reducing experimental neurosis in cats, when anxiety is no longer evident in response to one item on the hierarchy, the patient moves up to the next item and so on until he or she reaches the top of the hierarchy.

The first controlled study of systematic desensitization (Lang & Lazovik, 1963) was published less than 5 years after the publication of *Psychotherapy by Reciprocal Inhibition*, and numerous other studies followed shortly thereafter. Indeed, the pace of publication of information on systematic desensitization was so rapid that Gordon Paul, in a pair of chapters on the "Outcome of Systematic Desensitization" that were published in 1969, reviewed 75 papers reporting results on the efficacy of systematic desensitization administered to more than 1,000 patients by more than 90 different therapists. Of these studies, 20 were controlled experiments, 10 of which included control conditions to address the potential confounding of therapist characteristics and treatment techniques. In the summary of his review, Paul (1969) offered the following conclusion:

> The findings were overwhelmingly positive, and *for the first time in the history of psychological treatments, a specific therapeutic package reliably*

produced measurable benefits for clients across a broad range of distressing problems in which anxiety was of fundamental importance [italics added]. . . . Investigations of equal quality and scope have not been carried out with other treatment techniques considered appropriate for similar problems. . . . (p. 159)

In addition to his conclusions regarding the efficacy of systematic desensitization, Paul (1969) identified four areas for further research. First, he advocated studies "testing the limits" of systematic desensitization, in keeping with his earlier rhetorical question (Paul, 1967), "*What* treatment, *by whom*, is most effective for *this* individual with *that* specific problem, and under *which* set of circumstances?" (p. 111, italics in original). Second, he recommended conducting "process studies" that included outcome assessments in order to identify the mechanisms responsible for the efficacy of systematic desensitization. Third, he recommended "parametric studies" to standardize and better delineate the necessary and sufficient procedures to treat patients. Last, he recommended "the development of standardized assessment procedures with adequate reliability and validity" (p. 159).

Beyond Systematic Desensitization

Building on this strong beginning, research on systematic desensitization began to address several of the issues highlighted in Paul's recommendations. For example, the primary problem addressed in most of the randomized controlled trials (RCTs) in Paul's review involved simple animal phobias and social anxiety. By contrast, systematic desensitization did not seem to be as effective with individuals suffering from severe agoraphobia (e.g., Gelder & Marks, 1966) or obsessive–compulsive disorder (OCD; Cooper, Gelder, & Marks, 1965). Moreover, progress up the imaginal hierarchy was often greater than the progress obtained on behavioral tests (e.g., Barlow, Leitenberg, Agras, & Winczel, 1969; Lang, Lazovik, & Reynolds, 1965; Davison, 1968). Thus some of the limits to the efficacy of systematic desensitization were beginning to be identified.

Additional research into the mechanism of systematic desensitization did not always yield results in keeping with predictions that would be derived from the principle of reciprocal inhibition. Krapfl (1967, cited in Bandura, 1969), for example, found that starting at the top and working down the hierarchy was as effective as starting at the bottom and working up. In addition, although some studies found that pairing the feared images with relaxation was more effective than simply imagining them (e.g., Davison, 1968), other similarly designed studies did not find any benefit to including relaxation (e.g., McGlynn, 1973). Also problematic for the principle of reciprocal inhibition is the finding by Lang, Melamed, and Hart

(1970) that those individuals who most benefited from systematic desensitization displayed *greater* heart-rate reactivity in response to the feared scenes on early trials, one of the key observations in the development of Lang's (1977, 1979, 1984) bioinformational theory of aversive imagery and Foa and Kozak's (1986) theory of emotional processing (see Foa, Huppert, & Cahill, Chapter 1, this volume).

During this same period of time (late 1960s into the mid-1970s), other researchers began to investigate alternative procedures to promote fear reduction that also involved exposure to fear-evoking stimuli but were conducted in ways that clearly violated the theoretical boundary conditions of reciprocal inhibition theory. Referred to as implosive therapy (e.g., Stampfl & Levis, 1967) or imaginal and *in vivo* flooding (e.g., Emmelkamp & Wessels, 1975), these approaches sought to intentionally elicit moderate to high intensity levels of anxiety for prolonged periods of time while preventing any attempts to escape and without employing any programmed coping responses, with the goal of achieving habituation or extinction of the fear response. These procedures, which were antithetical to the "start low and go slow" approach inherent in systematic desensitization, were found to be effective not only for simple phobias but also for agoraphobia (e.g., Agras, Leitenberg, & Barlow, 1968; Leitenberg, Agras, Edwards, Thompson, & Wincze, 1970) and OCD (Meyer, 1966; Meyer & Levy, 1973), problems for which systematic desensitization had been of limited use. Moreover, even in the case of specific fears, variations of prolonged imaginal and *in vivo* exposure without relaxation were found as effective as or more effective than systematic desensitization (e.g., Bandura, Blanchard, & Ritter, 1969).

To this point, there has been an implicit distinction between the stimuli that elicit fear or anxiety and the fear or anxiety response that is elicited. Yet, during this same time period, there was a growing recognition that the core fear of individuals with agoraphobia was not of the various avoided situations, such as crowded public places or confined spaces per se. Rather, they are attempting to avoid the sensations associated with the kind of intense physiological and emotional response now known as a panic attack that may occur in such situations. In other words, people with agoraphobia have, as one influential reanalysis of agoraphobia (Goldstein & Chambless, 1978) put it, acquired a fear of fear.

Although such a conceptualization tends to blur the distinction between stimulus and response, it does help to account for the observation that several seemingly unrelated procedures—such as repeated lactate infusions or inhalation of carbon dioxide (both known to induce acute panic in vulnerable individuals; e.g., Bonn, Harrison, & Reese, 1971; Haslam, 1974), vigorous physical exercise such as running (Orwin, 1973), and imaginal exposure to fear-evoking images that are "irrelevant" to the target complaint (e.g., imagining being eaten by a tiger when the target complaint is agoraphobia; Watson & Marks, 1971)—have all been associated with symptom reduction. The practical outgrowth of this and similar conceptualizations of panic and agoraphobia, such as Clark's (1986) theory of catastrophic misinterpretation of sensations theory and Reiss and McNally's (1985) theory of anxiety sensitivity, has been the development of interoceptive exposure procedures—such as intentional rapid breathing, spinning in a chair, rapid stair stepping, or breathing through a straw—that are designed to voluntarily induce sensations similar to those experienced during a panic attack, such as hyperventilation, dizziness, sweating, tachycardia, and difficulty breathing. These procedures are a central component in contemporary cognitive behavioral treatment programs for panic disorder and agoraphobia (see Allen & Barlow, Chapter 10, this volume).

Summary

As this brief history illustrates, considerable progress was made in understanding the nature and treatments of pathological anxiety during the 1960s and 1970s that has served as a strong foundation for the continued advances that have occurred during the 1980s, 1990s, and into the first decade of the 21st century. The influence of this research can easily be seen in many of the chapters of this volume, which illustrate that many of the basic procedures pioneered during this early period continue to serve as the foundation for contemporary cognitive-behavioral programs for the treatment of anxiety. For example, a variation of systematic desensitization continues to be used in the treatment of generalized anxiety disorder (see Behar & Borkovec, Chapter 11). Imaginal and/or in vivo exposure are central components in treatment packages for social phobia (see Davidson, Chapter 7), for OCD in adults (see Simpson & Liebowitz, Chapter 8) and in children (see March & Franklin, Chapter 9), and for posttraumatic stress disorder (see Hembree & Feeny, Chapter 12). Interoceptive exposure has become a hallmark of cognitive-behavioral programs in the treatment of panic disorder (see Allen & Barlow, chapter 10). At the same time that advances were being made in the development and assessment of therapy procedures to treat pathological anxiety, progress was also being made in improving our conceptual understanding of how these procedures worked. In particular, theoretical explanations for the efficacy of CBT began to shift from the notion of extinguishing or inhibiting simple conditioned responses to incorporating more complex cognitive concepts (e.g., fear structures; Lang, 1977) and to viewing treatment as promoting emotional processing (Rachman, 1980; Foa & Kozak, 1986; see also Foa, Huppert, & Cahill, Chapter 1, this volume). In the next section of this chapter, we review the advances that have been made since 1980 and summarize the current status of the field before making recommendations for future research in the final section.

RECENT ADVANCES AND CURRENT STATUS
(POST-DSM-III)

Clear Diagnostic Criteria

One of broadest changes affecting the entire field of mental heath was the publication in 1980 of the third edition of the *Diagnostic and Statistical Manual of the American Psychiatric Association* (DSM-III, American Psychiatric Association, 1980), which marked a substantial change in format in an effort to improve diagnostic validity and reliability. DSM-III introduced clear lists of signs and symptoms needed to diagnose disorders, with the intention of reducing diagnostic heterogeneity and improving reliability. With each subsequent revision of the DSM (American Psychiatric Association, 1987, 1994), our diagnostic categories have been further refined, and many look to the fifth edition for additional refinements (or, perhaps, a more radical reshaping) in our classification of these disorders. During the DSM-III field trials, initial reliability estimates were obtained for the Axis I disorders, with agreement clearly improved from earlier versions of the DSM, with kappas ranging from .68 to .72 (Spitzer, Forman, & Nee, 1979; Williams & Spitzer, 1980).

Reliability studies based on DSM-III-R criteria have also generally shown good interrater agreement. DiNardo, Moras, Barlow, Rapee, and Brown (1993) reinterviewed 267 patients using the Anxiety Disorders Schedule—Revised (ADIS-R), and coefficients for interrater agreement were fair to quite good for current diagnoses of anxiety disorders: generalized anxiety disorder, .53, social phobia, .66; panic disorder with agoraphobia, .71; posttraumatic stress disorder, .55; simple phobias, .63; and OCD, .75. In another reliability study conducted by Mannuzza et al. (1989) using the Schedule for Affective Disorders and Schizophrenia (SADS), kappas were generally good, with some exceptions. For the anxiety disorders, kappas were: generalized anxiety disorder, .27; social phobia, .68; panic disorder with agoraphobia, .81; panic, .79; simple phobias, .29; and OCD, .91.

Studies of the DSM-IV have generally shown good to excellent reliability for the majority of diagnostic categories as well (e.g., Brown, DiNardo, Lehman, & Campbell, 2001). Thus, with the development of clearer diagnostic criteria for the anxiety disorders, diagnostic reliability has improved; concomitantly, our measures have improved, and assessment and treatment outcome have by extension also become considerably easier. With clear treatment targets and reliable and valid measures, we are able to track progress and to examine treatment outcome systematically across sites and disorders.

Measures

As described, with the development of clear, measurable diagnostic criteria, assessment of the anxiety disorders improved as well. Assessment utilizing reliable and valid measures allows for accurate differential diagnosis, more precise treatment planning, and specific measurement of treatment outcome. Although a comprehensive review of empirically based measures for the anxiety disorders is beyond the scope of this chapter (for excellent reviews, see Antony, Orsillo, & Roemer, 2001; and Keane & Riggs, Chapter 6, this volume), we highlight several disorder-specific measures and measures of underlying constructs thought to be particularly relevant to anxiety. For example, the Beck Anxiety Inventory (BAI; Beck, Epstein, Steer, & Brown, 1988) and the State–Trait Anxiety Inventory (STAI; Spielberger, Gorsuch, Lushene, Vagg, & Jacobs, 1983) are both well-validated self-report measures of general anxiety that are used commonly by clinicians and researchers alike.

More specific measures have been developed and validated across the anxiety disorders as well. In terms of the assessment of PTSD, for example, the Posttraumatic Stress Diagnostic Scale (PDS; Foa, Cashman, Jaycox, & Perry, 1997) is a widely utilized, validated self-report measure of PTSD that yields both a DSM-IV PTSD diagnosis and a measure of PTSD severity. Psychometrically sound interview measures of PTSD exist as well and are widely used, including the Clinician-Administered PTSD Scale (CAPS; Blake et al., 1995) and the PTSD Symptom Scale—Interview (PSS-I; Foa, Riggs, Dancu, & Rothbaum, 1993). The assessments of OCD, panic disorder, and social phobia have been improved by the validation of brief self-report measures such as the Obsessive–Compulsive Inventory (OCI; Foa, Kozak, Salkovskis, Coles, & Amir, 1998), the Panic and Agoraphobia Scale (PAS; Bandelow, 1999), the Mobility Inventory for Agoraphobia (MI; Chambless, Caputo, Jasin, Gracely, & Williams, 1985), and the Brief Social Phobia Scale (BSPS; Davidson et al., 1997) respectively. Clinician-rated scales have been validated for these anxiety disorders as well, including the Yale–Brown Obsessive Compulsive Scale (Y-BOCS; Goodman et al., 1989), the Panic Disorder Severity Scale (PDSS; Shear et al, 1992), and the Liebowitz Social Anxiety Scale (LSAS; Liebowitz, 1987). These measures have increased our ability to detect symptom change over the course of treatment and have been used in many of the treatment studies discussed in previous chapters and later in this chapter.

Development of Effective Psychosocial and Pharmacological Treatments for All Anxiety Disorders

There now exist controlled studies illustrating the efficacy of psychosocial treatments (in particular, cognitive-behavioral therapy) across the anxiety disorders (cf., Barlow, 2002; Foa, Franklin, & Moser, 2002; Nathan & Gorman, 2002). Pharmacological interventions have also been shown to be generally efficacious (e.g., Nathan & Gorman, 2002). In the case of posttraumatic stress disorder (PTSD), for example, a series of randomized controlled trials evaluating cognitive-behavioral interventions have demonstrated both short- and long-term improvements following such treatments (e.g., Foa et al., 2004; Foa et al., 1999; Foa, Rothbaum, Riggs, & Murdock, 1991; Marks, Lovell, Noshirvani, Livanou, & Thrasher, 1998; Resick, Nisith, Weaver, Astin, & Feuer, 2002). With long-term follow-up, results suggest that approximately 60–70% of patients are PTSD-diagnosis-free (see Foa & Rothbaum, 2003). Evidence has also begun to accumulate regarding the efficacy of serotonin reuptake inhibitors (SRIs) in the treatment of PTSD, with both sertraline and paroxetine being shown to be superior to placebo (Brady et al., 2000; Davidson et al., 2001; Marshall, Beebe, Oldham, & Zaninelli, 2001) and both approved by the Food and Drug Administration (FDA) for use with PTSD. As Jonathan Davidson reviewed in Chapter 7 in this volume, efficacious psychosocial and pharmacological treatments for social phobia have become increasingly available. For example, in a large controlled trial comparing group CBT and phenelzine, about 75% of those who completed treatment evidenced significant improvements (Heimberg et al., 1998). Similarly, a recently published randomized controlled trial comparing group CBT, fluoxetine, and their combination with placebo showed response rates of about 50% for all active conditions, with no added benefit for combination treatment (Davidson et al., 2004).

With regard to panic disorder with agoraphobia, a meta-analysis of 43 controlled studies showed average effect sizes across treatments of .88 for CBT plus interoceptive exposure, .68 for CBT alone, .56 for combination treatment, and .47 for pharmacotherapy (Gould, Otto, & Pollack, 1995). In the largest combined panic treatment study to date, panic control therapy (PCT; Barlow & Craske, 2000) and imipramine were combined and compared with each treatment alone, with a pill placebo, and with PCT plus a pill placebo. Results showed that after 12 weeks both monotherapies were superior to placebo, as were both combined treatments (Barlow, Gorman, Shear, & Woods, 2000). Following the 6-month maintenance phase, whereas all active treatments remained superior to placebo, the combination of PCT and imipramine showed somewhat better outcomes than the other treatments (Barlow et al., 2000). Interestingly, however, 6 months after all treatments were stopped, those who had benefited from imipramine (singly or in combination with PCT) no longer showed treatment benefits, and thus PCT emerged as the most efficacious (at this time point) and the most durable treatment.

Similarly, effective psychosocial and pharmacological interventions exist for OCD. Most recently (and relevant to this book), Foa, Liebowitz, and their colleagues completed a randomized controlled study comparing exposure and response prevention (EX/RP), clomipramine, and their combination with placebo. At posttreatment, all active treatments were superior to placebo, and conditions that included EX/RP were superior to clomipramine but did not differ from one another (Foa et al., 2005). At follow-up, again the groups that received EX/RP showed superior results to those for clomipramine alone but did not differ from one another (Simpson et al., 2004). Moreover, a recent meta-analysis concluded that behavioral and cognitive-behavioral therapy and a range of pharmacological interventions were on average efficacious for the treatment of OCD (Eddy, Dutra, Bradley, & Westen, 2004). Individual therapies (e.g., EX/RP), clomipramine, and SSRIs were most helpful across multiple measures of outcome.

With this body of evidence regarding the efficacy of these treatments across the anxiety disorders, researchers are now poised to begin to grapple with different sorts of research questions, such as: Which treatments are best for whom? How can we disseminate efficacious interventions so that they are more widely available? How can research effectively inform clinical practice? These questions will likely shape the next generation of investigations into treatment for the anxiety disorders.

FUTURE DIRECTIONS

As just summarized and as detailed in the earlier chapters of this book, clearly a great deal of progress has been made in the development and empirical evaluation of theory-driven treatments for anxiety disorders. We now have data from multiple randomized controlled trials conducted in different centers all over the world to guide us with respect to making clinical recommendations for treatment of these disorders in adults, and these trials consistently support the use of CBT protocols. Moreover, the study of combined treatments (CBT + SRIs especially) has grown considerably in the last 10 years in particular, and although these data do not support the position that combined treatment is generally superior to CBT monotherapy, it does appear that CBT and pharmacotherapy are compatible and that there may be some circumstances and disorders for which combined treatment is superior (for reviews, see Foa, Franklin, & Moser, 2002; Otto, Smits, & Reese, 2005). The pediatric literature on the treatment of anxiety disorders is also growing, and there is now a published randomized controlled trial that examined CBT, sertraline, and combined treatment versus pill placebo for pediatric OCD (Franklin, Foa, & March, 2003; Pediatric OCD Treatment Study Team, 2004). Despite the seemingly exponential growth in the evidence base for CBT, however, many challenges remain for clinical researchers to address. We discuss several of these challenges in detail and provide recommendations regarding future research that would continue to keep the field moving forward.

Treatment of Partial Responders and Nonresponders

CBT, pharmacotherapy, and combined treatments have all been shown to be efficacious for anxiety disorders, yet the outcomes for all of these treatments do not appear to be universal nor complete. It also appears that at least a subset of patients with anxiety disorders is nonresponsive to the best-studied therapy regimens. What, then, should be done to help partial responders and nonresponders achieve more satisfactory outcomes with respect to both symptom reduction and psychosocial functioning? On probabilistic grounds, patients who have been partially responsive to SRIs for OCD may be expected to have a poorer response to another singular treatment in the same class, with perhaps a threefold lower chance of responding on a third SRI compared with a treatment-naive patient (March & Ollendick, 2004). Augmentation with CBT would appear to be a logical next step clinically, and indeed the recently completed randomized controlled trial (RCT), in which PTSD patients received sertraline followed by random assignment to continued medication plus CBT augmentation or continued medication only, supports the efficacy of this strategy, particularly for partial responders (Rothbaum et al., 2004). Two multicenter RCTs in OCD that specifically focus on SRI partial responders are currently under way that involve Center for the Treatment and Study of Anxiety (CTSA) faculty and collaborators. The first of these (principal investigators: E. B. Foa, CTSA, and M. R. Liebowitz, Columbia University) is an adult study in which patients who have evidenced a partial response to an adequate trial of SRI are randomly assigned to twice-weekly EX/RP or stress management training (SMT). The second study is on children and adolescents (principal investigators: M. E. Franklin, CTSA; J. S. March, Duke University; and H. L. Leonard, Brown University), and involves random assignment of SRI partial responders to 12 weeks of medication management only (MM), MM + CBT delivered by a psychologist ("two-doctor combined" treatment), or MM plus a brief CBT protocol called Instructions in CBT (I-CBT), which is delivered by the same psychiatrist who also conducts MM ("one-doctor" combined treatment). Logically, then, it could also be the case that CBT partial responders may be improved by adding pharmacotherapy; this possibility is also under study with adult PTSD patients at the CTSA in conjunction with Duke University (principal investigator: J. R. T. Davidson), Massachusetts General Hospital (principal investigator: M. Pollack), and San Diego State University (principal investigator: M. Stein). All of the approaches to developing combined treatments described previously involve combining two treatments, one psychological and the other pharmacological, that have each been found separately to be an effective treatment for the condition of interest. It is assumed that the treatments operate through different mechanisms, and it is the hope that combined treatments will produce additive effects. An alternative approach to combined treatment is to select a pharmacological agent that enhances the mechanisms underlying psychological treatment. Basic research has shown that the glutaminergic N-methyl-D-aspartate (NMDA) receptors are involved in the learning that occurs during Pavlovian conditioning and extinction. In particular, although the medication d-cycloserine (DCS), an NMDA partial agonist, has no known anxiolytic effects by itself, it has been shown to enhance the extinction of conditioned fear in animals (e.g., Walker, Ressler, Lu, & Davis, 2002). Similarly, in humans, DCS has been recently been shown to enhance the efficacy of virtual reality exposure therapy for acrophobia (Ressler et al., 2004; see also Rothbaum, Chapter 13, this volume). These studies and others like them may help to clarify what treatment strategies to use when a patient remains symptomatic despite having received an empirically supported treatment.

Treatment Dropouts and Tolerability of Treatment

As discussed in the earlier chapters of this book, most CBT protocols for anxiety disorders require direct confrontation of feared stimuli, thoughts, and, in the case of prolonged exposure therapy (PE) for PTSD in particular, traumatic memories. Accordingly, concerns about patients' ability to comply with these treatments have been raised, and some have suggested that PE in particular may not be as well tolerated as other forms of treatment (e.g., Pitman et al., 1991). However, a reanalysis of 25 controlled PTSD studies that included data on dropout indicated comparable attrition rates for PE and other exposure treatments (20%), cognitive therapy or stress inoculation training (22%), and eye movement desensitization and reprocessing (EMDR; 19%; Hembree et al., 2003). Notably, all three of these active treatments evidenced higher dropout rates than various control conditions (11%). Although 20% is comparable to other anxiety disorder RCTs and, on average, lower than other treatments for PTSD (e.g., SRI pharmacotherapy), it remains an issue that at least one in five patients in most studies fail to complete active treatment. Concern about this issue has led to recent treatment development efforts aimed at reducing the CBT dropout rates and also at improving compliance within CBT protocols. In particular, several research groups (e.g., Tolin, Maltby, Diefenbach, & Worhunsky, 2004; Westra & Dozois, 2004) including Foa, Simpson, and Liebowitz and collaborators in adult OCD have begun to incorporate and study motivational interviewing (MI) techniques in CBT packages for anxiety disorders. Based on the principles developed and described by Miller and Rollnick (2002) for use with patients with alcohol and other substance abuse or dependence, MI aims to help therapists "roll with resistance" and assist patients in making informed choices about whether or not to make change efforts, instead of having therapists attempt to impose the choices on ambivalent patients. Further development in this area is much needed, especially randomized controlled trials directly comparing MI-enhanced CBT protocols with standard CBT protocols.

Generalizability of Findings from RCTs

As we have reviewed, in the past 20 years the number of RCTs examining CBT and other treatments for anxiety disorders has grown substantially, and presumably their collective results can be used to inform clinical practice. However, some have questioned the degree to which RCT findings gathered from carefully screened patient samples are generalizable to clinical practice (e.g., Persons & Silberschatz, 1998), as well as whether or not manualized treatments can actually be delivered in clinical settings (e.g., Westen, in press; Westen, Novotny, & Thompson-Brenner, 2004). Such criticisms are extremely informative, because the degree to which they are shared by the very practitioners who see most anxious patients clinically may affect the ultimate utility of RCT findings. It is incumbent on those of us who develop and study these treatments to address these concerns, and accordingly several studies within the anxiety disorders have been done in order to determine the clinical, or "real world," effectiveness of CBT protocols that have been found efficacious in RCTs. A good deal of this kind of work has already been done in OCD. The efficacy of EX/RP already having been established (for a review, see Franklin & Foa, 2002), several recent studies have now explored its effectiveness in less restrictive samples (Franklin, Abramowitz, Kozak, Levitt, & Foa, 2000) and in clinical practice settings (Rothbaum & Shahar, 2000; Warren & Thomas, 2001) in which EX/RP experts either provided or closely supervised all of the treatment. Their collective findings suggest that EX/RP also yields very positive outcomes with patients treated outside the context of RCTs, although the direct involvement of experts in treatment delivery limits the degree to which they can inform us about treatment provider effects. Thus this issue was explored in a subsequent study in which outcomes of clinical psychology interns and highly experienced EX/RP therapists were compared and shown to be comparable at posttreatment (Franklin, Abramowitz, Bux, Zoellner, & Feeny, 2002); notably, random assignment was not employed, the interns were supervised by experts, and there were pretreatment differences such that the patients treated by the highly experienced therapists had on average more severe symptoms at pretreatment.

Dissemination

Dissemination of CBT beyond the confines of academic centers of expertise is a major research initiative that has yet to be fully embraced, although there have been some encouraging studies conducted within the anxiety disorders. A pediatric OCD effectiveness study recently completed in middle Norway (Valderhaug, Gotestam, Larsson, & Piacentini, 2004) differs from the aforementioned EX/RP effectiveness studies in that access to the pediatric EX/RP expert was much more limited, in that the model included a training of supervisors element, and in that EX/RP was conducted by therapists who were not highly experienced with using the protocol with children and adolescents. Preliminary outcomes of EX/RP with 24 children and adolescents who completed open treatment were very encouraging and appear comparable to those achieved in pediatric OCD open trials conducted in expert clinics (e.g., Franklin et al., 1998; March, Mulle, & Herbel, 1994; Piacentini, Bergman, Jacobs, McCracken, & Kretchman, 2002; Wever & Rey, 1997), to RCT findings (de Haan, Hoogduin, Buitelaar, & Keijsers, 1998; Pediatric OCD Treatment Study Team, 2004), and with adult OCD patients (e.g., Foa et al., 2005). Studies such as this one represent a critical next step in determining the extent to which EX/RP and other CBT protocols can be taught and then implemented in more representative clinical settings. Along these lines, a recently completed RCT examining PE and PE plus cognitive restructuring (PE + CR) for adult PTSD also included an effectiveness element: Approximately half of the patients were treated at the CTSA, and half were treated by master's-level counselors at a rape counseling center. Notably, comparable PE and PE + CR outcomes were found between the CTSA experts and the master's-level counselors, supporting the transportability of CBT to more representative clinical settings (Foa et al., in press). Similarly encouraging outcomes have been found in dissemination studies for panic disorder in a community mental health center (Wade, Treat, & Stuart, 1998) and with exposure therapy for social anxiety disorder in a general medical practice setting (Blomhoff et al., 2001). Studies will soon be needed that vary the presence and also the intensity of expert supervision in order to more fully explore the boundaries of effective CBT implementation.

CONCLUDING REMARKS

The purpose of this book was to provide a venue in which many leaders in the field of anxiety treatment and research could synthesize and summarize the accomplishments realized over the past several decades, as well as outline an agenda for the future. One theme that reverberates throughout the book and, indeed, throughout the field more broadly is the influence and contribution of emotional processing theory (Foa & Kozak, 1986). This collective body of work has been critically important in propelling the field forward and has helped build the evidence base to the point at which anxiety disorders are now often cited as a particular area within psychology and psychiatry in which much has already been learned about how best to help patients with these conditions. There is much left to do, however: For example, treatment response is still neither universal nor complete; many questions pertaining to biological and psychological mechanisms of action have yet to be addressed; and, despite typical onset of these disorders during childhood or adolescence, the pediatric treatment literature continues to lag behind the adult literature. Answers to many of these remaining problems are being pursued by the researchers and authors in this volume, and hopefully the progress in these key areas will further enhance the evidence base and spawn new theoretical developments that will be of great importance to improving our understanding and decreasing the suffering of the millions of people worldwide who either have or are vulnerable to anxiety disorders.

REFERENCES

Agras, W. S., Leitenberg, H., & Barlow, D. H. (1968). Social reinforcement in the modification of agoraphobia. *Archives of General Psychiatry, 19*, 423–427.

American Psychiatric Association. (1980). *Diagnostic and statistical manual of mental disorders* (3rd ed.). Washington, DC: Author.

American Psychiatric Association. (1987). *Diagnostic and statistical manual of mental disorders* (3rd ed., rev.). Washington, DC: Author.

American Psychiatric Association. (1994). *Diagnostic and statistical manual of mental disorders* (4th edition). Washington, DC: Author.

Antony, M. M., Orsillo, S. M., & Roemer, L. (2001). *Practitioner's guide to empirically based measures of anxiety.* New York: Kluwer Academic/Plenum.

Bandelow, B. (1999). *Panic and Agoraphobia Scale (PAS).* Seattle, WA: Hogrefe & Huber.

Bandura, A. (1969). *Principles of behavior modification.* New York: Holt, Rinehart & Winston.

Bandura, A., Blanchard, E. B., & Ritter, B. (1969). The relative efficacy of desensitization and modeling approaches for inducing behavioral, affective, and attitudinal changes. *Journal of Personality and Social Psychology, 13*, 173–199.

Barlow, D. H. (2002). *Anxiety and its disorders: The nature and treatment of anxiety and panic* (2nd ed.). New York: Guilford Press.

Barlow, D. H., & Craske, M. G. (2000). *Mastery of your anxiety and panic (MAP-3): Client workbook for anxiety and panic* (3rd ed.). San Antonio, TX: Graywind/ Psychological Corporation.

Barlow, D. H., Gorman, J. M., Shear, M. K., & Woods, S. W. (2000). Cognitive-behavioral therapy, imipramine, or their combination for panic disorder: A randomized controlled trial. *Journal of the American Medical Association, 283*, 2529–2536.

Barlow, D. H., Leitenberg, H., Agras, W. S., & Winczel, J. P. (1969). The transfer gap in systematic desensitization: An analogue study. *Behaviour Research and Therapy, 7*, 191–196.

Beck, A. T., Epstein, N., Steer, R. A., & Brown, G. (1988). An inventory for measuring clinical anxiety: Psychometric properties. *Journal of Consulting and Clinical Psychology, 56*, 893–897.

Blake, D. D., Weathers, F. W., Nagy, L. M., Kaloupek, D. G., Gusman, F. D., & Charney, D. S., et al. (1995). The development of a Clinician-Administered PTSD Scale. *Journal of Traumatic Stress, 8*, 75–90.

Blomhoff, S., Haug, T. T., Hellstrom, K., Holme, I., Humble, M., & Wold, J. E. (2001). Randomised controlled general practice trial of sertraline, exposure therapy and combined treatment in generalised social phobia. *British Journal of Psychiatry, 179*, 23–30.

Bonn, J. A., Harrison, J., & Rees, W. L. (1971). Lactate-induced anxiety: Therapeutic implications. *British Journal of Psychiatry, 119*, 468–470.

Brady, K., Pearlstein, T., Asnis, G. M., Baker, D., Rothbaum, B., Sikes, C. R., & Farfel, G. M. (2000). Efficacy and safety of Zoloft treatment of posttraumatic stress disorder: A randomized controlled trial. *Journal of the American Medical Association, 283*, 1837–1844.

Brown, T. A., Di Nardo, P. A., Lehman, C. L., & Campbell, L. A. (2001). Reliability of DSM-IV anxiety and mood disorders: Implications for classification of emotional disorders. *Journal of Abnormal Psychology, 110*, 49–58.

Chambless, D. L., Caputo, G. C., Jasin, S. E., Gracely, E. J., & Williams, C. (1985). The Mobility Inventory for Agoraphobia. *Behaviour Research and Therapy, 23*, 35–44.

Clark, D. M. (1986). A cognitive approach to panic. *Behaviour Research and Therapy, 24*, 461–470.

Cooper, J. E., Gelder, M. G., & Marks, I. M. (1965). Results of behavior therapy in 77 psychiatric patients. *British Medical Journal, 1*, 1222–1225.

Davidson, J., Foa, E. B., Huppert, J. D., Keefe, F. J., Franklin, M. E., Compton, J. S., et al. (2004). Fluoxetine, comprehensive cognitive behavioral therapy, and placebo in generalized social phobia. *Archives of General Psychiatry, 61*, 1005–1013.

Davidson, J., Pearlstein, T., Londborg, P., Brady, K. T., Rothbaum, B., Bell, J., et al. (2001). Efficacy of sertraline in preventing relapse of posttraumatic stress disorder: Results of a 28-week double-blind, placebo-controlled study. *American Journal of Psychiatry, 158*, 1974–1981.

Davidson, J. R. T., Miner, C. M., De Veaugh-Geiss, J., Tupler, L. A., Colket, J. T., & Potts, N. L. S. (1997). The Brief Social Phobia Scale: A psychometric evaluation. *Psychological Medicine, 27*, 161–166.

Davison, G. C. (1968). Systematic desensitization as a counterconditioning process. *Journal of Abnormal Psychology, 73*, 91–99.

de Haan, E., Hoogduin, K. A., Buitelaar, J. K., & Keijsers, G. P. (1998). Behavior therapy versus clomipramine for the treatment of obsessive–compulsive disorder in children and adolescents. *Journal of the American Academy of Child and Adolescent Psychiatry, 37*, 1022–1029.

Di Nardo, P. A., Moras, K., Barlow, D. H., Rapee, R. M., & Brown, T. A. (1993). Reliability of DSM-III-R anxiety disorder categories using the Anxiety Disorders Interview Schedule—Revised (ADIS-R). *Archives of General Psychiatry, 50*, 251–256.

Eddy, K. T., Dutra, L., Bradley, R., & Westen, D. (2004). A multidimensional meta-analysis of psychotherapy and pharmacotherapy for obsessive–compulsive disorder. *Clinical Psychology Review, 24*, 1011–1030.

Emmelkamp, P. M. G., & Wessels, H. (1975). Flooding in imagination vs. flooding *in vivo*: A comparison with agoraphobics. *Behaviour Research and Therapy, 13,* 7–15.

Foa, E. B., Cashman, L., Jaycox, L. H., & Perry, K. (1997). The validation of a self-report measure of PTSD: The PTSD Diagnostic Scale. *Psychological Assessment, 9,* 445–451.

Foa, E. B., Dancu, C. V., Hembree, E. A., Jaycox, L. H., Meadows, E. A., & Street, G. P. (1999). A comparison of exposure therapy, stress inoculation training, and their combination for reducing PTSD in female assault victims. *Journal of Consulting and Clinical Psychology, 67,* 194–200.

Foa, E. B., Franklin, M. E., & Moser, J. (2002). Context in the clinic: How well do CBT and medications work in combination? *Biological Psychiatry, 52,* 989–997.

Foa, E. B., Hembree, E. A., Cahill, S. P., Rauch, S. A., Riggs, D. S., Feeny, N. C., et al. (in press). Prolonged exposure for PTSD with and without cognitive restructuring: Outcome at academic and community clinics. *Journal of Consulting and Clinical Psychology.*

Foa, E. B., & Kozak, M. J. (1986). Emotional processing of fear: Exposure to corrective information. *Psychological Bulletin, 99,* 20–35.

Foa, E. B., Kozak, M. J., Salkovskis, P. M., Coles, M. E., & Amir, N. (1998). The validation of a new obsessive–compulsive disorder scale: The Obsessive–Compulsive Inventory. *Psychological Assessment, 10,* 206–214.

Foa, E. B., Liebowitz, M. R., Kozak, M. J., Davies, S. O., Campeas, R., Franklin, M. E., et al. (2005). Treatment of obsessive–compulsive disorder by exposure and ritual prevention, clomipramine, and their combination: A randomized, placebo-controlled trial. *American Journal of Psychiatry, 162,* 151–161.

Foa, E. B., Riggs, D. S., Dancu, C. V., & Rothbaum, B. O. (1993). Reliability and validity of a brief instrument for assessing post-traumatic stress disorder. *Journal of Traumatic Stress, 6,* 459–473.

Foa, E. B., & Rothbaum, B. O. (2003). Posttraumatic stress disorder. *Psychiatric Annals, 33,* 11–12.

Foa, E. B., Rothbaum, B. O., Riggs, D. S., & Murdock, T. B. (1991). Treatment of posttraumatic stress disorder in rape victims: A comparison between cognitive-behavioral procedures and counseling. *Journal of Consulting and Clinical Psychology, 59,* 715–723.

Franklin, M. E., Abramowitz, J. S., Bux, D. A., Zoellner, L. A., & Feeny, N. C. (2002). Cognitive-behavioral therapy with and without medication in the treatment of obsessive–compulsive disorder. *Professional Psychology: Research and Practice, 33,* 162–168.

Franklin, M. E., Abramowitz, J. S., Kozak, M. J., Levitt, J., & Foa, E. B. (2000). Effectiveness of exposure and ritual prevention for obsessive–compulsive disorder: Randomized compared with non-randomized samples. *Journal of Consulting and Clinical Psychology, 68,* 594–602.

Franklin, M. E., & Foa, E. B. (2002). Cognitive-behavioral treatment of obsessive–compulsive disorder. In P. E. Nathan & J. M. Gorman (Eds.), *A guide to treatments that work* (2nd ed., pp. 367–386). Oxford, UK: Oxford University Press.

Franklin, M. E., Foa, E. B., & March, J. S. (2003). The Pediatric OCD Treatment Study (POTS): Rationale, design and methods. *Journal of Child and Adolescent Psychopharmacology, 13*(Suppl. 1), 39–52.

Franklin, M. E., Kozak, M. J., Cashman, L. A., Coles, M. E., Rheingold, A. A., & Foa, E. B. (1998). Cognitive-behavioral treatment of pediatric obsessive–compulsive disorder: An open clinical trial. *Journal of the American Academy of Child and Adolescent Psychiatry, 37*, 412–419.

Gelder, M. G., & Marks, I. M. (1966). Severe agoraphobia: A controlled prospective trial of behaviour therapy. *British Journal of Psychiatry, 112*, 309–319.

Goldstein, A. J., & Chambless, D. L. (1978). A reanalysis of agoraphobia. *Behavior Therapy, 9*, 47–59.

Goodman, W. K., Price, L. H., Rasmussen, S. A., Mazure, C., Fleischmann, R. L., Hill, C. L., et al. (1989). The Yale–Brown Obsessive Compulsive Scale: I. Development, use, and reliability. *Archives of General Psychiatry, 46*, 1006–1011.

Gould, R. A., Otto, M. W., & Pollack, M. H. (1995). A meta-analysis of treatment outcome for panic disorder. *Clinical Psychology Review, 15*, 819–844.

Haslam, M. T. (1974). The relationship between the effect of lactate infusion on anxiety states, and their amelioration by carbon dioxide inhalation. *British Journal of Psychiatry, 125*, 88–90.

Heimberg, R. G., Liebowitz, M. R., Hope, D. A., Schneier, F. R., Holt, C. S., Welkowitz, L. A., et al. (1998). Cognitive behavioral group therapy vs. phenelzine therapy for social phobia. *Archives of General Psychiatry, 55*, 1133–1141.

Hembree, E. A., Foa, E. B., Dorfan, N. M., Street, G. P., Kowalski, J., & Tu, X. (2003). Do patients drop out prematurely from exposure therapy for PTSD? *Journal of Traumatic Stress, 16*, 555–562.

Jacobson, E. (1938). *Progressive relaxation.* Chicago: University of Chicago Press.

Jones, M. C. (1924). A laboratory study of fear: The case of Peter. *Journal of Genetic Psychology, 31*, 308–315.

Lang, P. J. (1977). Imagery in therapy: An information processing analysis of fear. *Behavior Therapy, 8*, 862–886.

Lang, P. J. (1979). A bio-informational theory of emotional imagery. *Psychophysiology, 16*, 495–512.

Lang, P. J. (1984). Cognition in emotion: Concept and action. In C. Izard, J. Kagan, & R. Zajonc (Eds.), *Emotion, cognition and behavior* (pp. 193–206). New York: Cambridge University Press.

Lang, P. J., & Lazovik, A. D. (1963). Experimental desensitization of a phobia. *Journal of Abnormal and Social Psychology, 66*, 519–525.

Lang, P. J., Lazovik, A. D., & Reynolds, D. J. (1965). Desensitization, suggestibility and pseudotherapy. *Journal of Abnormal Psychology, 70*, 395–402.

Lang, P. J., Melamed, B. G., & Hart, J. (1970). A psychophysiological analysis of fear modification using an automated desensitization procedure. *Journal of Abnormal Psychology, 76*, 220–234.

Leitenberg, H., Agras, W. S., Edwards, J. A., Thompson, L. E., & Wincze, J. P. (1970). Practice as a psychotherapeutic variable: An experimental analysis within single cases. *Journal of Psychiatric Research, 7*, 215–225.

Liebowitz, M. R. (1987). Social phobia. *Modern Problems in Pharmacopsychiatry, 22*, 141–173.

Mannuzza, S., Fryer, A. J., Martin, L. Y., Gallops, M. S., Endicott, J., Gorman, J. M., et al. (1989). Reliability of anxiety assessment: I. Diagnostic agreement. *Archives of General Psychiatry, 46,* 1093–1101.

March, J. S., Mulle, K., & Herbel, B. (1994). Behavioral psychotherapy for children and adolescents with obsessive–compulsive disorder: An open trial of a new protocol-driven treatment package. *Journal of the Ameerican Academy of Child and Adolescent Psychiatry, 33,* 333–341.

March, J. S., & Ollendick, T. H. (2004). Integrated psychosocial and pharmacological treatment. In T. H. Ollendick & J. S. March (Eds.), *Phobic and anxiety disorders in children and adolescents: A clinician's guide to effective psychosocial and pharmacological interventions* (pp. 141–174). New York: Oxford University Press.

Marks, I., Lovell, K., Noshirvani, H., Livanou, M., & Thrasher, S. (1998). Treatment of posttraumatic stress disorder by exposure and/or cognitive restructuring. *Archives of General Psychiatry, 55,* 317–325.

Marshall, R. D., Beebe, K. L., Oldham, M., & Zaninelli, R. (2001). Efficacy and safety of paroxetine treatment of chronic PTSD: A fixed dosage, multicenter placebo-controlled study. *American Journal of Psychiatry, 158,* 1982–1988.

McGlynn, F. D. (1973). Graded imagination and relaxation as components of experimental desensitization. *Journal of Nervous and Mental Disease, 156,* 377–385.

Meyer, V. (1966). Modification of expectations in cases with obsessional rituals. *Behaviour Research and Therapy, 4,* 273–280.

Meyer, V., & Levy, R. (1973). Modification of behavior in obsessive–compulsive disorders. In H. E. Adams & P. Unikel (Eds.), *Issues and trends in behavior therapy* (pp. 77–136). Springfield, IL: Thomas.

Miller, W. R., & Rollnick, S. (2002). *Motivational interviewing* (2nd ed.). New York: Guilford Press.

Nathan, P. E., & Gorman J. M. (Eds.). (2002). *A guide to treatments that work* (2nd ed.). New York: Oxford University Press.

Orwin, A. (1973). "The running treatment": A preliminary communication on a new use for an old therapy (physical activity) in the agoraphobic syndrome. *British Journal of Psychiatry, 122,* 175–179.

Otto, M. W., Smits, J. A., & Reese, H. E. (2005). Combined psychotherapy and pharmacotherapy for mood and anxiety disorders in adults: Review and analysis. *Clinical Psychology: Science and Practice, 12,* 72–86.

Paul, G. L. (1969). Outcome of systematic desensitization: II. Controlled investigations of individual treatment, technique variations, and current status. In C. M. Franks (Ed.), *Behavior therapy: Appraisal and status* (pp. 105–159). New York: McGraw-Hill.

Pediatric OCD Treatment Study Team. (2004). Cognitive-behavioral therapy, sertraline, and their combination for children and adolescents with obsessive–compulsive disorder: The Pediatric OCD Treatment Study (POTS) randomized controlled trial. *Journal of the American Medical Association, 292,* 1969–1976.

Persons, J. B., & Silberschatz, G. (1998). Are results of randomized controlled trials useful to psychotherapists? *Journal of Consulting and Clinical Psychology, 66,* 126–135.

Piacentini, J., Bergman, R. L., Jacobs, C., McCracken, J. T., & Kretchman, J. (2002). Open trial of cognitive behavior therapy for childhood obsessive–compulsive disorder. *Journal of Anxiety Disorders, 16,* 207–219.

Pitman, R. K., Altman, B., Greenwald, E., Longpre, R. E., Macklin, M. L., Poire, R. E., & Steketee, G. S. (1991). Psychiatric complications during flooding therapy for posttraumatic stress disorder. *Journal of Clinical Psychiatry, 52,* 17–20.

Rachman, S. (1980). Emotional processing. *Behaviour Research and Therapy, 18,* 51–60.

Reiss, S., & McNally, R. J. (1985). Expectancy model of fear. In S. Reiss & R. R. Bootzin (Eds.), *Theoretical issues in behavior therapy* (pp. 107–121). San Diego, CA: Academic Press.

Resick, P. A., Nishith, P., Weaver, T., Astin, M. C., & Feuer, C. A. (2002). A comparison of cognitive processing therapy, prolonged exposure, and a waiting condition for the treatment of posttraumatic stress disorder in female rape victims. *Journal of Consulting and Clinical Psychology, 70,* 867–879.

Ressler, K. J., Rothbaum, B. O., Tannenbaum, L., Anderson, P., Graap, K., Zimand, E., et al. (2004). Cognitive enhancers as adjuncts to psychotherapy: Use of D-cycloserine in phobics to facilitate extinction of fear. *Archives of General Psychiatry, 61,* 1136–1144.

Rothbaum, B. O., Foa, E. B., Davidson, J. R. T., Cahill, S. P., Compton, J., Connor, K., & Astin, M. (2004). *Augmentation of sertraline with prolonged exposure in the treatment of PTSD.* Unpublished manuscript.

Rothbaum, B. O., & Shahar, F. (2000). Behavioral treatment of obsessive–compulsive disorder in a naturalistic setting. *Cognitive and Behavioral Practice, 7,* 262–270.

Shear, M. K., Brown, T. A., Sholomskas, D. E., Barlow, D. H., Gorman, J. M., Woods, S. W., & Cloitre, M. (1992). *Panic Disorder Severity Scale (PDSS).* Pittsburgh, PA: University of Pittsburgh School of Medicine, Department of Psychiatry.

Sherrington, C. S. (1961). *The integrative action of the nervous system.* New Haven, CT: Yale University Press. (Original work published 1906)

Simpson, H. B., Liebowitz, M. R., Foa, E. B., Kozak, M. J., Schmidt, A. B., Rowan, V., et al. (2004). Post-treatment effects of exposure therapy and clomipramine in obsessive–compulsive disorder. *Depression and Anxiety, 19,* 225–233.

Spielberger, C. D., Gorsuch, R. L., Lushene, R., Vagg, P. R., & Jacobs, G. A. (1983). *Manual for the State–Trait Anxiety Inventory (Form Y).* Palo Alto, CA: Mind Garden.

Spitzer, R. L., Forman, J. B., & Nee, J. (1979). DSM-III field trials: I. Initial interrater diagnostic reliability. *American Journal of Psychiatry, 136,* 815–817.

Stampfl, T. G., & Levis, D. J. (1967). Essentials of implosive therapy: A learning-theory-based psychodynamic behavioral therapy. *Journal of Abnormal Psychology, 72,* 496–503.

Tolin, D. F., Maltby, N., Diefenbach, G. J., & Worhunsky, P. (2004, November). Motivating treatment-refusing OCD patients. In D. J. A. Dozois (Chair), *Motivational interviewing and related strategies for the treatment of anxiety and depression.* Symposium conducted at the annual meeting of the Association for Advancement of Behavior Therapy, New Orleans, LA.

Valderhaug, R., Gotestam, K. G., Larsson, B., & Piacentini, J. C. (2004, May). *An open clinical trial of cognitive behaviour therapy for childhood obsessive–compulsive disorder in regular outpatient clinics.* Paper presented at the SOGN Centre Conference on Pediatric Anxiety Disorders in Children and Adolescents, Oslo, Norway.

Wade, W. A., Treat, T. A., & Stuart, G. L. (1998). Transporting an empirically supported treatment for panic disorder to a service clinic setting: A benchmarking strategy. *Journal of Consulting and Clinical Psychology, 66,* 231–239.

Walker, D. L., Ressler, K. J., Lu, K. T., & Davis, M. (2002). Facilitation of conditioned fear extinction by systemic administration or intra-amygdala infusions of D-cycloserine as assessed with fear-potentiated startle in rats. *Journal of Neuroscience, 22,* 2343–2351.

Warren, R., & Thomas, J. C. (2001). Cognitive-behavior therapy of obsessive–compulsive disorder in private practice: An effectiveness study. *Journal of Anxiety Disorders, 15,* 277–285.

Watson, J. B. (1913). Psychology as the behaviorist views it. *Psychological Review, 20,* 158–177.

Watson, J. B., & Rayner, R. (1920). Conditioned emotional reactions. *Journal of Experimental Psychology, 3,* 1–14.

Watson, J. P., & Marks, I. M. (1971). Relevant and irrelevant fear in flooding: A cross-over study of phobic patients. *Behavior Therapy, 2,* 275–293.

Westen, D. (in press). Efficacious laboratory-validated treatments are generally not transportable to clinical practice. In J. C. Norcross, L. E. Beutler, & R. F. Levant (Eds.), *Evidence-based practices in mental health: Debate and dialogue on the fundamental questions.* Washington, DC: American Psychological Association.

Westen, D., Novotny, C. M., & Thomson-Brenner, H. (2004). The empirical status of empirically supported psychotherapies: Assumptions, findings, and reporting in controlled clinical trials. *Psychological Bulletin, 130,* 631–663.

Westra, H. A., & Dozois, D. J. A. (2004, November). Motivational interviewing as a prelude to group CBT for anxiety: A randomized trial. In D. J. A. Dozois (Chair), *Motivational interviewing and related strategies for the treatment of anxiety and depression.* Symposium conducted at the annual meeting of the Association for Advancement of Behavior Therapy, New Orleans, LA.

Wever, C., & Rey, J. M. (1997). Juvenile obsessive–compulsive disorder. *Australian and New Zealand Journal of Psychiatry, 31,* 105–113.

Williams, J. B. W., & Spitzer, R. L. (1980). DSM-III field trials: Interrater reliability and list of project staff and participants. In American Psychiatric Association, *Diagnostic and statistical manual of mental disorders* (3rd ed.). Washington, DC: American Psychiatric Association.

Wolpe, J. (1958). *Psychotherapy by reciprocal inhibition.* Stanford, CA: Stanford University Press.

Index

n indicates note

ACC. *See* Anterior cingulate cortex
Acrophobia, 229–230, 239–240
Activation, 7, 41
ADIS-C. *See* Anxiety Disorders Interview Schedule for Children
ADIS-IV. *See* Anxiety Disorders Interview Schedule of DSM-IV
ADIS-R. *See* Anxiety Disorders Schedule—Revised
AgCQ. *See* Agoraphobic Cognitions Questionnaire
Agoraphobia. *See also* Panic disorder with agoraphobia
  assessment tools, 103
  conceptualization of, 249
  defined, 167
  habituation and, 9
  interoceptive exposure therapy, 250
  panic disorder and, 100
  social reinforcement strategies and, 167–168
Agoraphobic Cognitions Questionnaire (AgCQ), 103
Alcohol abuse, 118
Alien abduction phenomenon, 84–86
Alprazolam, 119
Amygdala
  brain target areas, 58
  defense system and, 57, 58
  emotional encoding and, 29
  fear activation and, 7, 18–19
Anger, 117
Anhedonia, 69
Anterior cingulate cortex (ACC), 20, 30
Anticonvulsants, 119–120, 120
Anxiety/Anxiety disorders. *See also specific disorders*
  assessment methods, 92
  definitions of, 91, 170
  depression and, 70–71
  distinguished from fear, 91
  DSM-III and, 251
  emotional processing theory on, 171

fear structure and, 5–6
  measures, 251–252
  memory bias for threatening information, 26–28
  relationship to panic, 170
  response channels, 91–92
  John Watson's case studies and, 245–246
Anxiety Disorders Clinic, 132, 133, 141, 142
Anxiety Disorders Interview Schedule for Children (ADIS-C), 148, 150
Anxiety Disorders Interview Schedule of DSM-IV (ADIS-IV), 63, 70, 92
Anxiety disorder spectrum, 62–73
Anxiety Disorders Schedule—Revised (ADIS-R), 251
Anxiety sensitivity, 169
Anxiety Sensitivity Index (ASI), 70, 102, 169
Anxiety Sensitivity Profile, 102
Anxiolytics, 120
Articulated thought, 105
ASI. *See* Anxiety Sensitivity Index
Assessment measures, 251–252. *See also individual measures*
Assessments
  obsessive–compulsive disorder, 105–107
  panic disorder, 100–103
  pediatric obsessive–compulsive disorder, 148–151
  posttraumatic stress disorder, 92–100
  social phobia, 103–105
Atenolol, 120
Attention, decreased, 10
Attentional narrowing, 46
Atypical antipsychotics, 120
Atypical nueroleptics, 120
Autobiographical memory, 41–42, 46
"Autonoetic awareness," 41
Avoidance, cognitive, 80–83, 182–183

BAI. *See* Beck Anxiety Inventory
BAT. *See* Behavioral avoidance test

BDD. *See* Body dysmorphic disorder
BDI. *See* Beck Depression Inventory
Beck Anxiety Inventory (BAI), 223, 252
Beck Depression Inventory (BDI), 223, 224
Behavioral approach tests, 92, 105
Behavioral avoidance test (BAT), 238
Behavioral Inhibition Scale (BIS), 29
Benton Visual Retention Test, 139
Benzodiazepines
   panic disorder treatment and, 173
   social phobia treatment and, 118–119,
      120, 121
Beta blockers, 120
Between-session habituation, 9, 10
BIS. *See* Behavioral Inhibition Scale
Body dysmorphic disorder (BDD), 108
Body Sensations Interpretation
   Questionnaire, 102
Body Sensations Questionnaire (BSQ), 102
Body Vigilance Scale (BVS), 103
Brain. *See also* Amygdala
   action of CBT and SSRIs in, 122–123
Brief Social Phobia Scale (BSPS), 105, 125,
   252
Brofaromine, 119
Bromazepam, 118, 119
BSPS. *See* Brief Social Phobia Scale
BSQ. *See* Body Sensations Questionnaire
Buproprion, 218
Buspirone, 120, 121
BVS. *See* Body Vigilance Scale

Cambridge Neuropsychological Test
   Automated Battery (CANTAB), 139
CANTAB. *See* Cambridge
   Neuropsychological Test Automated
   Battery
CAPS. *See* Clinician-Administered PTSD
   Scale
Carbon dioxide, 167
Catastrophic Cognitions Questionnaire, 103
Catastrophizing, 176
CBGT. *See* Cognitive-behavioral group
   therapy
CCBT. *See* Comprehensive CBT
CDI. *See* Children's Depression Inventory
Center for the Treatment and Study of
   Anxiety (CTSA), 132, 133, 141, 142,
   255
CGT. *See* Complicated grief therapy
Childhood sexual abuse, 79–84
Children's Depression Inventory (CDI), 150
Children's OCD Impact Scale (COIS), 150
Children's Yale–Brown Obsessive–
   Compulsive Scale (CY- BOCS), 148,
   149, 156, 159
Citalopram, 123
Claustrophobia, 235
Clinical Global Impression-Improvement
   Scale, 125, 134, 135, 138, 223
Clinician-Administered PTSD Scale (CAPS),
   95–96, 99, 100, 252

Clomipramine, 159
   in treatment of OCD, 132–138, 141–
      143, 253–254
Clonazepam, 118–119, 120, 122, 173
Cognitive avoidance, 80–83, 182–183
Cognitive-behavioral group therapy
   (CBGT), 117, 125
Cognitive-behavioral therapy (CBT)
   complicated grief therapy and, 219
   Comprehensive CBT, 18, 123–126
   dissemination of, 257–258
   DSM-III and, 251
   exposure and, 123
   historical overview, 246–250
   measures, 251–252
   neurobiological mechanisms, 122–123
   panic disorder and, 172–177
   pediatric obsessive–compulsive disorder
      and, 147
   PTSD treatments and outcome studies,
      201–205
   randomized clinical trials and, 257
   social phobia treatment and, 116–117,
      122–123
   treatment dropouts and, 256–257
   treatment of partial responders and
      nonresponders, 255–256
   John Watson's case studies and, 245–246
Cognitive restructuring, 116
Cognitive therapy
   generalized anxiety disorder and, 187–
      192
   in pediatric OCD treatment, 152–153
   in PTSD treatment, 202–203, 204–205
COIS. *See* Children's OCD Impact Scale
Complicated grief, 215–218
Complicated grief therapy (CGT)
   development of, 218–221
   outcome studies, 222–224
   therapist training, 221–222
Comprehensive Cognitive Behavioral
   Therapy (CCBT), 18, 123–126
Compulsive Activity Checklist, 109
Context, trauma memory and, 42
Coping, dual process model of, 220
CTSA. *See* Center for the Treatment and
   Study of Anxiety
Cue-driven reexperiencing, 42, 50n
CY-BOCS. *See* Children's Yale–Brown
   Obsessive–Compulsive Scale

D-Cycloserine (DCS), 239–240, 256
Daily Panic Attack and Anxiety Record
   (DPAAR), 175
DCS. *See under* Cycloserine
Decreased attention, 10
Deese–Roediger–McDermott paradigm,
   80
Defense system, 56, 57, 58, 59
Depression
   anxiety and, 70–71
   exposure processing theory and, 18

Depression (*continued*)
  generalized anxiety disorder and, 192
  OCD and, 106, 107
  social phobia and, 118, 125
  startle potentiation study and, 68–69, 70–71
Diagnostic and Statistical Manual of the American Psychiatric Association (DSM-III), 251
Diagnostic Interview Schedule (DISC), 150
Directed-forgetting experiments, 81–83
DISC. *See* Diagnostic Interview Schedule
Distraction, in exposure therapy, 10
Dopamine transporter protein, 121
DPAAR. *See* Daily Panic Attack and Anxiety Record
Dropouts, 256–257
DSM-III. *See* Diagnostic and Statistical Manual of the American Psychiatric Association
Dysfunctional Attitudes Scale, 187
Dysthymia, OCD and, 106

Elevated autonomic response, 168
Embarrassment, 14
EMDR. *See* Eye movement desensitization and reprocessing
Emotional encoding
  of fear-related information, 25–36
  human fear system and, 29–30
  instructional control over, 30–32
  memory bias for threatening information, 26–28, 35
  persistence of training effects, 34–35
  startle magnitude and, 28–29
  training via practice, 32–34, 35
Emotional imagery, 60–62
Emotional processing, 4–5, 6, 7
Emotional processing theory
  activation and, 7
  depression and, 18
  exposure therapy, 7–10, 171 (*See also* Exposure/Exposure therapy)
  on fear and anxiety, 171
  fear structure modification, 6–7
  fear structures, 5–6, 123
  historical background, 4–5
  neuroscience and, 18–19
  panic disorder and, 172–173
  PTSD and, 199–200
  questions for further examination, 18–19
  on social anxiety disorder, 14–16
  trauma recovery, 11–13
Exposure and response prevention (EX/RP)
  OCD treatment, 132–138, 141–143, 253–254
  pediatric OCD treatment, 151–155, 156, 157, 161, 162, 257–258
  randomized clinical trials and, 257
Exposure/Exposure therapy. *See also* Imaginal exposure; Prolonged exposure therapy
  cognitive-behavioral therapy and, 123

cognitive modifications, 7–8
complicated grief therapy and, 218–219, 220–221
definitions of, 8
distraction, 10
emotional processing theory and, 7–10, 171
fear of flying and, 232–235
habituation, 8–10
interoceptive, 175–176, 250
panic disorder and, 170–171, 172–173
in PTSD treatment, 201, 204
social anxiety disorder and, 17–18
social phobia treatment and, 116
EX/RP. *See* Exposure and response prevention
Extinction, 6, 153, 172
Eyeblink, 59
Eye movement desensitization and reprocessing (EMDR), 203, 204, 205

"False" memories, 84–86
Family, pediatric OCD treatment and, 154, 155
Fear
  assessment methods, 92
  contextual factors and, 170
  distinguished from anxiety, 91
  emotional processing theory on, 171
  evolutionary perspective, 59
  response channels, 91–92
  two-stage theory of, 182
Fear and avoidance hierarchy, 176
Fearfulness, 61–63
Fear image, 4
"Fear of embarrassment," 14
Fear of fear, 169
Fear structures
  anxiety disorders and, 5–6
  emotional processing theory and, 123
  erroneous evaluations, 8
  Lang's concept of, 4
  modifying pathological associations in, 6–7
  normal and pathological, 5
  pathological elements characterizing, 7
  in PTSD, 12, 40–41
  of social anxiety disorder, 14–16
  trauma recovery and, 13
Fear Survey Schedule (FSS), 69
Fear system, 29–30, 35
Fluoxetine, 124, 159, 253
Fluvoxamine, 118, 159
Flying, fear of, 230–235
fMRI. *See* Functional magnetic resonance imaging
Frost Indecisiveness Scale, 109
FSS. *See* Fear Survey Schedule
Functional magnetic resonance imaging (fMRI), 29

Gabapentin, 119–120
GAD. *See* Generalized anxiety disorder

Generalized anxiety disorder (GAD)
  characterization of, 181–183
  in a diagnostic spectrum, 61–62
  nonadaptive behavior treatments, 186–187
  nonadaptive cognition and treatment strategies, 187–192
  nonadaptive emotional experiencing and treatment strategies, 192–193
  nonadaptive patterns of awareness, 183–184
  nonadaptive physiological functioning, 185
  relaxation methods, 185–186
  self-monitoring, 184
  startle potentiation study and, 65, 66, 67, 70, 71, 72
Generalized social phobia, 115, 124–126
Glutaminergic N-methyl-D-aspartate (NMDA), 256
Graded exposure, 152
Grief. See Complicated grief
Grief interventions, 217–218

Habituation, 8–10, 25
Helplessness, 72–73
Hippocampus, 29
Hoarding, 107
Homographs, 32, 33–34
Hyperhidrosis, 117
Hypochondrasis, 108

ICG. See Inventory of Complicated Grief
IES-R. See Impact of Event Scale—Revised
Imagery, 190–191
Imaginal exposure, 250
  in complicated grief therapy, 218, 219, 220–221
  in PTSD treatment, 201, 206–207
  social phobia treatment and, 126
  use and effects of, 8
Imaginal flooding, 249
Imaginal revisiting, 221
Imagination inflation, 190
Imipramine, 173–174, 253
Immobility, defensive, 57
Impact of Event Scale—Revised (IES-R), 97–98
Implosive theory, 249
Intelligence, as risk factor for PTSD, 45
Intent-to-treat (ITT) model, 160
Interoceptive conditioning, 169
Interoceptive exposure
  description of, 175–176
  and panic attack with agoraphobia, 250
Interpersonal and emotional processing, 186–187
Interpersonal psychotherapy
  augmentation studies, 218
  complicated grief therapy and, 223
  integrating with cognitive-behavioral techniques, 219–221
  social phobia and, 117

Intrinsic motivation, 192
Inventory of Complicated Grief (ICG), 217, 218, 223
In vivo exposure, 8, 250
  complicated grief therapy and, 219, 221
  in panic disorder treatment, 172–173
In vivo flooding, 249
ITT model. See Intent-to-treat model

"Learned helplessness," 72–73
Learning theory, 172
Liebowitz Social Anxiety Scale (LSAS), 105, 252
Life Events Checklist, 99
Likert scale, 98, 99
Lorazepam, 173
LSAS. See Liebowitz Social Anxiety Scale

Major depressive disorder (MDD), 217, 218
MAOIs. See Monoamine oxidase inhibitors
MAP-3. See Mastery of Your Anxiety and Panic, 3rd Edition
MASC. See Multidimensional Anxiety Scale for Children
MASQ. See Mood and Anxiety Symptom Questionnaire
Mastery of Your Anxiety and Panic, 3rd Edition (MAP-3), 174
Maudsley Obsessive–Compulsive Inventory (MOCI), 109
MDD. See Major depressive disorder
Meaning propositions, 84
Medical histories, 151
Memory
  anxiety disorders and, 26–28, 35
  "false," 84–86
  recovered, 84
Mississippi Scale for Combat-Related PTSD, 98, 100
Mobility Inventory for Agoraphobia, 103, 252
MOCI. See Maudsley Obsessive–Compulsive Inventory
Moclobemide, 119
Modeling, in pediatric OCD treatment, 153
Monoamine oxidase inhibitors (MAOIs), 119, 121
Mood and Anxiety Symptom Questionnaire (MASQ), 68
Mood disorders, social phobia and, 117–118
Motivation, intrinsic, 192
Motivational enhancement therapy, 220
Motivational interviewing, 256
Multidimensional Anxiety Scale for Children (MASC), 150
Muscle relaxation. See Progressive muscle relaxation

Negative affect, 70–71
Negative Thoughts about the Self scale, 48, 49

Neuroimaging, 29–30, 35
NMDA. *See* Glutaminergic
  N-methyl-D-aspartate
Nongeneralized social phobia, 118, 120
Nonresponders, 255–256
Norepinephrine transporter protein, 121
Nortriptyline, 218, 223
"Nowness," 41, 42, 43

Obsessive–compulsive disorder, pediatric
  assessment, 148–151
  CBT treatment, 147
    application guidelines, 151–155
    EX/RP techniques and, 151–155, 156,
      157, 161, 162, 257–258
    outcome studies, 156–158
    Pediatric OCD Treatment Study, 158–
      160
    research areas, 161–162
  prevalence, 147
Obsessive–compulsive disorder (OCD)
  assessment strategies, 108–109
  characterization, 105–106
  differential diagnosis, 107–108
  EX/RP and SRI treatment
    augmentation study, 140–142
    key findings regarding, 132–133, 142–
      143
    residual impairment study, 138–140
    vs. clomipramine, 133–138, 253–254
  features of, 106–107
  imaginal exposure and, 8
  memory for threatening events and, 26
  psychosocial and pharmacological
    interventions, 253–254
  social phobia and, 104
  treatment dropouts, 256
  treatment of partial responders, 255
Obsessive–Compulsive Inventory (OCI),
  109, 252
Obsessive Thoughts Questionnaire, 109
OCD. *See* Obsessive–compulsive disorder
OCI. *See* Obsessive–Compulsive Inventory
Olanzapine, 120
Ondansetron, 120
Overactivation, 7

Padua Inventory (PI), 109
PANDAS, 151
Panic, relationship to anxiety, 170
Panic and Agoraphobia Scale (PAS), 103,
  252
Panic attacks
  conditioning experiences, 169–170
  in panic disorder, 101–102, 166–167
Panic disorder. *See also* Panic disorder with
    agoraphobia
  assessment strategies, 102–103
  characterization, 100
  differential diagnosis, 101–102
  fear structure and, 6
  features of, 100–101, 166
  interoceptive exposure and, 250

panic attacks in, 101–102, 166–167
Panic Disorder Severity Scale (PDSS), 252
Panic disorder with agoraphobia (PDA)
  cognitive-behavioral therapy and, 172–
    177
  comorbidity and, 71
  conditioning experiences, 169–170
  in a diagnostic spectrum, 61–62
  emotional processing theory and, 172–
    173
  emotion provocation, 170–171
  exposure and, 170–171, 172–173, 250
  future research directions, 177–178
  initial studies on, 167–168
  intensive treatment program, 177
  psychopharmacological interventions,
    173–174
  psychosocial and pharmacological
    interventions, 253
  startle potentiation study and, 65, 66,
    67, 69, 71, 72
  treatment approaches, 171–174
  vulnerabilities to developing, 168–169
Paroxetine, 118, 121, 122, 123, 218, 223,
  253
Partial responders, 255–256
PAS. *See* Panic and Agoraphobia Scale
PCL. *See* PTSD Checklist
PDA. *See* Panic disorder with agoraphobia
PDS. *See* Posttraumatic Diagnostic Scale
PDSS. *See* Panic Disorder Severity Scale
Pediatric autoimmune neuropsychiatric
  disorders associated with streptococcal
  infection (PANDAS), 151
Pediatric obsessive–compulsive disorder. *See*
  Obsessive–compulsive disorder,
  pediatric
Pediatric OCD Treatment Study (POTS),
  158–160, 161
Personal goals technique, 220
Phenelzine, 119, 120, 253
Phobias, specific
  comorbidity and, 71
  in a diagnostic spectrum, 61–62
  startle potentiation study and, 65, 66,
    67, 69, 70, 71, 72
PI. *See* Padua Inventory
PMR. *See* Progressive muscle relaxation
Posttraumatic Cognitions Inventory, 48,
  49
Posttraumatic Diagnostic Scale (PDS), 99,
  252
Posttraumatic stress disorder (PTSD)
  assessment strategies, 94–100
  CBT approaches to, 200–203
  CBT outcome studies, 203–205
  childhood sex abuse survivors and, 81–
    82, 84
  complicated grief and, 215, 216,
    217
  diagnostic criteria, 197–198
  differential diagnosis, 94
  early conceptualizations of, 199

emotional processing theory and, 199–200
exposure therapies and, 8, 11–13, 204, 205–208, 235–237
fear structure and, 6, 12, 40–41
features of, 93–94
obsessive–compulsive behavior and, 107–108
onset *vs.* maintenance of symptoms, 40
pharmacological interventions, 252–253
predictors, 39, 42, 48–50
prevalence, 92–93, 198, 235
research overview, 208–209
role of schemas, beliefs, and appraisals in, 47–48, 49
trauma memories and, 40–47
treatment dropouts and, 256
treatment of partial responders, 255
virtual reality exposure therapy and, 235–237
POTS. *See* Pediatric OCD Treatment Study
Pregabalin, 119, 120
Probability overestimation, 176
Progressive muscle relaxation (PMR), 185–186
Prolonged exposure/exposure therapy
complicated grief therapy and, 219, 221
PTSD treatment and, 204, 205–208
Propranolol, 121
PSS-I. *See* PTSD Symptom Scale—Interview
Psychodrama, 220
Psychotherapy, interpersonal. *See* Interpersonal psychotherapy
PTSD Checklist (PCL), 99–100
PTSD Symptom Scale—Interview (PSS-I), 96, 252
Public speaking anxiety, 238–239

Quality of Life Enjoyment and Satisfaction Scale, 139
Randomized controlled trials (RCTs), 257
Rape survivors, 13, 44
RCTs. *See* Randomized controlled trials
Reactivity, 168
Recall. *See* Voluntary recall
Reciprocal induction, 246–248
Recovered memory, 84
Relapse, social phobia treatment and, 120–121
Relaxation, 152, 185–186
Repetitive behavior, 106–108
Responsibility Attitudes Scale, 109
Responsibility Interpretations Questionnaire, 109
Reversible and selective inhibitors of MAO type A (RIMA), 119, 120
Rey–Osterrieth Complex Figure Test, 139
RIMA. *See* Reversible and selective inhibitors of MAO type A
Rituals
OCD and, 106–108
prevention, 153

Rodents, fear of, 239
Rumination, 107, 183
SAD. *See* Social anxiety disorder
SADS. *See* Schedule for Affective Disorders and Schizophrenia
"Safety behaviors," 15
Satanic cults, 86n
Schedule for Affective Disorders and Schizophrenia (SADS), 251
Schizophrenia, 108
SCID. *See* Structured Clinical Interviews for DSM-IV
SCID-II. *See* Structured Clinical Interview for DSM-IV Axis II Personality Disorders
Selective serotonin reuptake inhibitors (SSRIs)
neurobiological mechanisms, 122–123
in SAD treatment, 118
in treatment of social phobia, 121, 122
Self-control desensitization (SCD), 186, 189
Self-monitoring, 184
Self-report questionnaires, for PTSD, 97–100
Self-Statements during Public Speaking Scale (SSPS), 105
Separation distress, 217
Serotonin-norepinephrine reuptake inhibitors (SNRIs), 118
Serotonin reuptake inhibitors (SRIs). *See also specific medications*
CBT augmentation and, 255
OCD treatment and, 132–138, 141–143
pediatric OCD treatment and, 159, 161
PTSD treatment and, 253
Sertraline, 121, 122, 148, 158–160, 253, 254, 255
Shaping, in pediatric OCD treatment, 153
SIAS. *See* Social Interaction Anxiety Scale
Simple phobia, 106
SIP. *See* Structured Interview for PTSD
SIT. *See* Stress inoculation training
Sleep paralysis, 85
SMT. *See* Stress management training
SNRIs. *See* Serotonin-norepinephrine reuptake inhibitors
Social Adjustment Scale, 139
Social anxiety disorder (SAD). *See also* Social phobia
fear structure, 14–16
treatment of, 17–18
virtual reality exposure therapy and, 238–239
Social Interaction Anxiety Scale (SIAS), 105
Social phobia
assessment strategies, 104–15
broad treatment approaches, 116
characterization and features of, 103–104
cognitive-behavioral therapy and, 116–118
comorbidity and, 71, 117–118, 125
comprehensive CBT treatment study, 123–126
in a diagnostic spectrum, 61–62
differential diagnosis, 104

Social phobia (*continued*)
  fear structure and, 6
  historical views of, 115
  instructional control over, 30–32
  management goals, 115–116
  OCD and, 106, 108
  pharmacotherapy and psychosocial
    treatments compared, 121–123
  pharmacotherapy, 118–121, 253
  psychosocial treatment approaches, 116–
    118
  startle potentiation study and, 65, 66,
    67, 71, 72
  virtual reality exposure therapy and,
    238–239
Social Phobia and Anxiety Inventory (SPAI),
  105
Social Phobia Scale (SPS), 105
Social reinforcement strategies, panic
  disorder and, 167–168
"Social Sciences Citation Index, The," 78
Social skills training
  comprehensive CBT and, 123–124
  in treatment of social phobia, 116
Space-alien-abductee phenomenon, 84–86
SPAI. *See* Social Phobia and Anxiety
  Inventory
Specific phobias. *See* Phobias, specific
Spider phobia, 235
SPS. *See* Social Phobia Scale
SRIs. *See* Serotonin reuptake inhibitors
SSPS. *See* Self-Statements during Public
  Speaking Scale
SSRIs. *See* Selective serotonin reuptake
  inhibitors
STAI. *See* State–Trait Anxiety Inventory
Startle magnitude, 28–29
Startle potentiation study, anxiety disorder
  spectrum and, 62–73
Startle reflex, 56, 59–60
State–Trait Anxiety Inventory (STAI), 252
Stimulus control techniques, 187
Streptococcal-precipitated OCD, 151
Stress inoculation training (SIT), 201–202,
  204, 205
Stress management training (SMT), 141
Stroop paradigm, 80
Structured Clinical Interview for DSM-IV
  Axis II Personality Disorders
  (SCID-II), 70
Structured Clinical Interviews for DSM-IV
  (SCID), 92, 95, 139, 217
Structured diagnostic interviews, 94–97
Structured Interview for PTSD (SIP), 96–97
Substance abuse disorders, 106
Sudden infant death syndrome, 13
Symptom induction test, 175
Systematic desensitization
  historical overview, 167, 247–249
  predictors of successful treatment, 4

Texas Safety Maneuver Scale (TSMS), 103

Thought–Action Fusion Scale, 109
Thought listing, 105
Tic disorders, 108
Tolstoy, Leo, 60
Toronto Alexithymia Scale, 192
Tourette's syndrome, 108
Trauma
  cognitive avoidance and, 80–83
  natural recovery from, 11–13
Trauma memories
  exposure therapy and, 11–12
  PTSD and, 40–47
  studies in childhood sexual abuse, 79–84
Trauma narratives
  natural recovery from trauma and, 12–
    13
  PTSD and, 44, 45, 46
Traumatic dissociative amnesia, 81
Traumatic distress, 217
Traumatic grief, 216
TSMS. *See* Texas Safety Maneuver Scale

Venlafaxine-XR, 118
Vietnam veterans
  PTSD and, 235
  virtual reality exposure therapy, 236–237
Virtual reality exposure therapy (VRE)
  acrophobia and, 229–230, 239–240
  advantages and disadvantages, 240–241
  claustrophobia and, 235
  combined with medication, 239–240
  D-cycloserine and, 256
  efficacy of, 241–242
  emotional processing therapy and, 227,
    228–229, 241
  fear of flying and, 230–235
  future research areas, 241
  physical symptoms of anxiety during,
    229
  PTSD and, 235–237
  social phobia and, 238–239
  spider phobia and, 235
  technology of, 228
Virtual Vietnam, 236–237
Voluntary recall, 43–47

WASI. *See* Wechsler Abbreviated Scale of
  Intelligence
Wechsler Abbreviated Scale of Intelligence
  (WASI), 139
Wisconsin Card Sorting Test, 139
Within-session habituation, 9–10
Work and Social Adjustment Scale, 224
Worry, 182–183
Worry-free-zones, 187
Worry outcome diaries, 189–190

Yale–Brown Obsessive Compulsive Scale
  (Y-BOCS), 109, 133–134, 135, 137,
    141, 252
Y-BOCS. *See* Yale–Brown Obsessive
  Compulsive Scale